Advanced Epidemiologic Methods for the Study of Rheumatic Diseases

Editor

SINDHU R. JOHNSON

RHEUMATIC DISEASE CLINICS OF NORTH AMERICA

www.rheumatic.theclinics.com

Consulting Editor
MICHAEL H. WEISMAN

May 2018 • Volume 44 • Number 2

ELSEVIER

1600 John F. Kennedy Boulevard • Suite 1800 • Philadelphia, Pennsylvania, 19103-2899
http://www.theclinics.com

RHEUMATIC DISEASE CLINICS OF NORTH AMERICA Volume 44, Number 2
May 2018 ISSN 0889-857X, ISBN 13: 978-0-323-61050-6

Editor: Lauren Boyle
Developmental Editor: Casey Potter

Rheumatic Disease Clinics of North America (ISSN 0889-857X) is published quarterly by Elsevier Inc., 360 Park Avenue South, New York, NY 10010-1710. Months of issue are February, May, August, and November. Business and editorial offices: 1600 John F. Kennedy Boulevard, Suite 1800, Philadelphia, PA 19103-2899. Periodicals postage paid at New York, NY and additional mailing offices. Subscription prices are USD 355.00 per year for US individuals, USD 706.00 per year for US institutions, USD 100.00 per year for US students and residents, USD 419.00 per year for Canadian individuals, USD 880.00 per year for Canadian institutions, USD 465.00 per year for international individuals, USD 880.00 per year for international institutions, and USD 230.00 per year for Canadian and foreign students/residents. To receive student/resident rate, orders must be accompanied by name of affiliated institution, date of term, and the *signature* of program/residency coordinator on institution letterhead. Orders will be billed at individual rate until proof of status received. Foreign air speed delivery is included in all *Clinics* subscription prices. All prices are subject to change without notice. **POSTMASTER:** Send address changes to *Rheumatic Disease Clinics of North America,* Elsevier Health Sciences Division, Subscription Customer Service, 3251 Riverport Lane, Maryland Heights, MO 63043. **Customer Service: 1-800-654-2452 (US and Canada). From outside of the US and Canada: 314-447-8871. Fax: 314-447-8029. For print support, e-mail: JournalsCustomerService-usa@elsevier.com. For online support, e-mail: JournalsOnline Support-usa@elsevier.com.**

Reprints. For copies of 100 or more of articles in this publication, please contact the Commercial Reprints Department, Elsevier Inc., 360 Park Avenue South, New York, New York, 10010-1710; Tel.: +1-212-633-3874, Fax: +1-212-633-3820, and E-mail: reprints@elsevier.com.

Rheumatic Disease Clinics of North America is covered in *MEDLINE/PubMed (Index Medicus), Current Contents/Clinical Medicine, Science Citation Index, ISI/BIOMED,* and *EMBASE/Excerpta Medica.*

Contributors

CONSULTING EDITOR

MICHAEL H. WEISMAN, MD
Cedars-Sinai Chair in Rheumatology, Director, Division of Rheumatology, Professor of Medicine, Cedars-Sinai Medical Center, Distinguished Professor, David Geffen School of Medicine at UCLA, Los Angeles, California, USA

EDITOR

SINDHU R. JOHNSON, MD, PhD
Assistant Professor, Division of Rheumatology, Department of Medicine, Toronto Western Hospital, Mount Sinai Hospital, Institute of Health Policy, Management and Evaluation, University of Toronto, Toronto, Ontario, Canada

AUTHORS

DORCAS E. BEATON, BScOT, PhD
Institute for Work & Health, University of Toronto, Toronto, Ontario, Canada

SUSANNE M. BENSELER, MD, PhD
Department of Paediatrics, Alberta Children's Hospital, Cumming School of Medicine, University of Calgary, Calgary, Alberta, Canada

JOSEPH BEYENE, PhD
Professor, McMaster University, Hamilton, Ontario, Canada

ELIZA F. CHAKRAVARTY, MD, MSc
Associate Member, Clinical Immunology Research Program, Oklahoma Medical Research Foundation, Oklahoma City, Oklahoma, USA

MEGAN CLOWSE, MD, MPH
Associate Professor, Medicine, Duke University School of Medicine, Durham, North Carolina, USA

CHARLES F. DILLON, MD, PhD
Silver Spring, Maryland, USA

LISA ENGEL, MScOT, PhD
University Health Network, Toronto, Ontario, Canada

LAUREN ERDMAN, MSc
Genetics and Genome Biology, Department of Computer Science, The Hospital for Sick Children, University of Toronto, Toronto, Ontario, Canada

GUY FAULKNER, PhD
Professor, Canadian Institutes of Health Research, Public Health Agency of Canada, Chair, Applied Public Health, The University of British Columbia, Vancouver, British Columbia, Canada

BRIAN M. FELDMAN, MD, MSc, FRCPC
Pediatric Rheumatologist, Department of Pediatrics, Division of Rheumatology, Faculty of Medicine, Professor, Institute of Health Policy, Management and Evaluation, Dalla Lana School of Public Health, University of Toronto, Senior Scientist, Child Health Evaluative Sciences, The Hospital for Sick Children, Toronto, Ontario, Canada

ANNA GOLDENBERG, PhD
Scientist, Genetics and Genome Biology, Assistant Professor, Department of Computer Science, The Hospital for Sick Children, University of Toronto, Toronto, Ontario, Canada

JOHN T. GRANTON, MD
Professor, Divisions of Respirology and Critical Care Medicine, Department of Medicine, Toronto General Hospital, University Health Network, Toronto, Ontario, Canada

LU HAN, PhD
Department of Medical Imaging, University of Toronto, Toronto, Ontario, Canada

GILLIAN A. HAWKER, MD, MSc
Professor, Institute of Health Policy, Management and Evaluation, University of Toronto, Division of Rheumatology, Department of Medicine, Women's College Hospital, Toronto, Ontario, Canada

GLEN S. HAZLEWOOD, MD, PhD
Assistant Professor, Departments of Medicine and Community Health Sciences, University of Calgary, Calgary, Alberta, Canada

SINDHU R. JOHNSON, MD, PhD
Assistant Professor, Division of Rheumatology, Department of Medicine, Toronto Western Hospital, Mount Sinai Hospital, Institute of Health Policy, Management and Evaluation, University of Toronto, Toronto, Ontario, Canada

ROBERT B.M. LANDEWÉ, MD
Professor, Amsterdam Rheumatology and Clinical Immunology Center, Amsterdam, The Netherlands; Zuyderland Medical Center Heerlen, Heerlen, The Netherlands

LILY SIOK HOON LIM, MBBS, MRCPCH, FRCPC, PhD
Clinician Scientist, Department of Pediatrics, Rady Faculty of Health Sciences, University of Manitoba, Winnipeg, Manitoba, Canada

LISA M. LIX, PhD
Professor, Department of Community Health Sciences, Rady Faculty of Health Sciences, University of Manitoba, Winnipeg, Manitoba, Canada

JOHN D. PAULING, BMedSci, BMBS, PhD, FRCP
Royal National Hospital for Rheumatic Diseases, Royal United Hospitals Bath, Senior Lecturer, Consultant Rheumatologist, Department of Pharmacy and Pharmacology, University of Bath, Bath, United Kingdom

JANET E. POPE, MD, MPH, FRCPC
Division Head, Rheumatology, Professor of Medicine, Western University, St. Joseph's Health Care, London, Ontario, Canada

ELEANOR PULLNAYEGUM, PhD
Senior Scientist, Child Health Evaluative Sciences, The Hospital for Sick Children, Associate Professor, Public Health Sciences, University of Toronto, Toronto, Ontario, Canada

LESLEY ANN SAKETKOO, MD, MPH
Associate Professor of Medicine, Division of Pulmonary Medicine and Critical Care, Tulane University School of Medicine, Lung Center, New Orleans Scleroderma and Sarcoidosis Patient Care and Research Center, University Medical Center, Comprehensive Pulmonary Hypertension Center, New Orleans, Louisiana, USA

JULIA F. SIMARD, ScD
Assistant Professor, Epidemiology, Health Research and Policy, Immunology and Rheumatology, Medicine, Stanford School of Medicine, Stanford, California, USA

SAMANTHA STEPHENS, PhD
Research Fellow, Neurosciences and Mental Health, Pediatric M.S., Neuroinflammatory Disorders Program, Center for Brain and Mental Health, Peter Gilgan Centre for Research and Learning, The Hospital for Sick Children, Toronto, Ontario, Canada

GEORGE A. TOMLINSON, PhD
Associate Professor, Institute of Health Policy, Management and Evaluation, Dalla Lana School of Public Health, University of Toronto, Department of Medicine, Division of Support, Systems and Outcomes, Toronto General Hospital Research Institute, Toronto General Hospital, Toronto, Ontario, Canada

ZAHI TOUMA, MD, FACP, FACR, PhD
University Health Network, University of Toronto, Toronto, Ontario, Canada

MARK S. TREMBLAY, PhD
Director Healthy Active Living and Obesity Research, CHEO Research Institute, Professor of Pediatrics, Faculty of Medicine, University of Ottawa, Ottawa, Ontario, Canada

PASCAL N. TYRRELL, PhD
Assistant Professor, Departments of Medical Imaging and Statistical Sciences, University of Toronto, Toronto, Ontario, Canada

DÉSIRÉE VAN DER HEIJDE, MD
Professor, Leiden University Medical Center, Leiden, the Netherlands

EVELYNE VINET, MD, PhD
Assistant Professor, Divisions of Rheumatology and Clinical Epidemiology, McGill University Health Centre, Montreal, Quebec, Canada

MICHAEL H. WEISMAN, MD
Professor of Medicine Emeritus, Division of Rheumatology, Cedars-Sinai Medical Center, Distinguished Professor Emeritus, David Geffen School of Medicine at UCLA, Los Angeles, California, USA

ANDRÉANNE N. ZIZZO, MD, MSc, FRCPC
Pediatric Gastroenterologist, Department of Pediatrics, Division of Gastroenterology and Hepatology, Western University, Children's Hospital, London Health Sciences Centre, London, Ontario, Canada

Contents

Foreword: The Brave New World of Rheumatic Disease Research Today xiii

Michael H. Weisman

Preface: Advanced Epidemiologic Methods for the Study of Rheumatic and Musculoskeletal Diseases xv

Sindhu R. Johnson

Minimal Clinically Important Difference: A Review of Outcome Measure Score Interpretation 177

Lisa Engel, Dorcas E. Beaton, and Zahi Touma

Clinicians, researchers, and outcome stakeholders have the crucial, albeit difficult, task of quantifying when a person or group experiences important change or difference on any given outcome measure, often in response to a specific intervention. The minimal clinically important difference (MCID) provides this quantified value of change/difference for a measure. There are many methods for MCID derivation, which can result in multiple values for the same measure. Thus, it is important for potential users of MCID values to be aware of the nuances of MCID development and cautions for interpreting values. This article outlines MCID-related definitions, methods, and guidelines.

Alternative Design and Analytical Techniques for Longitudinal Rheumatology Studies: Improved Understanding of Outcomes 189

Lily Siok Hoon Lim, Brian M. Feldman, and Lisa M. Lix

Longitudinal cohort designs (with three or more measurement occasions) are invaluable to investigate between- and within-individual variation in outcomes. However, traditional longitudinal designs require a lengthy implementation and data collection period and impose a substantial burden on participants and investigators. The authors discuss alternative longitudinal designs, including planned missing data designs and retrospective cohort studies with secondary data, which require a shorter period for data accrual and reduce participant burden while maintaining statistical power. They also discuss analysis strategies to maximize data use and produce unbiased estimates of treatment effectiveness, including models for recurrent or multistate events and time-varying covariates.

Propensity Score Methods for Bias Reduction in Observational Studies of Treatment Effect 203

Sindhu R. Johnson, George A. Tomlinson, Gillian A. Hawker, John T. Granton, and Brian M. Feldman

A challenge to the use of observational data to study treatment effects is the issue of confounding. Noncomparability of exposed and nonexposed subjects can lead to biased estimation of the treatment effect. The

meta-analyses. Examples of different randomized trials in rheumatic diseases are provided to understand the methods for trials and the rationale for outcomes within trials. Insights from meta-analyses and systematic literature reviews, including network meta-analyses within rheumatology treatment, are provided. Ethical considerations, sample size calculations, and types of randomized controlled trials are discussed.

"Big Data" in Rheumatology: Intelligent Data Modeling Improves the Quality of Imaging Data **307**

Robert B.M. Landewé and Désirée van der Heijde

Analysis of imaging data in rheumatology is a challenge. Reliability of scores is an issue for several reasons. The signal to noise ratio of most imaging techniques is rather unfavorable (too little signal in relation to too much noise). Optimal use of all available data may help increasing the credibility of imaging data, but knowledge of complicated statistical methodology and the help of skilled statisticians are required. Clinicians should appreciate the merits of sophisticated data modeling and liaise with statisticians to increase the quality of imaging results, as proper imaging studies in rheumatology imply more than a supersensitive imaging technique alone.

Strategies for Dealing with Missing Accelerometer Data **317**

Samantha Stephens, Joseph Beyene, Mark S. Tremblay, Guy Faulkner, Eleanor Pullnayegum, and Brian M. Feldman

Missing data are a universal research problem that can affect studies examining the relationship between physical activity measured with accelerometers and health outcomes. Statistical techniques are available to deal with missing data; however, available techniques have not been synthesized. A scoping review was conducted to summarize the advantages and disadvantages of identified methods of dealing with missing data from accelerometers. Missing data pose a threat to the validity and interpretation of trials using physical activity data from accelerometry. Imputation using multiple imputation techniques is recommended to deal with missing data and improve the validity and interpretation of studies using accelerometry.

Use of Administrative Databases to Assess Reproductive Health Issues in Rheumatic Diseases **327**

Evelyne Vinet, Eliza F. Chakravarty, Julia F. Simard, and Megan Clowse

Administrative databases, registers, and other sources of big data can be interesting sources to address important research questions on reproduction in women with rheumatic diseases. There are many different types of administrative datasets worldwide, and it is important to understand the type of data present and unavailable in each dataset, validity and potential misclassification of data, and the ability to link maternal data with infant data. This article discusses the advantages and methodological issues associated with administrative database use for the conduct of observational studies on reproductive issues in women with rheumatic diseases.

Measuring Patient Preferences: An Overview of Methods with a Focus on Discrete Choice Experiments **337**

Glen S. Hazlewood

There is increasing recognition of the importance of patient preferences and methodologies to measure them. In this article, methods to quantify patient preferences are reviewed, with a focus on discrete choice experiments. In a discrete choice experiment, patients are asked to choose between 2 or more treatments. The results can be used to quantify the relative importance of treatment outcomes and/or other considerations relevant to medical decision making. Conducting and interpreting a discrete choice experiment requires multiple steps and an understanding of the potential biases that can arise, which are reviewed in this article with examples in rheumatic diseases.

Cluster and Multiple Correspondence Analyses in Rheumatology: Paths to Uncovering Relationships in a Sea of Data **349**

Lu Han, Susanne M. Benseler, and Pascal N. Tyrrell

Rheumatic diseases encompass a wide range of conditions caused by inflammation and dysregulation of the immune system resulting in organ damage. Research in these heterogeneous diseases benefits from multivariate methods. This article describes and evaluates the current literature in rheumatology regarding cluster analysis and correspondence analysis. A systematic review showed an increase in studies making use of these 2 methods. However, standardization in how these methods are applied and reported is needed. Researcher expertise was determined to be the main barrier to considering these approaches, whereas education and collaborating with a biostatistician were suggested ways forward.

Applied Bayesian Methods in the Rheumatic Diseases **361**

Sindhu R. Johnson, George A. Tomlinson, John T. Granton, Gillian A. Hawker, and Brian M. Feldman

The use of applied Bayesian methods is increasing in rheumatology. Using the Bayes theorem, past evidence is updated with new data. Preexisting data are expressed as a prior probability distribution. New observations are expressed as a likelihood. Through explicit incorporation of preexisting data and new data, this process informs how this new information should change the way we think. In this article, the authors highlight the use of applied Bayesian methods in the study of rheumatic diseases.

RHEUMATIC DISEASE CLINICS OF NORTH AMERICA

FORTHCOMING ISSUES

August 2018
Medical practice challenges for the Rheumatologist
Herb Baraf, *Editor*

November 2018
Renal Involvement in Rheumatic Diseases
Andrew Bomback and Meghan E. Sise, *Editors*

February 2019
Best Practice and Challenges to the Practice of Rheumatology
Daniel J. Wallace and R. Swamy Venuturupalli, *Editors*

RECENT ISSUES

February 2018
Digestive and Hepatic Aspects of the Rheumatic Diseases
Liron Caplan, *Editor*

November 2017
Neurologic Manifestations of Rheumatic Diseases
John Imboden and Sarah E. Goglin, *Editors*

August 2017
Genomics in Rheumatic Diseases
S. Louis Bridges Jr and Carl D. Langefeld, *Editors*

ISSUE OF RELATED INTEREST

Neurologic Clinics, November 2016 (Volume 34, Issue 4)
Global and Domestic Public Health and Neuroepidemiology
David S. Younger, *Editor*

Foreword

The Brave New World of Rheumatic Disease Research Today

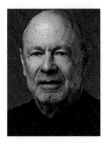

Michael H. Weisman, MD
Consulting Editor

Pick up any journal article today or review a grant that requests funding for innovative research in rheumatic diseases, and right away there is a methodologic challenge. As databases become larger and complex with observational cohorts more challenging due to patient protection and compliance fears, the need to interrogate data now requires new approaches. How do we begin to approach the racial and ethnic differences in our rheumatic diseases' susceptibility and severity keeping in mind the suspected interactions between genetic and environmental factors that are in play? The presence of publicly available "omics" data is now being matched to patient cohorts, substantially stretching our abilities to create new methodologic frameworks for proper analyses.

Clearly, we need to try to address these issues if we are going to meet the challenge of precision medicine and new therapeutic strategies. Dr Johnson was asked to plunge into this mix of applying new methods to the changing world of new data sources. She has assembled an impressive set of articles and expert opinion from international leaders as well as rising stars in the field. Topics range from the complexities of longitudinal data analysis to the analysis of qualitative data that could uncover new concepts previously hidden from view. After reading these articles, one should consider how we approach a journal article: the message from Dr Johnson suggests that we should begin with the materials and methods section before looking at anything else.

Michael H. Weisman, MD
Cedars Sinai Medical Center
David Geffen School of Medicine at UCLA, 1545 Calmar Court
Los Angeles, CA 90024, USA

E-mail address:
Michael.Weisman@cshs.org

Rheum Dis Clin N Am 44 (2018) xiii
https://doi.org/10.1016/j.rdc.2018.02.002
0889-857X/18/© 2018 Published by Elsevier Inc.

Preface

Advanced Epidemiologic Methods for the Study of Rheumatic and Musculoskeletal Diseases

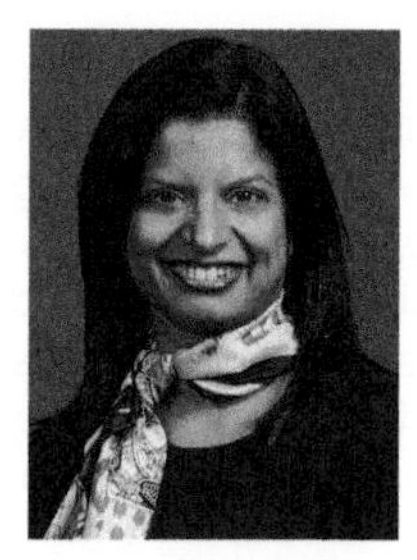

Sindhu R. Johnson, MD, PhD
Editor

While the practice of rheumatology is challenged by a variety of clinical questions encountered through the course of everyday patient care, research in rheumatology is challenged by issues related to bias, sample size, and data quality. Clinical epidemiology offers an array of "tools" to help address these challenges. This issue of the *Rheumatic Disease Clinics of North America* focuses on advanced epidemiologic methods for the study of the rheumatic and musculoskeletal diseases, including a range of novel study designs, methods, and analytic strategies.

The study design options discussed include systematic reviews, meta-analysis, network meta-analysis, randomized controlled trials, longitudinal observational cohorts (eg, accelerated cohort, two-method measurement approach, multiform design), and administrative data research. Methodologic and analytic strategies to efficiently use available data while generating unbiased estimates are presented. These strategies are considered in the settings of "big data," repeated measures longitudinal data, and data sets with limited sample size (as often encountered with rare systemic autoimmune rheumatic diseases).

This issue of the *Rheumatic Disease Clinics of North America* also addresses novel methods to identify similar groups of patients within datasets, including cluster analysis, multiple correspondence analyses, and similarity network fusion. Qualitative methods are also reviewed in this issue. Such methods are suited for clinical questions where investigators wish to explore an unknown phenomenon, evaluate the meaning of a concept, understand the phenomenon, or develop a new theory. In addition to reviewing qualitative methods, this issue contrasts them with quantitative methods, especially to highlight where these methods may be complementary or advantageous.

Rheum Dis Clin N Am 44 (2018) xv–xvi
https://doi.org/10.1016/j.rdc.2018.02.001

Understanding the value patients place on a health outcome is required for shared decision making and to inform policy decisions and treatment recommendations. In this issue, patient preferences and methodologies to measure them are reviewed, with a focus on discrete-choice experiments.

The challenge of handling missing data is another topic presented in this issue. Mechanisms of missingness, as well as strategies to deal with missingness, are summarized. The ability to measure and interpret change, whether it be at the individual level or group level, is also an important consideration. An overview and guidance on developing, reporting, interpreting, and applying values of minimal clinically important difference for outcome measures are presented.

Importantly, these articles include illustrative examples of these design, methodologic, and analytic strategies being applied in the rheumatology literature. These examples encompass a broad range of diseases in both adult and pediatric rheumatology.

Contributors to this issue include both global leaders and rising stars in clinical epidemiology. I would like to express my gratitude to each of the contributors for these excellent articles. It is hoped that this clinical epidemiology–themed issue of the *Rheumatic Disease Clinics of North America* will both educate consumers of the medical literature and inspire clinical researchers looking for new tools to address the methodologic challenges they face.

Sindhu R. Johnson, MD, PhD
Division of Rheumatology
Department of Medicine
Toronto Western Hospital
Ground Floor, East Wing
399 Bathurst Street
Toronto, Ontario M5T 2S8, Canada

Mount Sinai Hospital
Toronto, Ontario M5G 1X5, Canada

Institute of Health Policy
Management and Evaluation
University of Toronto
Toronto, Ontario M5S 1K7, Canada

E-mail address:
Sindhu.Johnson@uhn.ca

Minimal Clinically Important Difference

A Review of Outcome Measure Score Interpretation

Lisa Engel, MScOT, PhD[a], Dorcas E. Beaton, BScOT, PhD[b,c], Zahi Touma, MD, PhD[a,b,c,*]

KEYWORDS

• Reproducibility of results • Minimal important change • Change • Difference • Outcomes assessment • Methodology • Important

KEY POINTS

- Standardized health-related outcome measures require evidence for change and a way to interpret change within individuals or difference between groups.
- Values for the minimal clinically important difference (MCID) provide an option for the interpretation of meaningful change/difference.
- There are many methods for developing MCID values, but values can be influenced by sample characteristics and methods used for MCID quantification.
- Anchor-based methods using sensitivity and specificity analysis, such as receiver operating characteristic curve analysis, are recommended in the derivation of MCID to minimize misclassification of those who importantly change.

INTRODUCTION

Has the patient changed an important amount? How many people improved or deteriorated from an intervention? Did the intervention make a difference in the study? What value of change on a given measure is meaningful? These questions have challenged clinicians, researchers, funders, policymakers, and other health care stakeholders since the beginning of health-measurement science,[1] and before that in the education and psychology measurement fields.[2] The increase of standardized

[a] Toronto Western Hospital/University Health Network, 399 Bathurst Street, Room 1E-412, Toronto, Ontario M5T 2S8, Canada; [b] Institute of Health Policy, Management & Evaluation, University of Toronto; Health Sciences Building, 155 College Street, Suite 425, Toronto, Ontario M5T 3M6, Canada; [c] Institute for Work & Health, 481 University Avenue, Suite 800, Toronto, Ontario M5G 2E9, Canada
* Corresponding author. Centre for Prognosis Studies in the Rheumatic Diseases, Lupus Clinic, Toronto Western Hospital, East Wing, 1E-412, 399 Bathurst Street, Toronto, Ontario M5T 2S8, Canada.
E-mail address: zahi.touma@uhn.ca

Rheum Dis Clin N Am 44 (2018) 177–188
https://doi.org/10.1016/j.rdc.2018.01.011
0889-857X/18/

health-related outcome measures has increased the ability of clinicians and researchers to reliably and validly measure and evaluate outcomes.[3] Nevertheless, the issue of interpreting scores, or changes in scores, is an ongoing debate, although with more convergence appearing in recent years.[4,5] The idea of a minimal clinically important change (MCIC) or difference (MCID) is essential in understanding outcomes, both longitudinal change within individuals or cross-sectional difference between individuals, but there is continued questions regarding its development, interpretation, and application. Knowing the elements that create this controversy and then how to move through it will help readers to make the best use of this important threshold. Therefore, the *aim* of this review is to provide clinicians and researchers an overview and guidance on developing, reporting, interpreting, and applying values of MCID.

Minimal Clinically Important Difference Definition

In their seminal 1989 paper, Jaeschke and colleagues[6(p408)] defined MCID as "the smallest difference in score in the domain of interest which patients perceive as beneficial and which would mandate, in the absence of troublesome side effects and excessive cost, a change in the patient's management." Since its original definition, many variations have been proposed (**Table 1**), and variants now include concepts of important change to patients only, important change to other outcome stakeholders (eg, clinicians or researchers), worthwhile importance, risk reduction, or mean score differences between patients with ideal and less than ideal results.[7–9] The term minimal important difference (MID) is now often used to avoid a focus on the "clinical" importance of change. The authors use the term MCID because MCID terminology persists and is recognized. Furthermore, as seen in **Table 1**, polysemy (varying meanings for same term) and synonymy (same meaning for varying terms) complicate MCID literature.[9,10] Despite the variations in the name and the operational definitions, the general gist of MCID definitions is that it defines the lower threshold for change that is important to or valued by someone (eg, patients, health care providers, researchers conducting the study, funders, policymakers, or other stakeholders in the intervention outcomes), and ideally this change should surpass the boundaries of measurement errors/measurement variation to be interpreted as change.[7] Importantly, the concept has evolved to make a distinction between beneficial (improvement) and harmful (deterioration) change.[1,3,11,12]

Values of MCID can be determined for different settings or applications. Sometimes they are designed to offer insights for the interpretation of results in longitudinal evaluative observation studies and clinical trials (group-level applications), and in others, for clinical care and intervention decisions for patients (individual-level application). The values may differ depending on the application (discussed in more detail later). However, which level of application depends on how the MCID value is derived (ie, methods).[7,13,14]

For group-level applications, the MCID has been identified as a metric of clinical significance of the change, quite different from the statistical significance of group difference alone. In this application, it allows for interpretation of intervention efficacy and calculation of sample sizes for future evaluative studies or trials. Therefore, the MCID can offer important insights in situations where sample size and characteristics have driven the statistical significance to be too high, or too low, offering a means to interpret the change.[8,14–17]

In both individual and group-level applications, the MCID can be used to guide the threshold for meaning, rather than any statistical magnitude or significance of the change. It is a far more important threshold used to classify someone as improved (or responding to intervention), not improved (not responding to intervention), or harmed by an intervention (clinically important deterioration).

Table 1
Variations in minimal clinically important difference terminology in published literature

Term (Acronym)[a]	Definitions and/or Common Applications
Minimal clinically important difference (MCID)	Term discussed by Guyatt and colleagues[49] in 1987; Jaeschke and colleagues[6] in 1989 proposed MCID definition and initial methods. Wells and colleagues[12] in their review found MCID terminology to often be linked to important change based on patient viewpoint (perception).
Minimal important difference (MID)	Currently becoming the dominant terminology in literature (although MCID is still used). MID omits the "clinical" of MCID, where the anchor being used in the derivation of the change is not based on clinical judgment (eg, perceptions of clinicians or patients described in earlier MCID literature).[50] Therefore, MID could also be based on a change in a laboratory marker or a functional test such as pulmonary function test or 5-min walking test. Change in definition also expanded to include directions of beneficial and harmful important change.[50]
Minimal important change (MIC)	Used to emphasize a difference in terminology wherein "change" is longitudinal change within individuals and "difference" is cross-section differences between groups.[3] MIC is a change a patient considers important and therefore should be determined using patient-perspective anchor-based methods.[39,41]
Subjectively significant difference (SSD)	Introduced by Osoba and colleagues[51] in 1998 to emphasize patient-centered anchors.
Clinically important difference (CID)	CID reflects clinically important change that is not necessarily minimal.[29] The term is also used in contrast to Clinically important responder (CIR), where CID is the between-group difference considered clinically relevant (ie, as applied to a clinical intervention trial).[18]
Clinically important responder (CIR)	Amount of change an individual needs to report to consider they have experienced a meaningful improvement.[18] Terminology proposed to align more with patient-reported outcome measure development guidelines.[18,32]
MDC (minimal detectable change)	The amount of individual change needed to be achieved to differentiate from measurement error (random variation); argued that should not be a replacement for important change.[11,27,39,41]

[a] Also see King's 2011 review for evolution and nuances of MCID terminology.[9]

Minimal Clinically Important Difference Methods

A variety of methods have been proposed and used to quantify the MCID; however, each has its own merits and limitations. Other past reviews have reviewed and categorized these methods.[4,8,9,12,14,17,18]

The methods can be broadly described by 2 main approaches: anchor-based approaches and distribution-based approaches.[4,14,19] *Anchor-based approaches* use an external, tangible marker of change, termed the anchor, to identify the occurrence of change in the target concept of interest; for example, did a change in pain, function, or quality of life occur. These anchors become the critical part of the analysis. What constitutes an appropriate anchor of importance varies and is often debated.[8] Many anchors have been proposed, including other objective clinical measures or endpoints and, more commonly, subjective global indicator/impression of change (GIC; also sometimes termed global rating of change or global assessment rating) scales.[1,8,18,20]

When using a GIC anchor-based approach, the individual rates themselves (in the case of MCID from a patient perspective) or the patient in question (in the case of MCID from another outcome stakeholder or proxy perspective) on the GIC scale. This scale is usually balanced, allowing the respondent to state if they are better, the same, or worse using a Likert scale of varying number ranges.[14,21] A priori determination is made of what is to be considered an important change on this anchor, and after fielding it along with the questionnaires, the change score on the target questionnaire that relates to this threshold of important change on the anchor is calculated and reported as the MCID. Various thresholds and various statistical techniques can be found for this calculation.

Although anchor-based approaches provide the opportunity to define and quantify importance, they have been scrutinized because of their variability dependent on many factors (**Box 1**).[1,4,8,13,14,20–27] Furthermore, the use of subjective anchors like GIC scales have been criticized for their lack of reliability and validity evidence and the susceptibility to recall bias, response shift, and implicit theories of change.[3,8,28]

Distribution-based approaches use internal quantifications of statistical variability in the sample and magnitude of effect as a proxy to MCID quantification in the target measure of interest.[1,3,14] Other reviews and papers have listed distribution-based approach methods to include the one standard error of measurement (SEM), 0.5 standard deviation (SD), or change equivalent to 0.2 or 0.5 effect size. A distinction should be made between using these (ie, 1 SEM approach) as indicators of important change, and the use of related statistics around error (such as Guyatt's responsiveness index, the reliable change index, standard response difference [SRD], Bland and Altman's

Box 1
Factors influencing anchor-based minimal clinical (minimal clinically important difference) values for a given measure

Methods[3,4,18,21,24,27,28,43,44]

- Which methodological (difference between and/or changes within) and statistical approach
- Time between testing and influence on stability and recall bias, response shift, or implicit theories of change
- Direction of change to define importance (ie, improvement vs deterioration)
- Use of absolute versus relative change on target measure

Anchor[1,8,14,17,20,25,52]

- Anchor choice (eg, secondary measure/endpoint, global assessment rating)
- Whose perspective determines the change magnitude (eg, patient, family, caregiver, clinician, payer, society)
- Importance cutoffs on anchors (eg, any change vs small change vs moderate change) and whose perspective is used to determine minimal importance level from change magnitudes
- Statistical methods used to relate the anchor back to the change in score on the target instrument (eg, thresholds, ROC curve analysis)

Sample[4,5,8,21–24]

- Patient demographics such as age, gender, diagnosis
- Health issue acuity, level of disease activity (eg, mild vs severe), stability, and baseline status on measure
- Intervention (if any) received in MCID study

limits of agreement, and minimal/smallest detectable change [MDC/SDC]).[4,14,27,29] Although listed as distribution-base methods in past reviews, the authors argue that the last 5 listed are not distribution-based approaches to MCID approximation, but rather they are estimators of responsiveness or error.

Distributional approaches alone are less favored as an approach to MCID determination because of the lack of valuation of the importance of that change. Despite some reports of distribution-based quantifications providing values comparable to anchor-based values of MCID in some samples,[29] the use of mathematical analysis of sample distribution as a proxy for MCID is controversial and has been shown to be inconsistent; there are exceptions to the distribution-based hypotheses.[1,12,14,27,30] The remaining concern about the distribution-based approaches is that they do not verify concepts of important or meaningful change, therefore, are often not considered the ideal MCID approach.[14,27,30] Distribution-based approaches provide a starting point to determine the interpretation of change through defining the "noise" that must be surpassed in order to interpret the change as important.[14,31,32] At best distribution-based methods for MCID quantification are not encouraged as a sole method for MCID derivation,[21,32] despite their simplicity and continued utilization in MCID literature.[5,33]

A third approach less often used, *opinion-based approaches*, is where consensus-based methods, such as Delphi methods, are used to either quantify the MCID or choose the "final" MCID value from previously developed MCID values.[14] Whose opinion is used is based on experience, knowledge, or data. However, like anchor-based approaches, the MCID is again influenced by whose perspective is used.[31]

As well as the three approaches to MCID determination described earlier, another important consideration is the nature of the data itself. Many scores on the instruments are not pure "rulers" with the exact same difference reflected between each change in the scale (ie, for people with relatively good vs very poor health status), meaning the scales are not interval level data and are likely what is considered ordinal or ordered data. Some suggest that much of the variance in MCID determination is caused by this lack of interval level data and the solution to that is moving toward item response theory (IRT) scoring to the instruments. Once scored through either Rasch or through other forms of IRT, proponents would suggest that more consistency should be found in MCID values. Once the scoring is settled using these methods, the same approaches described earlier could be applied using these new scores rather than the simple sum of the responses to individual items and measurement error.[3] In MCID derivations from an IRT scoring perspective, the hierarchical Rasch score is used instead of the summed score, thereby using a scale that is interval rather than ordinal. Proponents of MCID using IRT-informed measures argue using an interval scale improves the mathematics and corrects for issues of MCID varying by baseline score seen in many ordinal-level measures (ie, where statistics requiring interval-level scoring are suboptimally applied).[34–36] Lee and colleagues[36] recently reported excellent agreement (κ statistical >0.74 [ranging between 0.71 and 0.93]) in the proportion of patients achieving MCID improvements between classical test theory (CTT)-informed distribution-based MCID values (ie, 1 SEM, 1.96 SEM, SRD) and IRT-informed MCID values.

However, limitations to IRT-informed approaches have also been identified. As the authors argued previously, distribution-based methods of MCID approximation do not actually address quantifying important change; therefore, the results from Lee and colleagues,[36] where they compared IRT-informed derivations of MCID values derived from distribution-based methods, need to be interpreted with caution. Furthermore, not all measures may be able to be IRT informed, as IRT-informed measures require a clear difficulty level gradient across items.[37] Last, there is very limited IRT-informed comparative MCID analysis available, and literature does not yet offer evidence to the necessity or superiority of IRT-informed MCID analysis. Rouquette and colleagues[35] found that an IRT-informed MCID approach is not necessarily superior when comparing the sensitivity, specificity, and the positive and negative predictive values of MCID derived from trait-level IRT-informed scaling to CTT-informed scaling using anchor-based approaches on the Medical Outcomes Study 36-item Short Form survey (SF-36). Therefore, the quantification of MCID using IRT-informed approaches instead of settling the MCID debate has instead emerged as a new area of debate where more research is needed, particularly comparative methods research.

Variable Minimal Clinically Important Difference Values: Recommendations and Cautions for Interpretation and Application

The MCID is a "variable concept," and there can be multiple MCID values for a given measure.[3(p256)] Not all methods result in comparable MCID values nor can values be applied universally.[4,30] Interpretation and application of MCID values require careful consideration.[4]

It is recommended that MCID values be based on anchor-based methods.[32,38,39] As previously identified, distribution-based methods do not estimate importance of change, but instead estimate the measure "noise" secondary to variability and measurement error.[7] Therefore, SEM or MDC/SDC values may only be useful to importance of change interpretation when used in conjunction with anchor-based MCID methods.[20,30,40] For example, the use of MDC/SDC values can provide information for interpreting anchor-based MCID values by answering if important change exceeds measurement error.[11,27,41]

Nevertheless, anchor-based approaches require 3 important steps (which the authors highlight in later discussion): deciding on the anchor, defining cutoffs, and choosing statistical approaches. As previously identified in **Box 1**, multiple factors in these steps can cause variations in MCID values for CTT-informed measures. These variations influence threshold value obtained for the MCID, and the correct interpretation and application of MCID require one to critically examine how an anchor-based MCID value was derived before application.[3,7,11,13] Caution should be used in applying MCID values without knowing exactly how they were derived.

Deciding on the anchor

An MCID value is influenced by choices of what the anchor is (ie, criterion measure), whose perspective is used on the anchor, and what is the direction of change on the anchor. As previously described, anchors can include an objective or subjective measure (although the use of objective measures is debated due to its perceived disconnect to the concept of important or meaningful change; subjective measures used are often GIC scales).[9,18] The anchor choice should be meaningful, easily interpretable, and related to the target concept/measure.[18]

When examining an MCID value, whose perspective was used needs to be evaluated. The quantification of change magnitude and/or importance can vary between the patient, family/caregivers/close others, clinicians, funders/payers, or society.[11,42] However, although often argued that MCID requires the patients' perspectives,[21] the evaluation of change may require nonpatient perspectives; it is dependent on the outcome being assessed. For example, decisions about important change not noticeable to a patient, such as outcomes of serologic signs that have no current symptoms but could relate to later health quality, may be best determined by anchors from the perspective of the clinician. In contrast, change in some outcomes that are reliant on the patients' subjective ratings, such as quality of life, are best judged by the patient.[21] Before applying an MCID value, the user needs to critically examine whether the anchor and perspective of the magnitude of change and importance value attached to the magnitudes of change make sense in the context of MCID use.

Users of MCID values also need to heed the original definition of MCID set forth by Jaeschke and colleageus[6] that highlights the importance of considering side effects and cost in addition to change when making intervention decisions. Current MCID methods, especially when using anchor-based GIC approaches, do not necessarily take these factors into account.[8] Further research is needed to identify methods for incorporating perspectives of important change in the context of side effects and costs.

Moreover, recent rheumatology research highlights the variations of MCID values based on the direction of change on the anchor analyzed.[33] Although the initial definition of MCID included only improvement or beneficial outcomes,[6] understanding both improvements and deteriorations is important to clinical outcomes. For example, in samples of adults with systemic lupus erythematosus, both Devilliers and colleauges[43] and McElhone and colleagues[44] found differences in MCID estimates for change based on deterioration versus improvement in the Lupus Quality of Life scale and the Medical Outcomes Study short form survey (SF-36) when using a mean-change response anchor-based approach informed by a GIC scale.

Defining cutoffs for important change on the anchor

Once an anchor is determined, someone then decides what parts of that anchor will be considered "important change" or "small and important change." For example, on the same 15-point GIC scale, Jaeschke and colleagues[6] defined "minimally important" as inclusive of almost the same, a little worse/better, and somewhat worse (ie, +/−1–3), whereas Juniper and colleagues[45] defined it as only encompassing the latter 2 (ie, +/−2–3). A different cutoff variation is that some studies use a cutoff of "a little change" to signal importance, whereas other studies use different magnitudes (eg, "moderate change"); each produces a different MCID value. For example, the identified cutoffs for SF-36 MCID values reported by Devilliers and colleagues[43] and McElhone and colleagues[44] differ. There is a lack of evidence and agreement as to optimal cutoff levels, and variations in MCID values will remain, whereas variation in cutoff exists.[21]

The decision of cutoffs is of paramount importance because it is defining what will become a criterion for a small but important change occurring and is in fact the valuing of that change as important.[21] Careful consideration should be given to who rates that importance: oftentimes it is left to the researcher or methodologist, who may or may not know if that is truly important change.

This arbitrary nature of cutoff determination has led some to question the predominance of current GIC anchors-based magnitudes of change (ie, how much are you worse or better) being translated to cutoff of values of importance.[21] Therefore, Terwee and colleagues[21] have suggested the validity of anchors should be improved and standardized by directly querying about the importance of change in the anchor item as an alternative to the currently used magnitude of change item originally proposed for MCID.[6]

Choosing the statistical approach to estimate minimal clinically important difference

Using various statistical approaches, the anchor scale is then compared with the target measure to quantify an approximation of the MCID. Different statistical approaches will also influence MCID quantification and application of MCID values.

Variations of anchor-based analysis include within-individuals (patients) mean change response, between-individuals/group minimum differences, bivariate/multivariate linear regression, bivariate/multivariate logistic regression, and sensitivity/specificity analysis.[4,8,13,14] Sensitivity/specificity analysis includes receiver operating characteristic (ROC) curve and area under the curve analysis methods; in this way, it is similar to diagnostic test validation studies, but where the anchor is categorically used as the comparator or gold-standard measure. MCID values based on ROC curve analysis are derived by identifying the most optimal level of both sensitivity and specificity (ie, [1 − sensitivity] + [1 − specificity]), which indicates a change score corresponding to the lowest amount of individual misclassification.[21] A variation of the ROC analysis and visual display is the visual anchor-based distribution method.[3,46] This method uses the anchor to divide and visually represent the anchor in 3 groups: the importantly improved, the not importantly changed, and importantly deteriorated.[46] For these 3 groups, the change distribution is then plotted for the given target outcome measure, and change for improvement and deterioration is analyzed separately (as discussed, these can differ).[33,46] Therefore, this visual display then provides more information for analyzing and determining the MCID values.

Which statistical methods are used, whether change within versus difference between versus difference between changes within, dictates the potential application of values (ie, group vs individual level).[12,38] Mean change response methods for anchor-based approaches have been criticized for their misclassification of some in the sample who will be deemed to not having changed because their level of change falls below the group mean, and therefore not appropriate for individual-level application.[21] Although MCID methods using group means can help in clinical trial change/difference interpretation (group level), they are not useful in clinical patient evaluation (individual level). Individual-level application often requires a greater magnitude of change to be confident change has occurred.[7] Therefore, ROC curve analysis is recommended for MCID values that are to be applied to individual level (eg, clinical patient intervention decisions).[21] Despite this recommendation, it has been found that there is less published literature using ROC methods, with much recent rheumatology research reporting MCID based on anchor-based group-level analysis such as mean change/response.[43,44,47]

Choosing the Minimal Clinically Important Difference Values to Use

Because the term MCID has variable conceptualizations, methods for quantification, and, subsequently, values pertinent to any particular measure used in any particular population/context, it is difficult to know which value to use for interpreting change when one measure may have many MCID values. Nevertheless, this is an important task especially when the MCID application has many potential implications. The misapplication of MCID values can have consequences to individual patient care or interventions research, for example, a clinician or payer deciding an intervention is not valuable based on a wrongful interpretation of MCID or using an incorrect MCID interpretation to determine clinical trial sample size or examine experimental effectiveness.

Multiple perspectives have been given on choosing the MCID value to use. As noted previously, anchor-based approaches using ROC curve analysis for MCID quantification are the recommended primary methods to determine MCID (with other methods viewed as supportive evidence for interpreting important change).[3,21,27,30] In this way, MCID is treated like a diagnostic test and minimizes misclassification. Nevertheless, a single standardized method and the optimal thresholds or cutoffs of importance for anchors have yet to be determined and from whose perspectives these are best determined.[4,27]

If other MCID methods and approaches are used, then the sensitivity and specificity of the MCID values should be evaluated for their sensitivity and specificity to check for accuracy in classification based on that MCID criterion.[33] Moreover, depicting the cumulative percentage of patients across all levels of intervention effect (change from baseline) using cumulative distribution function diagrams have been proposed as a way to improve the comparison of many values of MCID.[17] The diagrams plot the change score on the horizontal and the cumulative proportion of people exceeding these thresholds on the vertical. A diagram can be plotted for one or more groups. The MCIDs can be added as vertical lines and will demonstrate the impact of MCID variability on one group and between groups. These diagrams allow for the easy comparison of the percentage of patients that respond to interventions and achieve different MCID thresholds.

Presently, it is up to the consumer of the published literature (eg, clinician, researcher, funder, policymaker) to identify what type of MCID has been quantified and its appropriate application. In line with other reviews of MCID, the authors emphasize the need to view values of MCID as context specific and recommend caution in interpreting and applying any one value of MCID universally.[3,4,7,13,48] Critical appraisal of how each MCID value is derived is required to determine whether it is a useful and meaningful MCID value for the context of application.[13] Therefore, adequate and in-depth reporting of how MCID values are derived and their possible applications are critical to users to optimally appraising and apply MCID values.

The Future of Minimal Clinically Important Difference Methodology

As it stands, the topic of MCID continues to develop, and the debate over methods continues.[4,13,34] The breadth and depth of the topic of MCID determination direct us to more research into best practices. Increased standardization of MCID methods, including the anchors and cutoffs used, would allow for better comparison and pooling across studies.[21] The framework proposed in **Box 1** can guide the reporting of MCID development research to optimize the accuracy of MCID interpretation and subsequent application by MCID literature consumers.

Beaton and colleagues[7] in 2002 identified 6 main areas of future MCID methodology research to improve understanding of MCID meaning and generalizability of values, including further research into comparative MCID methods; subgroup analyses of the meaning of change (eg, different attributes and characteristics at baselines); and relative importance values for deterioration versus improvement.[7] However, from an examination of recent MCID literature, much of this research required to reach more resolution around MCID methods and interpretations remains to be done.[14] Furthermore, new methods for outcome measurement and MCID analysis, including the use of IRT informed measures, needs further research.

SUMMARY

Despite their publication more than 15 years ago, it still stands that "measurement of change is difficult and its interpretation is challenging."[7(p113)] Varied definitions of MCID leads to varied methods and interpretations where there is not one correct answer as to what is minimally important when considering change or difference for a particular outcome measure in a particular population.[12] What most matters when examining is the alignment between the purpose of the measure, the methods used to derive the MCID value, and the intended application of the MCID value. Without this correspondence, the risk of misinterpreting and misapplying MCID values is high. Although MCID is not a resolved topic yet, it is a methodological topic that gives further information in understanding the meaning of change.

REFERENCES

1. Guyatt GH, Osoba D, Wu AW, et al. Methods to explain the clinical significance of health status measures. Mayo Clin Proc 2002;77(4):371–83.
2. Cronbach LJ, Furby L. How we should measure "change": or should we? Psychol Bull 1970;74(1):68.
3. de Vet HC, Terwee CB, Mokkink LB, et al. Measurement in medicine: a practical guide. Cambridge: Cambridge University Press; 2011.
4. Wright A, Hannon J, Hegedus EJ, et al. Clinimetrics corner: a closer look at the minimal clinically important difference (MCID). J Man Manip Ther 2012;20(3): 160–6.
5. Smith-Forbes EV, Howell DM, Willoughby J, et al. Specificity of the minimal clinically important difference of the Quick Disabilities of the Arm Shoulder and Hand (QDASH) for distal upper extremity conditions. J Hand Ther 2016;29(1):81–8.
6. Jaeschke R, Singer J, Guyatt GH. Measurement of health status: ascertaining the minimal clinically important difference. Control Clin Trials 1989;10(4):407–15.
7. Beaton DE, Boers M, Wells GA. Many faces of the minimal clinically important difference (MCID): a literature review and directions for future research. Curr Opin Rheumatol 2002;14(2):109–14.
8. Copay AG, Subach BR, Glassman SD, et al. Understanding the minimum clinically important difference: a review of concepts and methods. Spine J 2007; 7(5):541–6.
9. King MT. A point of minimal important difference (MID): a critique of terminology and methods. Expert Rev Pharmacoecon Outcomes Res 2011;11(2):171–84.
10. Larsen KR, Voronovich ZA, Cook PF, et al. Addicted to constructs: science in reverse? Addiction 2013;108(9):1532–3.
11. Beaton DE, Bombardier C, Katz JN, et al. Looking for important change/differences in studies of responsiveness. OMERACT MCID Working Group. Outcome measures in rheumatology. Minimal clinically important difference. J Rheumatol 2001;28(2):400–5.
12. Wells G, Beaton D, Shea B, et al. Minimal clinically important differences: review of methods. J Rheumatol 2001;28(2):406–12.
13. Angst F, Aeschlimann A, Angst J. The minimal clinically important difference raised the significance of outcome effects above the statistical level, with methodological implications for future studies. J Clin Epidemiol 2017;82:128–36.
14. Rai SK, Yazdany J, Fortin PR, et al. Approaches for estimating minimal clinically important differences in systemic lupus erythematosus. Arthritis Res Ther 2015; 17(1):143.
15. Medina-Rosas J, Al-Rayes H, Moustafa AT, et al. Recent advances in the biologic therapy of lupus: the 10 most important areas to look for common pitfalls in clinical trials. Expert Opin Biol Ther 2016;16(10):1225–38.
16. Touma Z, Gladman DD. Current and future therapies for SLE: obstacles and recommendations for the development of novel treatments. Lupus Sci Med 2017;4(1).
17. Wyrwich K, Norquist J, Lenderking W, et al, Industry Advisory Committee of International Society for Quality of Life Research (ISOQOL). Methods for interpreting change over time in patient-reported outcome measures. Qual Life Res 2013; 22(3):475–83.

18. Coon CD, Cappelleri JC. Interpreting change in scores on patient-reported outcome instruments. Ther Innov Regul Sci 2016;50(1):22–9.
19. Rodrigues J, Mabvuure N, Nikkhah D, et al. Minimal important changes and differences in elective hand surgery. J Hand Surg Eur Vol 2015;40(9):900–12.
20. Revicki D, Hays RD, Cella D, et al. Recommended methods for determining responsiveness and minimally important differences for patient-reported outcomes. J Clin Epidemiol 2008;61(2):102–9.
21. Terwee CB, Roorda LD, Dekker J, et al. Mind the MIC: large variation among populations and methods. J Clin Epidemiol 2010;63(5):524–34.
22. Davis A, Perruccio A, Lohmander LS. Minimally clinically important improvement: all non-responders are not really non-responders an illustration from total knee replacement. Osteoarthritis Cartilage 2012;20(5):364–7.
23. de Vet HC, Foumani M, Scholten MA, et al. Minimally important change values of a measurement instrument depend more on baseline values than on the type of intervention. J Clin Epidemiol 2015;68(5):518–24.
24. Franchignoni F, Vercelli S, Giordano A, et al. Minimal clinically important difference of the disabilities of the arm, shoulder and hand outcome measure (DASH) and its shortened version (QuickDASH). J Orthop Sports Phys Ther 2014;44(1):30–9.
25. Kosinski M, Zhao SZ, Dedhiya S, et al. Determining minimally important changes in generic and disease-specific health-related quality of life questionnaires in clinical trials of rheumatoid arthritis. Arthritis Rheum 2000;43(7):1478–87.
26. Santanello N, Zhang J, Seidenberg B, et al. What are minimal important changes for asthma measures in a clinical trial? Eur Respir J 1999;14(1):23–7.
27. Turner D, Schünemann HJ, Griffith LE, et al. The minimal detectable change cannot reliably replace the minimal important difference. J Clin Epidemiol 2010; 63(1):28–36.
28. Norman G. Hi! How are you? Response shift, implicit theories and differing epistemologies. Qual Life Res 2003;12(3):239–49.
29. Norman GR, Sloan JA, Wyrwich KW. Interpretation of changes in health-related quality of life: the remarkable universality of half a standard deviation. Med Care 2003;41(5):582–92.
30. Beaton DE. Simple as possible? Or too simple?: possible limits to the universality of the one half standard deviation. Med Care 2003;41(5):593–6.
31. Lassere M, van der Heijde D, Johnson KR. Foundations of the minimal clinically important difference for imaging. J Rheumatol 2001;28(4):890–1.
32. U.S. Department of Health and Human Services Food and Drug Administration. Guidance for industry: patient-reported outcome measures: use in medical product development to support labeling claims. Fed Regist 2009;74:65132–3.
33. Nantes SG, Strand V, Su J, et al. Comparison of the Sensitivity to Change of the 36-Item Short Form Health Survey and the Lupus Quality of Life Measure Using Various Definitions of Minimum Clinically Important Differences in Patients With Active Systemic Lupus Erythematosus. Arthritis Care Res (Hoboken) 2018; 70(1):125–33.
34. Erdogan BD, Leung YY, Pohl C, et al. Minimal clinically important difference as applied in rheumatology: an OMERACT Rasch Working Group systematic review and critique. J Rheumatol 2016;43(1):194–202.
35. Rouquette A, Blanchin M, Sébille V, et al. The minimal clinically important difference determined using item response theory models: an attempt to solve the issue of the association with baseline score. J Clin Epidemiol 2014;67(4):433–40.

36. Lee MK, Yost KJ, McDonald JS, et al. Item response theory analysis to evaluate reliability and minimal clinically important change of the Roland-Morris Disability Questionnaire in patients with severe disability due to back pain from vertebral compression fractures. Spine J 2017;17:821–9.
37. Schünemann HJ, Akl EA, Guyatt GH. Interpreting the results of patient reported outcome measures in clinical trials: the clinician's perspective. Health Qual Life Outcomes 2006;4(1):62.
38. de Vet HC, Terluin B, Knol DL, et al. Three ways to quantify uncertainty in individually applied "minimally important change" values. J Clin Epidemiol 2010;63(1): 37–45.
39. de Vet HC, Terwee CB. The minimal detectable change should not replace the minimal important difference. J Clin Epidemiol 2010;63(7):804–5.
40. Terwee CB, Roorda LD, Knol DL, et al. Linking measurement error to minimal important change of patient-reported outcomes. J Clin Epidemiol 2009;62(10): 1062–7.
41. de Vet HC, Terwee CB, Ostelo RW, et al. Minimal changes in health status questionnaires: distinction between minimally detectable change and minimally important change. Health Qual Life Outcomes 2006;4(1):54.
42. Beaton D, Bombardier C, Katz J, et al. A taxonomy for responsiveness. J Clin Epidemiol 2001;54(12):1204–17.
43. Devilliers H, Amoura Z, Besancenot J-F, et al. Responsiveness of the 36-item short form health survey and the lupus quality of life questionnaire in SLE. Rheumatology 2015;54(5):940–9.
44. McElhone K, Abbott J, Sutton C, et al. Sensitivity to change and minimal important differences of the LupusQoL in patients with systemic lupus erythematosus. Arthritis Care Res (Hoboken) 2016;68(10):1505–13.
45. Juniper EF, Guyatt GH, Willan A, et al. Determining a minimal important change in a disease-specific quality of life questionnaire. J Clin Epidemiol 1994;47(1):81–7.
46. de Vet HC, Ostelo RW, Terwee CB, et al. Minimally important change determined by a visual method integrating an anchor-based and a distribution-based approach. Qual Life Res 2007;16(1):131–42.
47. Mills KA, Naylor JM, Eyles JP, et al. Examining the minimal important difference of patient-reported outcome measures for individuals with knee osteoarthritis: a model using the knee injury and osteoarthritis outcome score. J Rheumatol 2016;43(2):395–404.
48. Terwee C, Dekker F, Wiersinga W, et al. On assessing responsiveness of health-related quality of life instruments: guidelines for instrument evaluation. Qual Life Res 2003;12(4):349–62.
49. Guyatt G, Walter S, Norman G. Measuring change over time: assessing the usefulness of evaluative instruments. J Chronic Dis 1987;40(2):171–8.
50. Schünemann HJ, Guyatt GH. Commentary—goodbye M (C) ID! Hello MID, where do you come from? Health Serv Res 2005;40(2):593–7.
51. Osoba D, Rodrigues G, Myles J, et al. Interpreting the significance of changes in health-related quality-of-life scores. J Clin Oncol 1998;16(1):139–44.
52. Wu JS. "Important difference" for interpreting health-related quality of life outcome measures: important to whom? Support Care Cancer 2012;20:429–31.

Alternative Design and Analytical Techniques for Longitudinal Rheumatology Studies

Improved Understanding of Outcomes

Lily Siok Hoon Lim, MBBS, MRCPCH, FRCPC, PhD[a,*],
Brian M. Feldman, MD, MSc, FRCPC[b,c], Lisa M. Lix, PhD[d]

KEYWORDS

• Longitudinal cohorts • Planned missing data design • Longitudinal analysis

KEY POINTS

- Longitudinal cohort studies (with three or more measurement occasions) enable researchers to examine between- and within-individual variation, providing an improved understanding of disease evolution.
- Alternative longitudinal study designs, such as the accelerated cohort, two-method measurement approach, and multiform design, increase efficiency of longitudinal designs by reducing time to research output and participant burden, while maintaining statistical power.
- Longitudinally collected secondary data (eg, administrative data) can be used to create retrospective cohorts for study, also reducing the time to research output while offering a population-based perspective on the issue at hand.
- Statistical models that take account of time-varying factors (covariates, mediators, and confounders), such as the marginal structural model, allow for unbiased assessment of therapeutic effectiveness in real-world longitudinal cohorts.
- Recurrent events and multistate models maximize the yield of information pertaining to prognostic factors and incidence of health events during the disease course.

Disclosure: None of the authors has pertinent conflicts of interest.
[a] Department of Pediatrics, Rady Faculty of Health Sciences, University of Manitoba, 501F-715 McDermot Avenue, Winnipeg, Manitoba R3E 3P4, Canada; [b] Division of Rheumatology, The Hospital for Sick Children, 555 University Avenue, Toronto, Ontario M5G1X8, Canada; [c] Department of Pediatrics, Faculty of Medicine, Institute of Health Policy Management and Evaluation, Dana Lana School of Public Health, University of Toronto, Toronto, Ontario M5T 3M6, Canada; [d] Department of Community Health Sciences, Rady Faculty of Health Sciences, University of Manitoba, S113-750 Bannatyne Avenue, Winnipeg, Manitoba R3E 0W3, Canada
* Corresponding author.
E-mail address: llim@chrim.ca

Rheum Dis Clin N Am 44 (2018) 189–201
https://doi.org/10.1016/j.rdc.2018.01.001 rheumatic.theclinics.com

INTRODUCTION

Longitudinal cohort studies, in which individuals are followed over time and measurements of their health are repeatedly collected via primary data collection methods, are common in rheumatology. Cohorts may be defined for a specific disease (eg, rheumatoid arthritis) or group of diseases (eg, spondyloarthropathies). Longitudinal cohort studies may be conducted in a single center, or in multiple centers; the latter are favored to increase sample size for the study of rare rheumatic diseases (**Table 1**).

Longitudinal cohort studies enable researchers to investigate between- and within-individual variation.[1] They are powerful for examining the disease trajectory and factors that may influence it. However, longitudinal cohort studies have several limitations, including the lengthy duration of time required for patient follow-up, heavy respondent burden, potential for a high rate of attrition, and potential for substantial nonresponse bias.

This article reviews alternative study designs and analytical methods for longitudinal cohort studies with three or more measurement occasions. The focus is on methods that facilitate the investigation of the shape of the disease trajectory (ie, linear vs non-linear). With just two measurement occasions, only a linear trajectory can be investigated.[1] The alternative designs that are the focus of this article are accelerated cohort, two-method measurement (TMM) designs, and multiform designs.[2–6] Also considered are retrospective cohort studies, which rely on secondary data, such as administrative health data, instead of primary data collection. We review the general methodology of each of these designs and their limitations and strengths.

The alternative analytical techniques that we focus on include linear and non-linear models with time-varying covariates, marginal structural models, recurrent, and multi-state event models.[7–9] These longitudinal models allow researchers to use all available data from participants' disease courses. By using all data on events, such models allow the shape of disease trajectories to be modeled. Also, by using all data on

Table 1
Examples of national and international longitudinal cohorts

Disease	Name of Cohort	Geographic Base
Adult cohorts		
Rheumatoid arthritis	Corrona	United States
	Canadian early arthritis cohort (CATCH)	Canada
Systemic lupus erythematosus	SLE International Collaborating Clinics (SLICC)	Worldwide (predominantly North America)
	Grupo Latino Americano de Estudio del Lupus (GLADEL)	South America
Vasculitis	French Vasculitis Study Group	France/Belgium
	Canadian Vasculitis consortium (CanVasc)	Canada
Scleroderma	European Scleroderma Trials and Research Group (EUSTAR)	Europe/Americas
Inflammatory myositis	Canadian Inflammatory Myopathy Study (CIMS)	Canada
Pediatric cohorts		
Juvenile idiopathic arthritis	Childhood Arthritis and Rheumatology Research Alliance (CARRA)	United States/Canada
Systemic lupus erythematosus	CARRA	United States/Canada

covariates (baseline and time-varying), these techniques allow a more in-depth understanding of how and when covariates affect disease trajectory evolution. We discuss these approaches using examples from recent publications.[10–12]

At the outset, we note that missing data and attrition are common in longitudinal cohort studies. Depending on the type of missing data (ie, ignorable vs nonignorable), it can reduce statistical power and/or bias study conclusions.[13] Appropriate handling of missing data is therefore an integral part of the conduct of longitudinal studies.[4,14] However, we do not pursue an in-depth discussion about missing data because another article on this topic is found within this issue (See Samantha Stephens and colleagues' article, "Strategies for Dealing with Missing Accelerometer Data," in this issue.)

ALTERNATIVE LONGITUDINAL DESIGNS USING PRIMARY DATA

Planned missing data (PMD) designs with primary data collection include accelerated cohort, two-method, and multiform designs. These designs are efficient because they rely on strategically placed missing data, meaning that participants do not have the same measurement schedule.[3,6] Missing data in PMD designs are missing completely at random; accordingly, their absence does not result in biased study conclusions.[13,15] By reducing response burden on participants, PMD designs can potentially minimize loss to follow-up and nonresponse bias.[13,15]

Accelerated Cohort Design

The accelerated cohort design is a sequential multicohort design. It joins adjacent segments of longitudinal data obtained from different age cohorts to study the longitudinal outcome trajectory over their combined age range.[16] This design is appropriate for investigating age-specific or developmental changes. As an example, an investigator may be interested to examine disease trajectories of young adult patients (18–30 years) with childhood-onset systemic lupus erythematosus (cSLE), including the length of any periods of prolonged remission. Instead of recruiting patients at age 18 years and following them for 12 years, an accelerated cohort design involves recruitment of patients in overlapping age groups (eg, 18–21 years, 20–23 years, 22–25 years, 24–27 years). Each cohort is followed for 3 years (**Table 2**) so that information spanning the 12 years of young adulthood is collected.

Considerations when designing an accelerated cohort study include the number of cohorts, duration of follow-up, number of measurements, and amount of overlap.[2,17,18] The optimal combination depends on several factors. For a fixed number of participants, increasing the number of cohorts increases statistical power, although

Table 2
Classic longitudinal and accelerated cohort designs

X	X	X	X	X	X	X	X	X	X	Design 1
X	X	X	X	0	0	0	0	0	0	Design 2
0	0	X	X	X	X	0	0	0	0	
0	0	0	0	X	X	X	X	0	0	
0	0	0	0	0	0	X	X	X	X	
18	19	20	21	22	23	24	25	26	27	Ages of participants

Design 1 is the classic single cohort longitudinal design with a follow-up time of 10 y. Design 2 is an accelerated cohort design with four cohorts, overlapping by 2 y. Each cohort is followed for 3 y. X denotes occasions of measurements, 0 denotes data not collected.

there are diminishing returns with increasing number of cohorts.[2] Increasing follow-up more than 3 years may not result in a substantial increase in statistical power.[2] For a fixed number of measurements, power is increased with fewer measurements per person, regardless of the number of cohorts or amount of overlap.[2]

The accelerated cohort design has many advantages. With a shorter length of follow-up, this design reduces the burden on investigators and participants. In the scenario presented previously, it is easy to imagine that any loss to follow-up associated with the accelerated cohort design is reduced. This design shortens the time to research output, which reduces the likelihood that questions asked or results would be outdated by study completion. The duration of need for funding is shorter. Patient recruitment is often less onerous.

However, the accelerated cohort design is not without its limitations. The period of time available to measure within-individual change is short. Cumulative occurrences may not be possible to study unless additional design features are added, such as information about pertinent outcomes and possible prognostic factors up to the point of entry into the cohort or at least in the intercohort interval just before entry.[17] Immortal time bias is a potential threat to the validity of inference; only those individuals who have survived their disease can enter later age cohorts.[19] Investigators must carefully document the source population from which they drew their study cohort: that is, what proportion of all patients greater than 18 year old were recruited into the accelerated cohort and how those recruited into the cohort differ from those who did not enter into the study cohort. In using the accelerated cohort design in a disease population, these measures are essential to interpret the results.

Two-Method Measurement Design

The TMM design measures the construct of interest (covariate) with a valid but often costly reference measure, and a second measure that is less costly but often less valid. Both measures capture the same construct.

The TMM design borrows strength from the use of two or more methods of measurement. Given the same budget, it is more efficient (and hence has greater statistical power) than a study in which only the reference standard is used for data collection. If only the cheaper measure is used, more participants are measured (with increased power) but the validity of the results is reduced. Measuring a random subset of the study population with the expensive reference standard allows the researcher to calculate the response bias for the cheaper, less valid measure and to adjust for this bias.[4]

To illustrate, the TMM design can be used to investigate the effects of smoking on rheumatoid arthritis activity. The biased measure is patients' self-reported cigarette use, which is typically underreported because of perceived social undesirability. Unbiased measures include exhaled carbon monoxide and blood cotinine levels. For this design to work, there must be a measure of the cheaper tool and at least one measure of the expensive tool.[20,21] **Fig. 1** provides the model layout. In this model, smoking predicts disease activity. Smoking is measured by two cheap and two expensive measures. The cheap measures are associated with a response bias factor. Because the expensive measures are available, they can be used to estimate the response bias factor and separate out the parts of the cheap measures that measure the smoking construct. Structural equation models for longitudinal data can be used to define the response bias factor.[4,20,21] Structural equation models is a multivariate technique to model relationships between measured variables and latent (unmeasurable) constructs.[3,22]

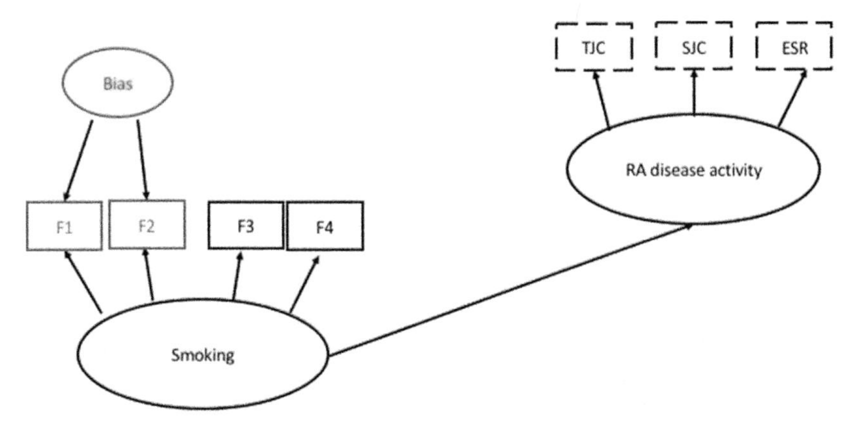

Fig. 1. An illustration of the response bias correction (structural equation) model. Ovals (*black border*) depict the covariate (smoking) and outcome (RA activity). Smoking (latent covariate) predicts RA disease activity (latent outcome). Small oval (*gray border*) denotes the bias response factor (Bias). Rectangles (*black and gray borders*) denote measures of the latent smoking variable. F1 and F2 are the biased self-reported measures. F3 and F4 are the gold standard measures. Dashed line rectangles denote the measures of the underlying latent construct of RA disease activity. ESR, erythrocyte sedimentation rate; RA, rheumatoid arthritis; SJC, swollen joint count; TJC, tender joint count.

The optimal total sample size to expensive measure ratio of a TMM design depends on cost ratio (number of cheap measures to one expensive measure), effect size of the construct of interest, and measure reliability.[4,5] Assume a fixed budget ($7200) and a cost for the cheap measure of $4 and for the expensive measure for $20 (5:1 cost ratio). If all participants receive both measures ($20 + $4), the total sample size is 300 ($7200/$24). **Table 3** shows the results for different scenarios.[4] The standard error

Table 3
Hypothetical data collection costs for two-measurement method (TMM) design where the cost ratio of expensive to cheap measure is 5:1, for a total cost of $7200

Total N	N Cheap	N Expensive	Standard Error	N_{eff}	N_{eff} Increase Factor
300	300	300	0.0543	300	—
600	600	240	0.0465	409	—
900	900	180	0.0422	495	—
1100	1100	140	0.0407	533	—
1200	**1200**	**120**	**0.0403**	**542**	**1.81**
1300	1300	100	0.0404	540	—
1500	1500	60	0.0425	489	—
1700	1700	20	0.0573	269	—

Bold line denotes the combination with the most precise standard error.

Total N denotes the total number of participants in a study. N cheap denotes the number studied with the cheap measure. N expensive denotes the number studied with the expensive measure. Standard error refers to that of the latent covariate, the smaller the better (more precise). N_{eff} denotes effective sample size, which refers to the equivalent sample size as though all were measured with the expensive measure. N_{eff} increase factor is the ratio of N_{eff}/N_{CD}, which denotes the power equivalent (for the TMM design) to testing a sample size of the corresponding longitudinal cohort design.

Adapted from Graham JW. Missing data: analysis and design. New York: Springer; 2012; with permission.

of the parameter estimate decreases to reach a nadir (ie, is most precise) when 1200 receive the cheap measure and 120 receive the expensive measure (ie, optimal PMD design). The effective sample size (N_{eff}) is 542, which means that measuring only 120 (out of 1200) participants with the expensive measure is equivalent to testing with 542 participants on both measures. If 542 participants were to be tested with the expensive measure alone, the cost would have been $10,840, and for both measures $13,008.

The N_{eff} increase factor (NIF) is the ratio of $N_{eff}/N_{complete\ data}$, which in this case for the most optimal study design is 1.81 (542/300). The optimal TMM design therefore allowed testing a hypothesis with a power equivalent to testing a sample size 1.81 times that of a longitudinal (complete data) cohort design.

Two factors affect the NIF: the cost ratio between the expensive and cheap measures and the effect size of the parameter estimate. If the expensive to cheap ratio is only 1.6 (small), the NIF is only 1.09, that is, 9% increase in N_{eff} compared with the longitudinal cohort design.[4] However, if the ratio is 10, which might be real in the case of expensive biomarkers, the NIF of the TMM design could increase to 1.96, that is, almost 200% increase over the longitudinal cohort design. Given the same cost ratio, the NIF is higher the smaller the effect size of the parameter estimate. Using the cost ratio of 10, if the effect size is 0.4, the NIF is 1.96 but if the effect size is 0.1, the NIF is 3.47. Therefore, for small effect sizes, using a TMM design can increase the effective sample size to approximately 3.5 times more than the longitudinal cohort design.

There are some limitations associated with using the TMM design. In real life, it may be hard to find a true unbiased measure as a reference standard, just a substantially less biased measure. This method is still applicable but the bias reduction can only be to the degree that the less biased reference standard is biased.[3] The TMM design is meant for inference at the group level and not at the individual level. The bias correction factor is meant for the latent construct and not for computing a correction to individual scores.[3]

Multiform Planned Missing Data

Often there are more questions to be asked than the participants are able to answer at each measurement occasion because of time constraints or attention drift. Instead of forgoing some questions altogether, the multiform design relies on the administration of different forms to different participants, allowing more questions to be asked of the entire cohort.[3,5]

Currently, many rheumatology cohorts try to minimize participant burden by measuring certain information only once per year. By adopting a multiform design, some of this information can potentially be collected during every visit without substantially overburdening participants. The information collected can then be tested more precisely for its effects on outcomes collected on every visit.

We illustrate this PMD design using the three-form (3F) design, the most common of the multiform designs.[4,5] All possible questions for participants are divided into four sets (X, A, B, C) (**Table 4**). An essential set of questions (X) that is most important for answering the central questions of the study is provided to every participant at every occasion. All other questions are distributed among three sets (A, B, C). Each participant is assigned to respond to one form (ie, XAB or XBC or XAC; see **Table 4**).

To illustrate, if there are 34 questions in X and 33 questions in each of A, B, and C, each participant would only be asked 100 questions. However, a total of 133 questions (overall) will be asked of the cohort. The 3F design therefore allows a 33% increase in the number of questions that can be asked when compared with a

Table 4
The 3-form design schedule

	Questionnaire ID and Number of Questions			
	X	A	B	C
Forms	34	33	33	33
1	1	1	1	0
2	1	0	1	1
3	1	1	0	1

1 denotes the data collection occasion, 0 denotes no data collection. Each form will collect data for questionnaire X, which contains core questions essential to address primary research questions. Forms A, B, C contain other questions of interest. At each study visit, one form (of 1–3) is administered to the participants. Each participant will answer two-thirds of all the questions in the study and have one-third of all questions missing (planned missing data).

single-form design. Following data collection, further processing is required using missing data models. For the models to accurately estimate the missing values, the correlation of items should be high (eg, >0.5).[4,23] It is suggested that items within a scale or questionnaire be split and redistributed among the three forms so that statistics are estimated with greater precision.[24] However for convenience, it might be easier to keep items within a scale on the same set.[4]

The 3F design can be extended to longitudinal studies. The strategy for assignment of forms depends on the study aims.[15] If the primary aim is to measure how single variables change during follow-up, then each participant should be given the same form across visits. If the primary aim is to test the relationships among questions, then a different form at each visit is preferred. Practically, the participants can be randomized at each visit to answer different forms.

There are some limitations associated with the multiform design.[15] The focus of research is at the group level; modern missing data techniques are used to facilitate the estimation of group-level parameters but cannot replace the missing data at an individual level. If the predicted effects are small, the correlation between items (in different sets) is weak, or the analysis requires large numbers, then the sample size requirements might be larger than for the longitudinal cohort design. Using modern missing data techniques requires the sample size to be sufficiently large to provide stable estimates of covariance (about 125).[3] With the 3F design, a conservative estimate of sample size is about 375 (3×125) to allow estimation of cross-set covariance.

Other variants include the six-form design and the 10-form design, which are more common than larger form designs.[4,25] With a fixed sample size, there are diminished returns with increased numbers of forms in terms of design complexity, amount of missing data, and statistical power.

ALTERNATIVE LONGITUDINAL DESIGN USING SECONDARY DATA

Administrative data are collected for managing and monitoring the health care system and not for research purposes. Examples of administrative data are records of physician billing claims, hospitalizations, and emergency department visits. These data are usually collected by the government to produce official statistics.[26] However, they are a potentially valuable resource for observational, longitudinal studies about chronic diseases. Rheumatologists are familiar with the use of administrative health care data for determining incidence and prevalence of various diseases and mortality.[27–29] However, the potential to use these data in novel ways is unlimited.

Longitudinal models can be applied to administrative data to answer questions about health care use trajectories.[30] For example, latent class analysis was used to identify different patterns of longitudinal health care (encounter) pathways during an episode of chronic obstructive pulmonary disease exacerbation and costs associated with different pathways.[31] These latent pathways were associated with different durations, types, and numbers of health care contacts and costs. By identifying patients' membership in different pathways, recommendations are derived about case management strategies to streamline episode management for those with the most severe disease and highest intensity health care use group. Combining longitudinal models with administrative data can leverage the availability of longitudinally collected data to clarify important outcomes of patients.

There are some unique advantages to using administrative data to measure outcomes and increase efficiency of research. The study population is likely be more representative as the extent of population coverage is close to 100%.[32,33] Even those individuals who might otherwise not participate in primary data collection studies are captured.[32] Administrative data is especially helpful when studying outcomes that occur after longer disease durations or older ages. This approach is helpful with detecting less common outcomes (although not rare because confidentiality considerations forbid report of very low numbers) faster than a study population recruited specifically for one study.

ALTERNATIVE LONGITUDINAL ANALYTICAL METHODS

In this section, we discuss several examples of newer (but less commonly used) longitudinal models that enable researchers to make full use of all available data. These models are used in longitudinal cohort studies to address long-term therapeutic outcomes (marginal structural modeling); recurrent events, such as flares of disease (recurrent event modeling); and progression through various stages of disease (multistate modeling). All of these models have in common the ability to evaluate time-varying (covariates, mediators, confounders) effects over the course of outcome evolution.

Marginal Structural Model

Rheumatologists are often interested in long-term outcomes of patients after treatment. Specifically, the researcher may seek to answer the question: "What treatment (eg, drug A vs drug B) is associated with better outcomes over time"? Although trials are important to establish efficacy and information about short-term outcomes (ie, commonly up to 24 months), most trials do not cover longer periods of time.

Therapeutic data from observational studies cannot be directly analyzed to determine unbiased therapeutic effects. There is likely confounding by indication, where sicker patients are treated differently than less sick patients. Treatments may be changed, augmented, or stopped and patients may leave (attrition), potentially resulting in a cohort that is no longer representative of the population by the end of follow-up. Many patients are treated with several medications (eg, steroids) that are constantly being adjusted based on information about disease activity and observed outcomes. These other treatments serve as time-varying confounders in that they are related to the outcomes and other covariates (eg, treatment of interest), and act as mediators, in that their past values influence the current observed outcomes. Standard statistical models assume that time-varying confounders of current and future treatments and outcomes are not affected by prior treatment. Therefore, in the presence of time-varying confounders that are affected by prior treatment (eg, steroids), even longitudinal models with time-varying variables cannot provide unbiased causal estimates.

Marginal structural models were developed to estimate causal treatment effects in the presence of treatment switching, time-varying confounders, and missing data.[34] The analysis has two steps. First, two sets of weights are calculated for each visit, one adjusts for treatment selection and another adjusts for attrition; these weights are multiplied to produce stabilized weights for each visit. Next, generalized estimating equations weighted with the stabilized weights are then used to estimate the treatment effect (as a time-varying factor) after adjusting for relevant baseline covariates.[35] Treatment history before each visit, baseline covariates, and time-varying covariates are incorporated into the computations of the treatment selection and attrition weights for each visit. Where time-varying factors (covariates and confounders) are strong predictors of treatment choice, observations are down-weighted because they are likely to be overrepresented in the cohort. These weights therefore create a pseudopopulation where treatment allocation is not confounded.[36–38] As prior treatment history is incorporated into the weights, they adjust for the relationship between current treatment and current and past confounding effects.

A recent study about cSLE nephritis used the marginal structural model.[12] The investigators tested the effectiveness of mycophenolate mofetil against other immunosuppressants for preserving renal function, as measured by glomerular filtration rates (GFR).[12] The investigators used marginal structural models to address confounding by indication, time-varying confounding, treatment switching, and concomitant treatments. Mycophenolate mofetil, compared with other immunosuppressants, increased overall GFR by 6%. This benefit was observable after the first 2 years of treatment and became significantly more pronounced over 4 to 6 years.

We showed in this section the application of marginal structural modeling to estimate unbiased long-term therapeutic outcomes in a longitudinal study. There are other strategies that can be used in similar situations to provide unbiased estimates of outcomes. Examples include longitudinal propensity score modeling and the instrumental variable approach.[39,40]

Recurrent Events Models

Many events in rheumatic diseases may be recurrent (eg, disease flares, remission, development of avascular necrosis). Although survival models are frequently used to model time to first event and the associated predictors, subsequent events are less frequently examined. Predictors of the first event may not be as strongly associated with subsequent events, and history of prior events may influence the occurrence of subsequent events.[7,41,42]

Some researchers have modeled recurrent events using generalized linear models with generalized estimating equations and nonlinear mixed-effects models, to account for repeated measurements on the same individuals. However, such approaches miss out on the opportunity to test hypotheses about the timing of events. Using recurrent event models, the researcher can ask what factors (baseline or time-varying) predict the occurrence of (multiple) events, and whether the same factors predict the occurrence of first versus subsequent events.[7,43]

Recurrent event analysis was compared with time-to-first-event analysis to evaluate the effect of sex on episodes of functional disability among elderly in a longitudinal study.[10] About 60% of participants did not have an event, 20% had one event, and another 20% more than one event. When evaluated with the first-event-only approach, women were found to be at a higher risk of developing bathing disability but not for other disability. However, when evaluated using recurrent event analysis, the effect of sex was even greater for bathing disability and became statistically significant for other disability. It is therefore obvious that the first-event-only approach is inadequate to evaluate the effects of prognostic factors. When the effect of previous disability episodes (in addition to other baseline and time-varying factors) is taken into consideration in recurrent event models for bathing disability and other disability, the effect of sex disappears. This further illustrates how incorporating all available longitudinal data (outcomes and time-varying covariates) in modeling can clarify the understanding of participants' disease trajectories.

Multistate Models

Some outcomes in rheumatic diseases may evolve through multiple stages (eg, extent of proteinuria or degree of renal impairment). The different stages may be reversible, that is, there could be several forward-backward transitions between adjacent states. However, this evolution through different stages has not been well-studied. More commonly, some kind of outcome categorization on a single occasion of ascertainment is used to study such outcomes. Such multistate events can be thought of as part a special case of recurrent events, where there are more than just two states (usually occurrence or nonoccurrence). Researchers could ask many questions in such a scenario: what disease states are cohort members in at various times of follow-up, what are the frequencies of transitions between reversible states, what are the probabilities of transitioning between states, what are the average duration of times spent in each state, what factors (baseline and time-varying) predict the transition between different states.[7,9,44]

The multistate event approach was recently used by the SLE international collaborating clinics to study longitudinal renal function outcomes (proteinuria, GFR) and to identify predictors of transitions between states (ie, worsening or improving).[11] It is now clear that with current management, renal functions in patients with SLE continue to improve up to 5 years after the initial presentation. The group was also able to identify predictors for different kinds of transitions (improvement and detriment) during follow-up.

Studying recurrent or multistate events can clarify the nature of the disease course. By knowing the different predictors of first and subsequent events, this information could potentially change the management approach to reduce patients' risks of an event, depending on whether they have had prior events. By the same measure, knowing the probabilities of transitioning to an improved or worsened state, and the duration of time spent in each of these states, can also dictate different risk management strategies of different urgencies for patients at different stages of disease evolution.

SUMMARY

We have shown in this review how alternative PMD designs are used to accelerate the time to research output, collect more information, and maintain or sometimes increase statistical power. We have also shown how advanced statistical models are used to provide estimations of unbiased treatment effects through adjustments of time-varying covariates, mediators, and confounders.[45] Methods that use all available disease course data allowing the modeling of recurrent events or multistate events were also presented.[7,9,41,42]

Longitudinal studies are especially valuable to study patients with rare diseases (like many rheumatic diseases) and their impact on health trajectory. It is challenging to accrue large cohorts without investments of substantial time, efforts, and commitments. Such studies are also important for informing the effectiveness of various management strategies in real-world settings, where patients have multiple comorbid conditions, suboptimal adherence, and other issues affecting control of their diseases; but this has been an underexplored potential. The methods we presented can help researchers maximize the yield of information from longitudinal studies.

The methods that we have focused on in this review are most helpful for researchers who are interested in a group-level view of the disease trajectory. This view is important for understanding the overall prognosis of a disease population and is an important piece of information for all stakeholders, including patients, physicians, and especially health care payers. However, this view does not take into account individual variation in outcomes relative to the overall population. If the researcher's main interest lies in understanding how individual variation affects patient outcomes, then the traditional longitudinal design and appropriate analysis strategies should be adopted. Developing more efficient longitudinal designs to model individual-level variation is an active area of research that should continue to be developed.

REFERENCES

1. Singer JD, Willett JB. Applied longitudinal analysis. New York: Oxford University Press; 2003.
2. Galbraith S, Bowden J, Mander A. Accelerated longitudinal designs: an overview of modelling, power, costs and handling missing data. Stat Methods Med Res 2017;26(1):374–98.
3. Garnier-Villarreal M, Rhemtulla M, Little TD. Two-method planned missing designs for longitudinal research. Int J Behav Dev 2014;38(5):411–22.
4. Graham JW. Missing data: analysis and design. New York: Springer; 2012.
5. Graham JW, Taylor BJ, Olchowski AE, et al. Planned missing data designs in psychological research. Psychol Methods 2006;11(4):323–43.
6. Wu W, Jia F, Rhemtulla M, et al. Search for efficient complete and planned missing data designs for analysis of change. Behav Res Methods 2016;48(3): 1047–61.
7. Amorim LD, Cai J. Modelling recurrent events: a tutorial for analysis in epidemiology. Int J Epidemiol 2015;44(1):324–33.
8. Robins JM, Hernan MA, Brumback B. Marginal structural models and causal inference in epidemiology. Epidemiology 2000;11(5):550–60.
9. Sutradhar R, Barbera L. A Markov multistate analysis of the relationship between performance status and death among an ambulatory population of cancer patients. Palliat Med 2014;28(2):184–90.
10. Guo Z, Gill TM, Allore HG. Modeling repeated time-to-event health conditions with discontinuous risk intervals: an example of a longitudinal study of functional disability among older persons. Methods Inf Med 2008;47(2):107.
11. Hanly JG, Su L, Urowitz MB, et al. A longitudinal analysis of outcomes of lupus nephritis in an International Inception Cohort using a multistate model approach. Arthritis Rheumatol 2016;68(8):1932–44.
12. Tian SY, Silverman ED, Pullenayegum E, et al. Comparative effectiveness of mycophenolate mofetil for the treatment of childhood-onset proliferative lupus nephritis. Arthritis Care Res (Hoboken) 2017.
13. Little RJ. Methods for handling missing values in clinical trials. J Rheumatol 1999; 26(8):1654–6.
14. Graham JW. Missing data analysis: making it work in the real world. Annu Rev Psychol 2009;60:549–76.

15. Rhemtulla M, Little T. Tools of the trade: planned missing data designs for research in cognitive development. J Cogn Dev 2012;13(4):425–38.
16. Nesselroade JR, Baltes PB. Longitudinal research in the study of behavior and development. New York: Academic Press; 1979.
17. Farrington DP. Longitudinal research strategies: advantages, problems, and prospects. J Am Acad Child Adolesc Psychiatry 1991;30(3):369–74.
18. Moerbeek M. The effects of the number of cohorts, degree of overlap among cohorts, and frequency of observation on power in accelerated longitudinal designs. Methodology 2011;7(1):11–24.
19. Rothman KJ, Greenland S, Lash TL, editors. Modern epidemiology. 3rd edition. Philadelphia: Lippincott Williams & Wilkins; 2008.
20. Kline RB. Software review: software programs for structural equation modeling: Amos, EQS, and LISREL. J Psychoeduc Assess 1998;16(4):343–64.
21. Kline RB. Principles and practice of structural equation modeling. New York: Guilford Publications; 2015.
22. Little TD. Longitudinal structural equation modeling. New York: Guilford Press; 2013.
23. Little TD, Rhemtulla M. Planned missing data designs for developmental researchers. Child Dev Perspect 2013;7(4):199–204.
24. Graham JW, Hofer SM, MacKinnon DP. Maximizing the usefulness of data obtained with planned missing value patterns: an application of maximum likelihood procedures. Multivariate Behav Res 1996;31(2):197–218.
25. Raghunathan TE, Grizzle JE. A split questionnaire survey design. J Am Stat Assoc 1995;90(429):54–63.
26. Supporting administrative data research in UK. What is administrative data and why use if for research. 2017. Available at: http://www.adls.ac.uk/about/. Accessed October 24, 2017.
27. Barnabe C, Joseph L, Belisle P, et al. Prevalence of systemic lupus erythematosus and systemic sclerosis in the First Nations population of Alberta, Canada. Arthritis Care Res (Hoboken) 2012;64(1):138–43.
28. Broten L, Avina-Zubieta JA, Lacaille D, et al. Systemic autoimmune rheumatic disease prevalence in Canada: updated analyses across 7 provinces. J Rheumatol 2014;41(4):673–9.
29. Ravi B, Croxford R, Austin PC, et al. The relation between total joint arthroplasty and risk for serious cardiovascular events in patients with moderate-severe osteoarthritis: propensity score matched landmark analysis. BMJ 2013;347:f6187.
30. van Dijk CE, Hoekstra T, Verheij RA, et al. Type II diabetes patients in primary care: profiles of healthcare utilization obtained from observational data. BMC Health Serv Res 2013;13(1):7.
31. Kuwornu JP, Lix LM, Quail JM, et al. Identifying distinct healthcare pathways during episodes of chronic obstructive pulmonary disease exacerbations. Medicine (Baltimore) 2016;95(9):e2888.
32. Roos LL Jr, Nicol JP, Cageorge SM. Using administrative data for longitudinal research: comparisons with primary data collection. J Chronic Dis 1987;40(1):41–9.
33. Raaschou P, Simard JF, Holmqvist M, et al, ARTIS Study Group. Rheumatoid arthritis, anti-tumour necrosis factor therapy, and risk of malignant melanoma: nationwide population based prospective cohort study from Sweden. BMJ 2013;346:f1939.

34. Hernan MA, Brumback BA, Robins JM. Estimating the causal effect of zidovudine on CD4 count with a marginal structural model for repeated measures. Stat Med 2002;21(12):1689–709.
35. Zeger SL, Liang KY, Albert PS. Models for longitudinal data: a generalized estimating equation approach. Biometrics 1988;44(4):1049–60.
36. Journal Citation Report. Available at: http://thomsonreuters.com/products_services/science/science_products/a-z/journal_citation_reports/. Accessed June 24, 2012.
37. Mansournia MA, Altman DG. Inverse probability weighting. BMJ 2016;352:i189.
38. Seaman SR, White IR. Review of inverse probability weighting for dealing with missing data. Stat Methods Med Res 2013;22(3):278–95.
39. Achy-Brou A, Griswold M, Frangakis C. Regression models on longitudinal propensity scores. Analysis of Observational Health Care Data Using SAS. Cary (NC): SAS institute; 2010. p. 263.
40. Newhouse JP, McClellan M. Econometrics in outcomes research: the use of instrumental variables. Annu Rev Public Health 1998;19:17–34.
41. Andersen PK, Gill RD. Cox's regression model for counting processes: a large sample study. The annals of statistics 1982;10(4):1100–20.
42. Prentice RL, Williams BJ, Peterson AV. On the regression analysis of multivariate failure time data. Biometrika 1981;68(2):373–9.
43. Austin PC, Lee DS, Fine JP. Introduction to the analysis of survival data in the presence of competing risks. Circulation 2016;133(6):601–9.
44. Meira-Machado L, de Uña-Álvarez J, Cadarso-Suárez C, et al. Multi-state models for the analysis of time-to-event data. Stat Methods Med Res 2009;18(2):195–222.
45. Faries DE, Obenchain R, Haro JM, et al. Analysis of observational health care data using SAS. Cary (NC): SAS Institute; 2010.

Propensity Score Methods for Bias Reduction in Observational Studies of Treatment Effect

Sindhu R. Johnson, MD, PhD[a,b,*], George A. Tomlinson, PhD[b,c,d], Gillian A. Hawker, MD, MSc[b,e], John T. Granton, MD[f,g], Brian M. Feldman, MD, MSc[b,c,h]

KEYWORDS

- Propensity score • Bias • Observational data • Scleroderma • Systemic sclerosis

KEY POINTS

- The absence of randomization in an observational study makes inferences about treatment effect susceptible to confounding by indication.
- Propensity score methods are a strategy to balance observed characteristics.
- Propensity score methods result in a pseudorandomization, facilitating exchangeability. This result allows for a less biased estimation of the effect of a treatment at each value of the propensity score.

Disclosure Statement: None of the authors have any commercial or financial conflicts of interest to disclose.
Dr S. Johnson has been awarded a Canadian Institutes of Health Research New Investigator Award. Dr G. Hawker is supported as the Sir John and Lady Eaton Chair of Medicine. Dr B. Feldman holds the Ho Family Chair in Autoimmune Disease Research.
[a] Division of Rheumatology, Department of Medicine, Toronto Western Hospital, Mount Sinai Hospital, Ground Floor, East Wing, 399 Bathurst Street, Toronto, Ontario M5T 2S8, Canada; [b] Institute of Health Policy, Management and Evaluation, University of Toronto, 155 College Street, Toronto, Ontario M5T 3M6, Canada; [c] Dalla Lana School of Public Health, University of Toronto, 155 College Street, Toronto, Ontario M5T 3M7, Canada; [d] Department of Medicine, Division of Support, Systems, and Outcomes, Toronto General Research Institute, Toronto General Hospital, Eaton North, 10th Floor, Room 235, 200 Elizabeth Street, Toronto, Ontario M5G 2C4, Canada; [e] Division of Rheumatology, Department of Medicine, Women's College Hospital, 76 Grenville Street, 8th Floor East, Room 815, Toronto, Ontario M5S 1B2, Canada; [f] Division of Respirology, Department of Medicine, Toronto General Hospital, University Health Network, MUNK Building, 11-1170, 200 Elizabeth Avenue, Toronto, Ontario M5G 2C4, Canada; [g] Division of Critical Care Medicine, Department of Medicine, Toronto General Hospital, University Health Network, MUNK Building, 11-1170, 200 Elizabeth Avenue, Toronto, Ontario M5G 2C4, Canada; [h] Division of Rheumatology, Department of Paediatrics, The Hospital for Sick Children, 555 University Avenue, Toronto, Ontario M5G 1X8, Canada
* Corresponding author. Division of Rheumatology, Toronto Western Hospital, Ground Floor, East Wing, 399 Bathurst Street, Toronto, Ontario M5T 2S8, Canada.
E-mail address: Sindhu.Johnson@uhn.ca

Rheum Dis Clin N Am 44 (2018) 203–213
https://doi.org/10.1016/j.rdc.2018.01.002
0889-857X/18/
rheumatic.theclinics.com

INTRODUCTION

Observational Data

The merits of observational data for the study of uncommon diseases have long been recognized.[1] Whereas the use of narrow inclusion criteria to select subjects for clinical trials can result in a more precise estimation of a treatment effect in a defined group of subjects, observational studies can evaluate the effect of a treatment in a wider population; a wider selection of subjects may result in a different estimate of treatment effect.[2] Thus, observational data may sometimes provide a better representation of the spectrum of real-world practice than conventional randomized trials.[3] Additionally, the use of observational data allows studies to have a longer duration of follow-up. This longer follow-up can yield an important understanding about long-term treatment effects as well as long-term adverse effects. Narrow inclusion criteria and a short follow-up have increasingly been recognized as limitations of clinical trials; there is, accordingly, great value in the use of observational studies, particularly observational cohorts or registries.[1]

Confounding

A challenge to the use of observational data to study treatment effects is the issue of confounding.[4] Confounding of a treatment effect occurs when there is a distortion of the estimated treatment effect on an outcome caused by the presence of another factor.[5] This factor (ie, confounder) must be (1) causally related to the outcome independently of the exposure and (2) associated with the exposure but not a consequence of exposure. The confounder can have a positive influence, increasing the measured treatment effect above what it would otherwise be, or it can have a negative influence, falsely lowering the measured treatment effect.[5] In its simple form, confounding can be considered a confusion or mixing of effects whereby the effect of an exposure is distorted because of the effect of another variable.[6,7]

Confounding by indication (also known as treatment selection bias or susceptibility bias) is a special and important form of confounding that threatens the use of observational data to make unbiased estimates of treatment effect.[5,8] In a randomized trial, the act of randomization ensures that treatment assignment is random. In an observational study, treatment assignment is not random and may be influenced by a variety of factors. Confounding by indication occurs when there is noncomparability between the study groups resulting from the way they were constructed.[5] Exposed and unexposed patients may differ systematically in important characteristics. These characteristics may include disease severity, comorbidity, prognosis, local practice patterns, health care access, and patient preferences.[9,10] Small differences between treatment groups in many covariates can accumulate into substantial overall differences.[3] It may be that these differences have a greater effect on the outcome than the intervention itself. Properly conducted randomized trials are not affected by confounding by indication. Confounding by indication needs to be considered when the interest of an analysis lies in the effect of a treatment that is given in the course of clinical care.

A more nuanced way of thinking about confounding by indication is the use of the counterfactual definition.[5,11] Savitz sets up the counterfactual concept as follows:

> *The ideal comparison group for the exposed group is the exposed group itself but under the condition of not having been exposed, an experience that did not, in fact, occur (thus it is counterfactual). If we could observe this experience (which we cannot), we would be able to compare the disease occurrence under the*

situation in which exposure has occurred to the counterfactual one in which everything else is the same except exposure was not present. Instead, we choose some other group...to provide an estimate of what the experience of the exposed group would have been absent the exposure...[11]

Thus, investigators are trying to estimate what they would have observed had the same individual been exposed and nonexposed at the same time—a difference that cannot be observed in reality.[12] When comparing different groups of subjects, the unexposed group may have other factors that influence the disease and make their disease experience an inaccurate reflection of the disease experience of the exposed had they not been exposed. This circumstance is referred to as *nonexchangeability* in that the exposed and nonexposed are not exchangeable, aside from the effect of the exposure itself.[5,11]

Random allocation of treatment exposure (randomization) on average removes the potential effect of confounding.[13] It is important to note, however, that randomization guarantees balance only on average but not in a particular trial.[9] Indeed, chance (random error) imbalance in baseline characteristics will occur. There may be some factors that might be causally related to the outcome that are imbalanced after randomization. However, this residual imbalance is *random imbalance* as opposed to *systematic imbalance*. The fact that there is no systematic direction to this imbalance allows us to use statistical inference to determine how likely our data, or more extreme data, are under the null hypothesis. In other words, what is the chance that imbalance due to random factors, and random variation in outcomes alone, has led to the results at least as unusual as the one that we see? Similarly, if there is imbalance of *unmeasured* influences on the outcome, the imbalance is random as opposed to systematic. Increasing the trial size can minimize the probability of imbalance occurring. In contrast, confounding in observational studies is not minimized as the study size increases.[5] Study design and analytical strategies are needed to address the potential effects of confounding.

Challenge for Clinical Researchers

The challenge for investigators is to develop and apply methods that will allow for the unbiased estimation of treatment effects with observational data, which approximate those that would be observed in a similarly sized clinical trial.[14] Indeed, investigators are encouraged to develop methods that will minimize bias to ensure the integrity of observational studies.[15] One potential methodological solution to the challenges of confounding by indication is the use of propensity score methods.

Propensity Score Methods

Interpreting data on the treatment effect involves consideration of the effect the treatment would have on a subject who did not receive it.[16] In observational studies, inferences are made by comparing exposed and nonexposed subjects. The noncomparability may result in a situation whereby the treatment group is systematically different from the comparator group in a way that distorts the estimation of the treatment effect. Direct comparisons of the 2 groups may be misleading and lead to a biased estimation of the treatment effect.[16]

The propensity score is a balancing score that can be used to compare groups, or pairs, that are not systematically different; a propensity score, thus, enables unbiased comparisons between groups.[16] It is defined as the conditional probability of exposure to treatment, given the observed covariates.[17] The propensity score can be estimated by regressing the treatment assignment on observed baseline characteristics using a logistic regression model (for example).

Formula 1. Propensity score

$$e(X) = P(Z = 1|X)$$

where $e(X)$ is the propensity score; Z is the exposure, where 1 is exposed, 0 is unexposed; X is a set of baseline characteristics, where X is $(X1 \ldots Xp)$; $P(Z = 1|X)$ is the probability of exposure given observed baseline characteristics.

Note: Each subject has a probability of exposure, where $0 < e(X) < 1$.

At an individual level, it is a measure of the likelihood that a person would have been treated considering their characteristics.[17] The propensity score summarizes all the relevant characteristics in a single composite score.[3,18] The propensity score can be used to ascertain if there is sufficient overlap in characteristics between the treatment and comparator groups to allow appropriate estimation of a treatment effect.[3] The propensity score can be used to create a design with balance. Most importantly, the use of the propensity score allows unbiased estimation of the causal effect of an exposure in the presence of confounding.[16,19] Subjects with a given propensity score will tend to have the same distribution of covariates. This distribution creates a pseudorandomized scenario allowing the unbiased estimation of the treatment effect at each value of the propensity score.[19]

Four Propensity Score Approaches

Table 1 shows 4 different methodological approaches that have been described for the application of the propensity score. The first approach involves matching treated and comparator subjects on the propensity score to create an individually matched sample. This method is typically used in a situation whereby there is a limited number of treated subjects and a larger number of comparator subjects.[17] Several matching methods have been proposed.[17] The easiest and most commonly used method is matching on the closest comparator, so long as the logit of the 2 propensity scores are no further apart than a predefined caliper width.[17] It has been recommended to use a caliper width of 0.2 to 0.25 of the standard deviation of the logit of the propensity score.[20,21] The treated subjects are randomly ordered. The first treated subject is matched to the closest comparator subject, and the pair is removed from the pool. This process is repeated until no further matches can be achieved within the defined caliper width.[17]

Once the matched sample has been created, it is recommended to use statistical methods appropriate for the analysis of the matched data when estimating the treatment effect and its statistical significance (eg, paired t-test, Wilcoxon signed ranks test).[22] Statistical testing should take into consideration the lack of independence of subjects within the propensity score matched pair.[23]

A second approach is subclassification (also called stratification) whereby treated and comparator subjects are divided by the propensity score into subclasses. Treated and comparator subjects who are in the same subclass are compared directly.[17] An estimate of the treatment effect is calculated either by a weighted average, pooling the treatment effects in each subclass, or by a single regression, with the subclass and treatment assignment as categorical predictor variables. Subclassification with 5 subclasses has been shown to remove up to 90% of the bias in the unadjusted estimate.[24]

A third approach is the inverse-probability-of-treatment weighted estimator (also called the marginal structural model approach). Weights are created that are

Table 1
Comparisons of propensity score methods

Method	Advantages	Disadvantages
Matching	Eliminates more bias from confounding by indication than stratification Transparency in comparing treated and comparator subjects Well-developed balance diagnostics Outcome is not specified in the model Allows estimation of risk differences and relative risk	Reduced sample size from discarding unmatched subjects Results in bias if there is a differential treatment effect in those who are matched vs those who are unmatched
Subclassification	Transparency in comparing treated and comparator subjects Permits use of the whole data set Can assess balance within each stratum	May not have adequate overlap May have very small cell sizes in some strata
Covariate adjustment	Permits use of the whole data set	Loses design comparability to a randomized trial: adjusting instead of comparing similar subjects May include treated subjects for whom there are no appropriate comparator subjects
Inverse probability weighting	Removes approximately equivalent amount of imbalance as matching Permits use of the whole data set.	Potential for decreased precision in estimated treatment effect

the inverse probability of the treatment actually received, that is, 1/e(X) in the treated group and 1/(1-e[X]) in the comparator group. This approach essentially creates the 2 groups (also referred to as pseudopopulations) that would have been observed if all subjects had been exposed and all subjects had not been exposed.[25] The estimated treatment effect is the difference in the weighted averages of the observed outcomes in the two groups. A criticism of this approach is that subjects with propensity scores near 0 or 1 can have extremely large weights; this results in a decreased precision in the estimate of the treatment effect (ie, very high variance and wide confidence intervals).[19] There are solutions that limit the weights to a maximum size (eg, 10) or multiply them by a factor to stabilize them.[26]

A fourth approach is the use of the propensity score in regression adjustment. With traditional multivariable modeling and a large data set, one could regress the outcome on baseline characteristics. However, in the setting of uncommon diseases, there are frequently insufficient numbers of subjects (and outcomes) to allow for a complex model with numerous variables. Using this approach, important subject characteristics are used to model the propensity score. The outcome is then regressed on the propensity score and an indicator for treatment assignment. The ability to include a complex model with many variables in the estimation of a propensity score, and then regress the outcome on the single propensity score, confers an important methodological advantage in the study of uncommon diseases.[16]

A criticism of this approach is the loss of the ability to mimic the design of a randomized trial. Matching, subclassification, and weighting remove confounding by design.[27]

Treatment assignment is independent of baseline characteristics in the matched sample, stratified sample, or weighted sample. The outcome is only assessed after confounding has been addressed. The use of the propensity score for regression adjustment requires the propensity score to be used in the same model as evaluation of the outcome. This lack of separation of the design and analysis is of concern for some critics.[20] Using the other 3 approaches, the propensity score is used in study design and the analysis is separate.[27] A comparison of the propensity methods highlighting their relative advantages and disadvantages[16,17,20] is summarized in **Table 1**.

Assessing Balance

After construction of a propensity score, the quality of balance achieved by the propensity score should be evaluated. The test of a good propensity score is the degree to which it results in the measured baseline characteristics being balanced between the treated and comparator subjects. If matching is used, it has been recommended that investigators describe the distribution of baseline characteristics in the two matched samples.[23] One method of assessing balance, after propensity score matching, is the evaluation of the standardized difference in each baseline characteristic. The standardized difference is the absolute difference in the sample means divided by an estimate of the pooled standard deviation of the variable. The standardized difference represents the difference in means between the two groups in units of standard deviation. A similar formula is used for determining the standardized differences for dichotomous variables.[28] When propensity score stratification is used, the standardized differences between treated and comparator subjects are calculated within each stratum.

Formula 2. Standardized difference for comparing means

$$d = \frac{(\overline{x}_{\text{treatment}} - \overline{x}_{\text{control}})}{\sqrt{\frac{s^2_{\text{treatment}} + s^2_{\text{control}}}{2}}}$$

where d is the standardized difference; $\overline{x}_{\text{group}}$ is the mean of baseline characteristic in the specified group; s^2_{group} is the variance of baseline characteristic in the specified group.

Formula 3. Standardized differences for comparing prevalences

$$d = \frac{(\widehat{p}_{\text{treatment}} - \widehat{p}_{\text{control}})}{\sqrt{\frac{\widehat{p}_{\text{treatment}}(1-\widehat{p}_{\text{treatment}}) + \widehat{p}_{\text{control}}(1-\widehat{p}_{\text{control}})}{2}}}$$

where d is the standardized difference; $\widehat{p}_{\text{group}}$ is the prevalence of baseline characteristic in the specified group.

The use of the standardized difference to assess balance is preferable to conventional significance testing, as it is not affected by the sample size and it is a property of the sample.[22] Diagnostics have also been proposed for when the propensity score is used for covariate adjustment (weighted conditional standardized difference). When imbalance occurs, it is suggested to modify the propensity score iteratively, in an attempt to achieve better balance.[22] When the inverse-probability-of-treatment weighted estimator approach is used, balance can be assessed by computing weighted summaries of subject characteristics in each group.[26]

As in a randomized trial, there may be some residual imbalance in measured baseline characteristics in the matched sample.[23] There is no gold standard criterion for assessing appropriate balance. It has been recommended that a standardized difference of 10% be used as a threshold for assessing balance.[28]

Threat of Unmeasured Confounding

A limitation to the use of observational data to make unbiased estimates of the treatment effect and a limitation of propensity score modeling is the threat of unmeasured confounders. Classically, only factors that have been measured can be accounted for in the design and analytical phases. Innovative strategies have been proposed to account for unmeasured confounding. These strategies include Bayesian bias analysis,[29] instrumental variable analysis,[30] and tracer analysis.[31] Conventionally, these strategies have been used in large data sets. Although they hold great promise for the study of uncommon diseases, how they operate in the setting of small samples is uncertain.

Propensity Score Use in Observational Data of an Uncommon Disease: An Example

Propensity score modeling is a bias-correcting method that may be useful in the setting of observational data on uncommon diseases. Propensity scores are traditionally used in large administrative data sets.[3] The use of propensity score methods in the setting of uncommon diseases, whereby the sample sizes are small, is less common. Using a small data set, one may not be able to find a suitable subject for propensity score matching. There is a risk of losing a substantial number of subjects when a suitable match cannot be found. The authors provide an illustrative example whereby propensity score methods were successfully used to study the effect of warfarin for improving survival in systemic sclerosis (SSc)–associated pulmonary arterial hypertension (PAH).[32]

SSc is an uncommon chronic disease characterized by fibrosis (of the skin, lungs, kidneys), vasculopathy (resulting in digital ulceration, gangrene, and PAH), and immune activation. It has an annual incidence of 2 to 10 per million and a prevalence of up to 290 per million.[33] A leading cause of death in patients with SSc is PAH.[34] Patients have shortness of breath, decreased exercise tolerance, progressive heart failure, and poor quality of life and die an untimely death. Right heart catheterization-based prevalence estimates of SSc-PAH range between 7% and 29%.[35–38] Untreated, SSc-PAH has a median survival of 12 months and 2-year, 3-year, and 5-year survival of 44%, 40%, and 4%.[39] Using modern treatments, survival has moderately improved with a median survival of 4 years and 2-year, 3-year, and 5-year survival of 72%, 67%, and 36%.[40]

Anticoagulation of patients with PAH has been recommended with the rationale that PAH has been characterized histologically by regions of in situ thrombosis and abnormalities in the coagulation cascade.[41–44] The authors' systematic review of the literature found that the evidence to support these recommendations is limited by methodological constraints and conflicting studies.[45] Although most SSc-PAH experts were guarded about the effect of warfarin, some experts think warfarin worsens survival (ie, confers harm), whereas others think that warfarin improves survival.[46]

The authors conducted a retrospective cohort study of 275 patients with SSc-PAH, 78 (28%) of whom received warfarin. Patients with warfarin-treated SSc-PAH had worse baseline measures of PAH severity and more use of PAH medications than unexposed patients with SSc-PAH (**Table 2**). This finding was suggestive of confounding by indication whereby sicker patients were exposed to warfarin. Simple comparisons of treated and untreated patients would have led to a biased estimation of the effect of warfarin. The differences in baseline characteristics between the treated and untreated groups were substantially reduced in the propensity score–matched SSc-PAH cohort. The largest standardized difference in the matched cohort was

Table 2
Systemic sclerosis–associated pulmonary arterial hypertension patient characteristics

	Unmatched n = 275		Matched n = 98		Absolute Standardized Difference	
Characteristics n (%)	**No Warfarin n = 197**	**Warfarin n = 78**	**No Warfarin n = 49**	**Warfarin N = 49**	**Unmatched n = 275**	**Matched n = 98**
Female sex	165 (84%)	66 (85%)	45 (92%)	44 (90%)	0.22	0.07
PAH characteristics at diagnosis						
mPAP mm Hg mean (SD)	39.0 (14.3)	46.8 (14.3)	38.8 (15.3)	42.5 (11.8)	0.54	0.27
WHO functional class III/IV	68 (35%)	36 (46%)	23 (47%)	23 (47%)	0.15	0
Moderate-severe RV enlargement	25 (13%)	25 (32%)	11 (22%)	13 (27%)	0.22	0.05
Moderate-severe RV hypokinesis	25 (13%)	25 (32%)	11 (22%)	13 (27%)	0.22	0.05
Comorbidities						
Cancer	21 (11%)	8 (10%)	7 (14%)	6 (12%)	<0.01	0.02
Coronary artery disease	27 (14%)	7 (9%)	6 (12%)	5 (10%)	0.05	0.02
Diabetes mellitus	10 (5%)	7 (9%)	4 (8%)	2 (4%)	0.04	0.04
Hyperlipidemia	11 (6%)	9 (12%)	6 (12%)	3 (6%)	0.06	0.06
Hypertension	55 (28%)	16 (21%)	16 (33%)	9 (18%)	0.09	0.06
Peripheral vascular disease	9 (5%)	4 (5%)	2 (4%)	3 (6%)	0.01	0.02
Ischemic stroke	7 (4%)	2 (3%)	2 (4%)	2 (4%)	0.01	0
Concomitant medications						
Calcium channel blocker	104 (53%)	33 (42%)	23 (47%)	23 (47%)	0.14	0
ER antagonist	35 (18%)	33 (42%)	9 (18%)	15 (31%)	0.29	0.14
PDE inhibitor	16 (8%)	5 (6%)	3 (6%)	5 (10%)	0.02	0.04
Prostaglandin analogue	10 (5%)	13 (17%)	4 (8%)	4 (8%)	0.12	0

Abbreviations: ER, endothelin receptor antagonist; mPAP, mean pulmonary artery pressure; PDE, phosphodiesterase; RV, right ventricular; SD, standard deviation; WHO, World Health Organization.

Reprinted from Johnson SR, Granton JT, Tomlinson GA, et al. Warfarin in systemic sclerosis- associated and idiopathic pulmonary arterial hypertension. A Bayesian approach to evaluating treatment for uncommon disease. J Rheumatol 2012;39(2):276–85; with permission.

27%, and a standardized difference greater than the recommended 10% was observed for 2 variables.[28] In a simulation, the authors found that in a randomized controlled trial (RCT) with 49 patients with SSc-PAH per group and 16 baseline characteristics, there is a 91% probability of observing an absolute standardized difference of 27% or greater and an almost 100% probability of observing at least 2 baseline characteristics with an absolute standardized difference of 10% or more. Therefore, the propensity score–matched cohort had differences in baseline covariates smaller than those that would be observed in an RCT of the same size. With closely matched samples, the estimated differences in outcomes between groups are less confounded.

SUMMARY

The use of observational data to make unbiased estimates of the treatment effect is challenged by confounding by indication. In the setting of the uncommon rheumatic disease, the challenge is compounded by small numbers of subjects. Propensity score methods are a strategy to balance observed characteristics to try to achieve exchangeability. That is, these are methods to produce groups that are functionally randomized.[5] Propensity score methods can facilitate causal inferences from observational data.[16]

REFERENCES

1. Bloom S. Registries in chronic disease: coming your way soon? Registries–problems, solutions and the future. Rheumatology (Oxford) 2011;50(1):4–5.
2. Bosco JL, Silliman RA, Thwin SS, et al. A most stubborn bias: no adjustment method fully resolves confounding by indication in observational studies. J Clin Epidemiol 2010;63(1):64–74.
3. Rubin DB. Estimating causal effects from large data sets using propensity scores. Ann Intern Med 1997;127(8 Pt 2):757–63.
4. Hughes MD, Williams PL. Challenges in using observational studies to evaluate adverse effects of treatment. N Engl J Med 2007;356(17):1705–7.
5. Savitz DA. Interpreting epidemiologic evidence. Strategies for study design and analysis. Oxford: Oxford University Press, Inc; 2003.
6. Rothman KJ, Greenland S. Modern epidemiology. 2nd edition. Philadelphia: Lippincott-Raven; 1998.
7. Last JM. A dictionary of epidemiology. 4th edition. New York: Oxford University Press; 2001.
8. Feinstein AR. Clinical epidemiology. The Architecture of clinical research. Philadelphia: W. B. Saunders Company; 1985.
9. Fletcher RH, Fletcher SW. Clinical epidemiology. The essentials. 4th edition. Baltimore (MD): Lippincott Williams and Wilkins; 2005.
10. Salas M, Hofman A, Stricker BH. Confounding by indication: an example of variation in the use of epidemiologic terminology. Am J Epidemiol 1999;149(11): 981–3.
11. Greenland S, Robbins JM. Identifiability, exchangeability, and epidemiologic confounding. Int J Epidemiol 1986;15:413–9.
12. Curtis LH, Hammill BG, Eisenstein EL, et al. Using inverse probability-weighted estimators in comparative effectiveness analyses with observational databases. Med Care 2007;45(10 Supl 2):S103–7.
13. Berry DA. Statistics: a Bayesian perspective. Belmont (CA): Wadsworth Publishing Company; 1996.
14. Feinstein AR. Scientific standards in epidemiologic studies of the menace of daily life. Science 1988;242(4883):1257–63.
15. Hudson M, Suissa S. Avoiding common pitfalls in the analysis of observational studies of new treatments for rheumatoid arthritis. Arthritis Care Res (Hoboken) 2010;62(6):805–10.
16. Rosenbaum PR, Rubin DB. The central role of the propensity score in observational studies for causal effects. Biometrika 1983;70(1):41–55.
17. D'Agostino RB. Tutorial in biostatistics. Propensity score methods for bias reduction in the comparison of a treatment to a non-randomized control group. Stat Med 1998;17:2265–81.

18. Rosenbaum PR, Rubin DB. Reducing bias in observational studies using subclassification on the propensity score. J Am Stat Assoc 1984;79(387):516–24.
19. Williamson E, Morley R, Lucas A, et al. Propensity scores: from naive enthusiasm to intuitive understanding. Stat Methods Med Res 2012;21(3):273–93.
20. Austin PC. Some methods of propensity-score matching had superior performance to others: results of an empirical investigation and Monte Carlo simulations. Biom J 2009;51(1):171–84.
21. Rosenbaum PR, Rubin DB. Constructing a control group using multivariate matched sampling methods that incorporates the propensity score. Am Stat 1985;39(1):33–8.
22. Austin PC. Propensity-score matching in the cardiovascular surgery literature from 2004 to 2006: a systematic review and suggestions for improvement. J Thorac Cardiovasc Surg 2007;134(5):1128–35.
23. Austin PC, Grootendorst P, Anderson GM. A comparison of the ability of different propensity score models to balance measured variables between treated and untreated subjects: a Monte Carlo study. Stat Med 2007;26(4):734–53.
24. Cochran WG. The effectiveness of adjustment by subclassification in removing bias in observational studies. Biometrics 1968;24(2):295–313.
25. Cole SR, Hernan MA. Constructing inverse probability weights for marginal structural models. Am J Epidemiol 2008;168(6):656–64.
26. Austin PC, Stuart EA. Moving towards best practice when using inverse probability of treatment weighting (IPTW) using the propensity score to estimate causal treatment effects in observational studies. Stat Med 2015;34(28):3661–79.
27. Rubin DB. The design versus the analysis of observational studies for causal effects: parallels with the design of randomized trials. Stat Med 2007;26(1):20–36.
28. Austin PC. Balance diagnostics for comparing the distribution of baseline covariates between treatment groups in propensity-score matched samples. Statist Med 2009;28:3083–107.
29. Streenland K, Greenland S. Monte Carlo sensitivity analysis and Bayesian analysis of smoking as an unmeasured confounder in a study of silica and lung cancer. Am J Epidemiol 2004;160:384–92.
30. Stukel TA, Fisher ES, Wennberg DE, et al. Analysis of observational studies in the presence of treatment selection bias: effects of invasive cardiac management on AMI survival using propensity score and instrumental variable methods. JAMA 2007;297(3):278–85.
31. Hackam DG, Mamdani M, Li P, et al. Statins and sepsis in patients with cardiovascular disease: a population-based cohort analysis. Lancet 2006;367(9508):413–8.
32. Johnson SR, Granton JT, Tomlinson GA, et al. Warfarin in systemic sclerosis-associated and idiopathic pulmonary arterial hypertension. A Bayesian approach to evaluating treatment for uncommon disease. J Rheumatol 2012;39(2):276–85.
33. Silman AJ. Scleroderma and survival. Ann Rheum Dis 1991;50(4):267–9.
34. Steen VD, Medsger TA. Changes in causes of death in systemic sclerosis, 1972-2002. Ann Rheum Dis 2007;66(7):940–4.
35. Salerni R, Rodnan GP, Leon DF, et al. Pulmonary hypertension in the CREST syndrome variant of progressive systemic sclerosis (scleroderma). Ann Intern Med 1977;86(4):394–9.
36. Ungerer RG, Tashkin DP, Furst D, et al. Prevalence and clinical correlates of pulmonary arterial hypertension in progressive systemic sclerosis. Am J Med 1983;75(1):65–74.

37. Mukerjee D, St George D, Coleiro B, et al. Prevalence and outcome in systemic sclerosis associated pulmonary arterial hypertension: application of a registry approach. Ann Rheum Dis 2003;62(11):1088–93.
38. Murata I, Takenaka K, Yoshinoya S, et al. Clinical evaluation of pulmonary hypertension in systemic sclerosis and related disorders. A Doppler echocardiographic study of 135 Japanese patients. Chest 1997;111(1):36–43.
39. Koh ET, Lee P, Gladman DD, et al. Pulmonary hypertension in systemic sclerosis: an analysis of 17 patients. Br J Rheumatol 1996;35(10):989–93.
40. Campo A, Mathai SC, Le Pavec J, et al. Hemodynamic predictors of survival in scleroderma-related pulmonary arterial hypertension. Am J Respir Crit Care Med 2010;182(2):252–60.
41. Johnson SR, Granton JT, Mehta S. Thrombotic arteriopathy and anticoagulation in pulmonary hypertension. Chest 2006;130(2):545–52.
42. Badesch DB, Abman SH, Simonneau G, et al. Medical therapy for pulmonary arterial hypertension: updated ACCP evidence-based clinical practice guidelines. Chest 2007;131(6):1917–28.
43. McLaughlin VV, Archer SL, Badesch DB, et al. ACCF/AHA 2009 expert consensus document on pulmonary hypertension a report of the American College of Cardiology Foundation Task Force on Expert Consensus Documents and the American Heart Association developed in collaboration with the American College of Chest Physicians; American Thoracic Society, Inc.; and the Pulmonary Hypertension Association. J Am Coll Cardiol 2009;53(17): 1573–619.
44. Galie N, Hoeper MM, Humbert M, et al. Guidelines for the diagnosis and treatment of pulmonary hypertension: the Task Force for the Diagnosis and Treatment of Pulmonary Hypertension of the European Society of Cardiology (ESC) and the European Respiratory Society (ERS), endorsed by the International Society of Heart and Lung Transplantation (ISHLT). Eur Heart J 2009;30(20):2493–537.
45. Johnson SR, Mehta S, Granton JT. Anticoagulation in pulmonary arterial hypertension: a qualitative systematic review. Eur Respir J 2006;28(5):999–1004.
46. Johnson SR, Granton JT, Tomlinson GA, et al. Effect of warfarin on survival in scleroderma-associated pulmonary arterial hypertension (SSc-PAH) and idiopathic PAH. Belief elicitation for Bayesian priors. J Rheumatol 2011;38(3):462–9.

US National Health and Nutrition Examination Survey Arthritis Initiatives, Methodologies and Data

Charles F. Dillon, MD, PhD[a,*], Michael H. Weisman, MD[b]

KEYWORDS

• Arthritis • National Health and Nutrition Examination Survey • Prevalence
• Prevention and control • Back pain • Neck pain

KEY POINTS

- The US National Health and Nutrition Examination Survey has collected US nationally representative arthritis examination, laboratory and radiographic data for more than 50 years.
- The collected data arthritis-related data are high quality and population based; data collection is designed to minimize sampling biases, and almost all data are publicly available.
- Although the data are most often used for basic scientific research, the primary purpose of the arthritis data collection is to support national-level public health prevention and control efforts.
- These data define the population arthritis prevalence; however, public health monitoring was never implemented to reduce arthritis incidence and to ensure early diagnosis and treatment of arthritis cases.
- Despite an impressive body of publications on the arthritis datasets, the bulk of the data remain unpublished; the extent of the existing data is outlined with guidelines for analysis.

INTRODUCTION

This article reviews population-based arthritis and musculoskeletal disease data available from the US National Health and Nutrition Examination Survey (NHANES) a major program initiative of the US National Center for Health Statistics (NCHS). The purpose is to provide the reader with a basic understanding of the NHANES survey design and

---

Disclosure Statement: The authors have no disclosures.
[a] 75 East Wayne Avenue # 302, Silver Spring, MD 20901, USA; [b] Division of Rheumatology, Cedars Sinai Medical Center, 1545 Calmar Court, Los Angeles, CA 90024, USA
* Corresponding author.
E-mail address: cfdillon1@gmail.com

Rheum Dis Clin N Am 44 (2018) 215–265
https://doi.org/10.1016/j.rdc.2018.01.010 rheumatic.theclinics.com
0889-857X/18/

capabilities, and to systematically review major NHANES accomplishments in the area of arthritis and musculoskeletal diseases. Currently available NHANES arthritis-related datasets are identified and guidelines for interpreting NHANES data and opportunities for data analysis and designing future NHANES studies are also presented.

US NATIONAL HEALTH AND NUTRITION EXAMINATION SURVEY OVERVIEW

NHANES is a US nationally representative cross-sectional health survey that simultaneously collects health interview and health examination data in addition to laboratory, radiologic, and imaging studies. Fielded first in the late 1950s as the US National Health Examination Survey (NHES), a national nutritional survey component was added in the early 1970s, hence the acronym NHANES. NHANES is unique in that it has provided high-quality national-level public health examination-based surveillance data for the most important high prevalence health conditions such as arthritis, hypertension, diabetes, chronic obstructive lung disease, osteoporosis, and obesity as well as for coronary heart disease major risk factors such as high cholesterol and smoking. Importantly, existing NHANES data and stored biospecimens are also routinely leveraged in retrospect to address and answer important health questions that arise years later, for example, the discovery of hepatitis C, human immunodeficiency virus, and hantavirus.

The early successful fielding of NHANES in the 1960s was a remarkable achievement. To accurately and efficiently produce nationally representative prevalence estimates, a staff of demographers and mathematical statisticians created a complex, multistage survey sampling design that included sequential elements of probability, stratification, and cluster sampling and new statistical methods and software were developed to support the complex data analysis required to produce prevalence estimates. Also, trained staff and infrastructure were developed to support national-scale mobile health center–based data collection, and field staff operational procedures developed to keep survey response rates at or above the nominal 70% benchmark for adequate random sampling survey response.[1]

NHANES has, therefore, functioned as the prototype national-level health examination survey and its successful fielding has provided proof of concept of the substantial public health benefits of national-level health examination surveillance data. The public health surveillance function of NHANES has 4 principal aims/goals: (a) situation assessment—to precisely define the overall burden of disease and risk factors on the public and to identify any key disparities in disease burden prevalence in major demographic subgroups (age, gender, race/ethnicity), (b) to acquire population-level surveillance data to support the primary prevention of disease in the first instance, (c) to support public health campaigns for secondary prevention of disease, that is, to monitor and control key factors critical to reducing long-term target organ damage and improving health outcomes, and (d) to provide a platform to conduct basic science studies on disease natural history and risk factors as well as critical methodologic studies required to support these goals.

NHANES national-level health examination survey data are relatively unique, both because of the innovative survey design, but also especially because the data collection is based on standardized active, in-person, examination-based surveillance rather than clinical case series or passive retrospective collection of medical records data. It, thus, represents a largely unbiased source of data for public health planning as well as for basic scientific research. NHANES is also unique in its degree of transparency: almost all data collected is well-documented and publicly available for the general scientific community to use. Historically, the lack of comparable survey data from countries other than the United States has meant that NHANES data have played a pivotal role in strategic global world international health planning. More recently, national-level health examination surveys have been successfully implemented in additional countries, notably the Canadian Health Measures Survey (Statistics Canada), KNHANES in South Korea, SA-NHANES in South Africa, and New York City HANES.

In essence, NHANES is a direct application of the classic public health primary and secondary disease prevention paradigm, that is, the population is the patient. In the arena of primary prevention, NHANES serologic survey data have been essential in guiding successful public health communicable infectious disease immunization control programs, most recently in the immunization campaign that significantly reduced US population cervical cancer risk from human papilloma virus.[2] Further, NHANES nutrition and nutritional biochemistry data have effectively supported nutritional programs to reduce rates of childhood and maternal anemia and population cholesterol levels. Also, NHANES detailed smoking data and cotinine biomonitoring provided risk assessment data for a US population–level reduction in cigarette smoking and for general population exposure to second hand smoke, which decreased from 80% in the 1990s to 25% in 2012.[3–5] Maternal health and childhood growth and development are a special NHANES focus, and NHANES blood lead level biomonitoring data was instrumental in documenting reductions in population exposure to airborne leaded gasoline down to levels considered safe for children's cognitive development.[6]

NHANES surveillance data have also been notably successful in guiding major secondary prevention programs. Here, NHANES data provide an ongoing monitoring of the population prevalence of rates of awareness of disease among those affected (to minimize undiagnosed cases), monitoring treatment rates to ensure those who need care are treated, as well as ongoing monitoring of disease control rates for those under treatment. A key example for secondary prevention is the role of NHANES blood pressure and prescription drug usage data in the successful decades-long national-level campaign to control hypertension on a population level so as to reduce hypertension-related morbidity and mortality.[7]

US NATIONAL HEALTH AND NUTRITION EXAMINATION SURVEY ARTHRITIS-RELATED DATA, RESULTS, AND MAJOR CONTRIBUTIONS

NHANES has now been fielded for more than 55 years and its contributions to arthritis and musculoskeletal research are substantial. The entirety of the NHANES published literature relevant to arthritis research generated from its data collections is extensive, making a full review well beyond the scope of the present article. A number of prior reviews of NHANES arthritis data have been written by NCHS and arthritis researchers at the National Institutes of Health, who designed and guided the early NHANES arthritis data collections,[8,9] as well as reviews by other scientists.[10] In addition, National Arthritis Data Workgroup reports that assess arthritis data insufficiency in the United States and specific data needs for future research highlight the major NHANES contributions to arthritis research in the context of significant contributions from other arthritis studies. This work in turn will help to place NHANES in context in relation to other scientific and public health work at those time periods.[11,12]

This article presents a focused analytical review of NHANES arthritis research, citing key work to explain how NHANES arthritis data have been collected, its current scope, and the major accomplishments to date. Arthritis data availability and gaps in current NHANES arthritis portfolio are highlighted. The overall framework for this review focuses on how existing NHANES arthritis data fit into a strategic approach to medical and public health efforts to define and effectively control arthritis and related diseases on a population level. This discussion directly highlights the strengths and limitations of NHANES arthritis data collections. Remarkably, a significant proportion of the publicly available NHANES arthritis data that have been collected remain unpublished. Also, prior analyses of NHANES arthritis datasets often do not reflect the population estimates that would be evaluated using modern disease classification criteria and modern statistical software for complex survey data, which was not always available to earlier researchers. A result is that the analysis of temporal trends in US arthritis prevalence, diagnosis, and treatment and impairment rates across the NHANES arthritis surveys remains largely unexplored. Because almost all NHANES arthritis data are publicly available online at the NHANES website for researchers to analyze, this review provides an orientation to NHANES arthritis data and basic guidelines to help researchers make full use of the NHANES datasets.

US NATIONAL HEALTH AND NUTRITION EXAMINATION SURVEY ESTIMATES FOR THE US POPULATION PREVALENCE OF THE PRINCIPAL RHEUMATIC DISEASES

This section reviews the data and basic results for NHANES arthritis-related surveys from 1960 to 2016. Historically, these NHANES surveys defined the US population prevalence for the major rheumatic and musculoskeletal diseases of public health concern, including osteoarthritis (OA), rheumatoid arthritis (RA), spondyloarthritis (SpA), and osteoporosis (**Table 1**). There has also been significant US population-level data collection on other topics, including gout, chronic back pain (including inflammatory back pain [IBP]) and chronic widespread pain (CWP). Logistically, individual NHANES surveys are called "survey cycles" because historically these data were collected in 3- to-6 year campaigns, between which NHANES was often out of the field for several years. In 1999, NHANES became a continuous survey—always in the field—with public data releases on a biannual basis. These data releases continue to be called "cycles." **Table 1** summarizes the specific NHANES arthritis data collection survey cycles.

EARLY ARTHRITIS STUDIES (1960 TO 1984)

NHANES arthritis survey data collection commenced in the early 1960s (NHES I) in partnership with the National Institute of Arthritis and Metabolic Disease. This survey was designed to provide the first US nationally representative prevalence estimates for OA and RA. Data collection included a medical history, physical examination, and radiologic studies of the hands and feet, as well as serology for rheumatoid factor.[13] Published OA results were only for radiographic disease, which was considered the standard OA metric at that time; although some OA-related health history and physical examination data were also collected. Radiographs were scored for OA according to the current Kellgren-Lawrence criteria at that time which rated OA severity on a 0 to 4 scale.[14] RA classification criteria used were the criteria of the American Rheumatism Association in that time frame based on interview, physical examination, serology, and radiographs.[15] Using an 8-point scoring system, RA cases were classified as probable (3–4 points), definite (5–6 points), or classic (7–8 points).

Detailed study results summary and data tables for OA and RA were published in 4 concise reports.[16–19] Radiographic OA was found in the hands or feet of 37% of the US adult population ages 18 to 79 years. There was a clear trend of increasing prevalence by age, ranging from 4% in the youngest adults to 85% among those 74 years and older. Moderate or severe radiographic OA (a Kellgren-Lawrence score of 3 or 4) occurred in 23% of OA cases. RA, defined as probable, definite, or classic by American

Table 1
NHANES arthritis and musculoskeletal disease data collections (1960-2014)

Survey Cycle	Years	Age Range	RA	OA	SpA	Axial Pain	Osteoporosis	Radiographs	Autoimmune Serology
NHES I	1960–62	18–79	X	x	—	—	—	Hands; feet	RF
NHES II	1963–65	6–11	—	—	—	—	—	Hand-wrist	—
NHES III	1966–70	12–17	—	—	—	—	—	Hand-wrist	—
NHANES I	1971–75	1–74	—	x	—	x	X-ray absorptiometry	Knees, AP pelvis, hand-wrist	—
NHANES II	1976–80	6 mo-74	—	x	—	x	—	Cervical, lumbar spine	—
Hispanic HANES	1982–84	6 mo-74	—	—	—	—	—	—	—
NHANES III	1988–94	≥2 mo	x	x	—	x	DEXA	Hand-wrist, knees	RF, ATA, TPO, EMA, TTG, anti-GAD65
Continuous NHANES	1999–2004	All ages	—	—	—	CWP	DEXA	—	ANA, ATA, TPO
Continuous NHANES	2005–06	All ages	—	—	—	—	DEXA	—	—
Continuous NHANES	2007–08	All ages	—	—	—	—	—	—	ATA, TPO
Continuous NHANES	2009–10	All ages	—	—	x	IBP	DEXA	—	ATA, TPO, EMA, TTG
Continuous NHANES	2011–12	All ages	—	—	—	—	DEXA	—	ATA, TPO, EMA, TTG
Continuous NHANES	2013–14	All Ages	—	—	—	—	DEXA	—	EMA, TTG

Notes: NHANES 2015 to 2016 data not yet publicly released; ATA TPO only measured in 2001 to 2002 in the NHANES 1999 to 2004 cycles.

Abbreviations: ANA, antinuclear autoantibodies; AP, anteroposterior; ATA, antithyroglobulin; CWP, chronic widespread pain; DEXA, dual-energy x-ray absorptiometry; EMA, anti-endomyselial; IBP, inflammatory back pain; NHANES, US National Health and Nutrition Examination Survey; NHES, US National Health Examination Survey; OA, osteoarthritis; RA, rheumatoid arthritis; RF, rheumatoid factor; SpA, spondyloarthritis; TPO, antithyroperoxidase; TTG, tissue transglutaminase.

Rheumatism Association criteria, was found in 0.9% of the US adult population ages 18 years and older. Definite RA was found in 2% of men ages 55 years and older and 3% of women 55 to 64 years; 5% of women ages 65 and older had definite disease. Overall, 30% of the cases identified exhibited 5 or more criteria and were classified as having as definite or classic disease. Useful additional perspective on the NHES I arthritis survey is provided in the 1989 National Arthritis Data Workgroup report.[9]

After the NHES I in 1960 to 1962, there was a hiatus in arthritis data collection as the survey turned to specifically define the status of children's health in the United States. The NHES II survey (1963–1965) studied children 6 to 11 years of age and NHES III (1966–1970) studied children ages 12 to 17 years of age, providing comprehensive-national level data for children's health, growth, and development. NHES II and III were both performed in the same geographic locations, and a one-third cohort of children was studied across the 2 survey cycles, demonstrating the feasibility of national-level longitudinal studies. Although joint disease was not a focus of NHES II and III, these studies as well as one subsequent NHANES survey cycle did obtain children's hand-wrist radiographs as a measure of skeletal maturation. NHANES I immediately followed these 2 surveys in 1971. It was a nationally representative survey of all ages that included for the first time a nutrition data component. Owing to a federal budget crisis and funding cuts, NHANES I was halted in midcourse, but as funding again became available, data collection recommenced and was completed by 1975 (ie, the NHANES I "augmentation" survey and focused study NHANES subsamples such as the NHANES I dermatology examination component).[20–22]

The principle focus of NHANES I arthritis-related data collection was OA of the knees and hips in Americans ages 25 to 74 years and knee radiographs and a single anteroposterior (AP) view of the pelvis and hips were obtained. The latter also permitted sacroiliac joint assessment. Data for radiographic OA used the same Kellgren-Lawrence criteria as the earlier NHES I OA survey. For the first time, a detailed interview arthritis questionnaire, the "Arthritis History Supplement," was fielded. This questionnaire was administered to participants who screened positive to a shorter arthritis data screening questionnaire in the household interview preceding the examination. The Arthritis History Supplement focused especially on knee, hip, and back pain symptomatology, but also included data collection on peripheral joints. Medical treatment, risk factor, and functional impairment data were also captured. Arthritis data collection also included a physician examination of the joints and spine. General NHANES I prevalence estimates for arthritis and site-specific musculoskeletal pain based on the interview and physician examination data have been published.[23–25] Some 12% of examined participants had OA on physician examination. NHANES I radiologic studies showed the radiographic OA prevalence of overall mild, moderate, and severe knee OA for those 25 to 74 years of age was 3.8%; the prevalence of moderate to severe OA was 0.9%. For knee OA, a clear trend of increasing prevalence with age was seen: in the 65- to 74-year-old age group, the overall OA prevalence was 13.8%, and the prevalence of moderate to severe findings was 4.6%. The overall prevalence of radiographic OA of the hips among males 25 to 74 years of age was 1.3% for mild to severe disease and 0.5% for moderate to severe disease, respectively. Overall radiographic hip OA estimates were not obtained for females, because pelvic radiographs were not taken in women of reproductive age. However, among men and women ages 55 to 74 years of age, the overall radiographic hip OA prevalence was 3.1% and the prevalence of moderate to severe radiographic disease was 1.4%. The 1989 National Arthritis Data Workgroup report provides additional perspective on context in relation to other contemporary arthritis surveys of that time period as well as the important relation of radiographic to symptomatic OA.[9]

After NHANES I, NHANES II (1976–1980) and Hispanic HANES (HHANES; 1982–1984) were fielded. HHANES (1982–1984) had a paucity of arthritis-related data; no arthritis radiologic studies and only very limited arthritis-related questionnaire content were obtained.[26] NHANES II, however, had significant arthritis-related data collection. Its primary focus was OA and specifically spinal disc degeneration, although questionnaire data on a wide variety of joint symptoms, prior medical treatments, and functional impairments was collected using a household interview questionnaire with essentially the same format as the NHANES I Arthritis History Supplement. NHANES II also fielded a physician physical examination and radiology studies that included single lateral views of the lumbar and cervical spine for men ages 25 to 74 years of age and women ages 50 to 74 years of age.[27] Data collection amounted to some 17,000 radiographs. The NHANES II radiology images were reported to have been read; however, these data were not released publicly.[9,28] However, the spinal radiographic images themselves have been digitized and are publicly available at the US National Library of Medicine's website for researchers' use.[29] These digital resources have not been used by the rheumatic disease research community with 1 recent exception: an OA epidemiology study that used a subsample of 500 films.[30]

THE US NATIONAL HEALTH AND NUTRITION EXAMINATION SURVEY III ARTHRITIS SURVEY (1988–1994)

The principal focus of NHANES III musculoskeletal disease survey was OA and RA in older Americans ages 60 years and above. NHANES III arthritis data collection used the same format as earlier survey cycles: an arthritis interview, physician examination, radiographic studies, and serology.[31] The arthritis interview instrument fielded had some overlap with its NHANES I and II predecessors, but content was revised and updated. This was the first NHANES arthritis survey to use pain diagrams in data collection. Radiologic images collected included hand-wrist films and non–weight-bearing knee radiographs. These studies were read using the Kellgren-Lawrence criteria as in NHANES I. Serum rheumatoid factor was also measured in this subpopulation. In phase 2 of NHANES III (1991–1994), the prevalence of knee OA was assessed in US adults ages 60 years or older.[32] The prevalence of overall (mild to severe) radiographic OA was 37%, and the prevalence of overall symptomatic radiographic OA was 12%. The overall radiographic knee OA prevalence was somewhat increased in women compared with men (42.1% vs 31.2%, respectively). Women had significantly more severe Kellgren-Lawrence grade 3 to 4 changes (12.9% vs 6.5% in men), yet symptomatic radiographic knee OA prevalence did not differ by gender. Knee joint replacements were read on these radiographs and at that time, an estimated 1.6% of older US adults had these implants.[33]

Readings for the set of NHANES III hand radiographs have not been performed so, unfortunately, there are no currently published NHANES III estimates for radiographic hand OA or RA. However, there has been NHANES work to digitize these radiographic images.[34] In the absence of this radiographic data, prevalence estimates from phase 2 of NHANES III (1991–1994) were published for hand OA based on arthritis interview and physician physical examination data using 1990 American College of Rheumatology (ACR) criteria.[35,36] Also, US prevalence for RA using the 1987 ACR criteria have been published based on NHANES III health interview, physician examination, and rheumatoid factor serology data.[37,38] Hand OA by physical examination was found to be widely prevalent among US adults ages 60 years and older. Almost 60% had examination evidence of Heberden's nodes, 30% with Bouchard's nodes, and 18% had first carpal–metacarpal joint deformities. The site-specific prevalence of symptomatic OA at these 3 locations was 5.4%, 4.7%, and 1.9%, respectively. Notably, women had significantly more first carpal–metacarpal joint deformities on examination than men (24% vs 10%). By ACR criteria, overall US symptomatic hand OA prevalence (at any hand joint location) was 8% (95% confidence interval, 6.5%–9.5%), an estimated 3 million persons.[36]

The NHANES III estimation of the US prevalence of RA by ACR criteria used 2 basic methods: first, a participant was classified as having RA if they met 3 of 6 the 1987 ACR criteria; second, the ACR classification tree algorithm was applied. A third method explored used NHANES III prescription medication data for RA disease-modifying drugs to augment the ACR classification tree algorithm. Overall US RA prevalence among older adults by all methods was similar and estimated at 2%. It should be noted that this estimates using the 2 ACR criteria are for the prevalence of clinically active RA. As such, the entire population burden of RA may not be captured. For example, RA cases in remission or with cases inactive or end-stage disease with joint deformity would not be included. The third case definition used was designed to account for the effect of disease-modifying antirheumatic drugs in reducing signs and symptoms of RA in those under active treatment (active RA cases under pharmacologic control). This modification did increase the number of active RA cases identified, but the increase was not sufficient to substantially increase active RA prevalence as compared estimates using the 2 standard ACR criteria.[37]

US NATIONAL HEALTH AND NUTRITION EXAMINATION SURVEY ARTHRITIS AND MUSCULOSKELETAL DISEASE SURVEYS (1999 TO 2010)

Two survey cycles, NHANES 1999 to 2004 and NHANES 2009 to 2010, had significant arthritis-related data collection.[39] These were nonradiologic surveys designed to provide prevalence estimates for arthritis-related syndromes not studied in previous NHANES surveys. NHANES 1999 to 2004 fielded an arthritis questionnaire aimed at defining the US population with CWP, a principal feature of fibromyalgia.[40] This data collection was designed to address the US prevalence of musculoskeletal pain at all body sites, although a few questions regarding nonmusculoskeletal pain were included. Oddly, the questionnaire was named the "Miscellaneous Pain Questionnaire," abbreviated as "MPQ." The MPQ questionnaire had 2 sections: a first that elicited detailed responses on pain occurring specifically in the joints, and a second section on non–joint-related musculoskeletal pain that had occurred within the previous 3 months lasting 1 day or longer. A detailed pain diagram was used for data collection similar to others in use at that time.[41] No musculoskeletal examination or any arthritis-specific radiographic studies were performed in the NHANES 1999 to 2004 survey cycle. Published results for the this dataset showed an estimated 3.6% of respondents ages 20 years or older met the 1990 ACR criteria for CWP.[42] The 50- to 59-year-old age group had the highest CWP rates (6%) and, based on a multivariate analysis, women had higher risk for CWP than men (odds ratio, 1.5; 95% confidence interval, 2.2–2.1).[43]

The NHANES 2009 to 2010 arthritis survey was designed to estimate the US prevalence of IBP and SpA among adults ages 20 to 69 years of age, IBP being a component of and often a precursor to the development of SpA. Coexistent peripheral arthritis and reactive arthritis were not studied.[44] The overall plan and elements of the IBP/SpA study were published previously.[45] An IBP/SpA questionnaire was developed specifically for IBP and SpA prevalence estimation, using cognitive testing and pilot studies to operationalize existing clinical questionnaires for administration in the population setting. A spinal pain diagram was used to screen for a history of chronic pain, aching, or stiffness at 5 specific axial locations (neck, upper, mid and lower back, and sacroiliac joint area). An additional detailed history was obtained for those with axial pain at any one of these axial sites. The instrument was designed specifically to provide population-based prevalence estimates for the original Calin and colleagues[46] and European Spondyloarthritis Study Group IBP criteria[47], as well as for 2 IBP criteria published by Rudwaleit and colleagues.[48] The more recently available Assessment of Spondyloarthritis International Society criteria for IBP and SPA were not included in the study because they were published after the study was already fielded.[49] The estimated US population prevalence of IBP according to the 4 criteria sets was: Calin and colleagues, 5%; European Spondyloarthropathy Study Group (ESSG), 5.6%; Rudwaleit and colleagues criteria 8a, 5.8%; and Rudwaleit and colleagues[50–52] criteria 7b, 6%.

The NHANES 2009 to 2010 arthritis data collection had 3 other components including questionnaire, examination, and laboratory data. First, an addition to the arthritis questionnaire data was fielded to estimate of the US population prevalence of SpA using the ESSG and Amor and colleagues[47,53] criteria. These data constituted lower bound prevalence estimates for SpA because not all criteria variables could be included in the study: no imaging studies were done and some other variables could not feasibly be captured in data collection. The ESSG SpA prevalence estimate data collection included all ESSG IBP criteria variables and 4 of the 7 additional ESSG SpA criteria elements. A lower percentage of Amor and colleagues[53] back symptom and SPA criteria were collected. The age-adjusted prevalence of definite and probable SpA by ESSG criteria were 1.4% and 0.9% by Amor and colleagues[54] criteria. Second, US population-based data for 3 standard spondyloarthritis-related body measures were obtained in the 2009 to 2010 data collection: the occiput-to-wall distance, thoracic expansion (chest expansion with inhalation), and the anterior lumbar flexion test (modified Schober test). All measurements were obtained by experienced, professional anthropometry technicians as a part on the ongoing NHANES anthropometry data collection. Population-based percentile reference values for these spinal mobility measures in a nationally representative sample of 5103 US adults 20 to 69 years of age have been published elsewhere.[55]

Finally, a 1-year survey was fielded in 2009 to assess the age-adjusted US prevalence of HLA-B27. This survey was the first nationally representative study of HLA-B27. The overall US prevalence was 6.1%, and varied from 7.5% (among non-Hispanic whites) to 3.5% among all other US races/ethnicities combined. Among Mexican Americans, the prevalence was 4.6%.[56] Remarkably, this study showed that, for US adults ages 20 to 49 years, the prevalence of the HLA-B27 allele was 7.3%, whereas for those ages 50 to 69 years, it was 3.6%, a significant difference. This study, however, was conducted with a relatively small 1-year NHANES sample (discussed elsewhere in this article), which did not support detailed HLA-B27 prevalence trends analysis. These study findings for a heritable trait are unexplained and are unprecedented in NCHS data collections. They have prompted follow-up research, which has shown increased HLA-B27 related mortality in large clinical samples; however, thus far, population-based HLA-B27 mortality studies have not been performed.[57,58]

A primary role of population-based studies like NHANES is to provide prevalence data for undiagnosed populations with a specific disease and to identify underserved populations. Clinically, SpA has traditionally been considered a disease of men and uncommon among women. However, a literature reviews of ankylosing spondylitis had questioned this assumption, and subsequently community-based surveys demonstrated equal prevalence in men and women.[59,60] On a general population level, the NHANES 2009 to 2010 data showed no evidence for a gender differential in the prevalence of IBP and SpA according to established case classification criteria, and no gender differentials in the prevalence of HLA-B27.[50,54,57]

US NATIONAL HEALTH AND NUTRITION EXAMINATION SURVEY RESULTS FOR OTHER MUSCULOSKELETAL DISORDERS

Chronic Axial Pain Data

Since the 1970s, many NHANES survey cycles have collected basic prevalence data on chronic neck and back pain and the cumulative data collection is extensive in scope. NHANES I (1971–1975) and NHANES II (1976–1980) collected extensive questionnaire data relating to the back and neck, as well as key joints in other parts of the body. Both surveys targeted the same participant age range (12–74 years) and fielded similar data questionnaire formats. Gate questions were given in the household interview and, if screening was positive for symptoms, a main questionnaire was administered. The NHANES I screener question asked whether there had ever been pain in the back, neck, hip, knee, or other joints on most days lasting at least a month; or joint swelling and pain or morning stiffness lasting at least a month. In NHANES II, the screener asked separate questions according to pain location. It used a pain duration criterion of 2 weeks for asking about back or neck pain, 6 weeks for other joint pain, and 1 month for painful joint swelling and joint/muscle stiffness. Both surveys contained a question on the duration of the longest pain episode to preserve time frame comparability in intersurvey prevalence estimates. Detailed data were collected at 4 spinal levels: the neck, upper, and mid and low back. NHANES II did not collect data on buttock pain, whereas NHANES I did as a part of the hip joint data collection. Detail was captured on number of years of symptoms, current pain status, the duration of the longest episode, aggravating factors for pain, patterns of pain radiation, stiffness, and the presence of rest pain or pain with sleeping. Also, injury history, the specific type of medical practitioner seen, medical diagnosis and therapy, medication use, prior surgeries, the use of assistive devices, any physical activity restrictions, any change in job status owing to the condition and the number of days of work lost. A self-reported severity rating for the condition was also captured.

NHANES III (1988–1994) collected much less back pain data and was primarily focused on supporting the newly introduced osteoporosis data collection. Participants ages 20 years and older were asked if they ever had back pain for at least 1 month, and if so whether this had been symptomatic during the previous 12 months. A pain diagram was then used to capture back pain location (upper, mid, or low back). This pain diagram did not include neck or buttock pain. Then, a question on prior history of spinal fracture was asked. Subsequent NHANES survey cycles with back pain data collection include the previously mentioned NHANES 1999 to 2004 CWP survey and the NHANES 2009 to 2010 IBP/SpA data collection.

There are not a great number of publications on the NHANES chronic axial pain datasets; however, basic prevalence and some descriptive data are available for these NHANES survey cycles. These datasets give broadly similar results, however, with some variation owing to differences in age ranges studied as well as variation in the data collection instruments. In NHANES I, the prevalence of back pain having lasted 1 month or more in in adults 25 to 74 years of age was 17.2% by questionnaire self-report and 15.2% by physician examination.[24] In NHANES II for this same age range, the prevalence of back pain lasting at least 2 weeks was estimated 13.8%.[61] For NHANES III, an overall back pain prevalence estimate for adults 60 years and older is 22%.[62] The published overall prevalence estimate for chronic back pain in the United States is also available from the detailed pain diagram used in the NHANES

1999 to 2004 MPQ questionnaire for CWP. For US adults ages 20 years and older, the prevalence of chronic back pain (defined as pain in the lower back, upper back, central spine area, or the posterior aspect of the shoulders or neck) was 10.1%.[43] In the NHANES 2009 to 2010 IBP/SpA, data collection, definition of back pain was anatomically wider than these studies, including the neck, the upper, mid, and lower back and the sacroiliac joint areas on the axial pain diagram. By this definition, the overall US prevalence of back pain lasting for at least 3 months in those 20 to 69 years of age was 19.2%.[50]

US NATIONAL HEALTH AND NUTRITION EXAMINATION SURVEY I SPINAL RADIOLOGY STUDIES

Radiographic Sacroiliitis

As mentioned, in NHANES I, AP pelvic radiographs were obtained for adult participants but not in women less than 50 years of age. In the set of film readings obtained, the overall prevalence of moderate to severe radiographic sacroiliitis (RS) for men ages 25 to 74 years was 0.7%. Among women ages 50 to 74 years, the overall prevalence was 0.3% (NADQ 2008 part 1)[11]. The highest prevalence of moderate to severe RS for both men and women was seen at the oldest ages: 65 to 74 years.[23] The absence of the ability to examine prevalence of RS in women less than 50 years of age seen here may have contributed to the ongoing notion that men substantially outnumber women with this disease. Nevertheless, differences in the radiographic phenotype between men and women might play a role in this ongoing controversy. Significantly in these data, of all of those with moderate to severe grades of RS, only 8% reported currently experiencing significant pain in their lower backs on most days for at least 1 month.[11] Some 46% of all those with moderate RS and 49% of those with severe RS had a history of prior medical treatment for joint problems. All cases of moderate RS reported a history of past treatment, but none currently, whereas 54% of those with severe RS reported current medical treatment, and 46% past therapy.[23]

Paget's Disease of the Pelvis

The US population prevalence of radiographic Paget's disease of bone in the pelvic region population was estimated by readings of the set of NHANES-I AP pelvic films made some 25 years after data the original data collection.[63] Only radiographic prevalence was studied; symptoms and examination data were not studied. The pelvis proper is likely the most common area involved in Page's disease; however, it can occur in any bone in the body. In the NHANES AP pelvis radiograph set, Paget's involvement was most commonly noted in the pelvis itself, but also seen in the lower lumbar vertebrae and the proximal femur. Fusion of the sacroiliac joint owing to Paget's disease was noted in 1 case. The overall US prevalence of Paget's disease was estimated at 0.7%. The peak prevalence was seen in the 65- to 74-year-old age group (2.3%). Men's and women's prevalences were similar except for the 65- to 74-year-old age group (a prevalence of 3.7% in men vs a prevalence of 1.3% among women). By race/ethnicity, the prevalence of pelvic region Paget's disease was equal in non-Hispanic whites and non-Hispanic blacks.

Spinal Scoliosis

Both the NHANES I (1971–1975) and II (1976–1980) performed PA and lateral chest radiographs as a part of their respiratory health component data collection, which also included questionnaire items, a chest physical examination, spirometry, and in NHANES I pulmonary diffusion capacity. The radiographic readings for scoliosis are included in the public dataset releases for both survey cycles (ie, a single nonquantitative, categorical reading for the presence or absence of a lateral curvature of the spine).[64] Because these were chest films, the lower lumbar region was not included on most of the radiographs, and lower lumbar pathology contributions to scoliosis could not be not assessed. The NHANES I data are published in a detailed analysis,[65] but the NHANES II data are unpublished. For NHANES I, the overall cross-sectional US prevalence of spinal scoliosis in adults aged 25 to 74 years was 8.3% and the prevalence among women was twice that in men (10.7% vs 5.6%, respectively). A quantitative spinal curve assessment substudy of some 600 films found a curvature of 10° or more in 70% of those classified as scoliotic. A variety of health and reproductive factors were examined in the study. The most significant associations seen were for delayed menarche (scoliotics, 38%; nonscoliotics, 31%) and a lower mean bone density by an older measurement method (distal radius radiographic absorptiometry; discussed elsewhere in this article).

US NATIONAL HEALTH AND NUTRITION EXAMINATION SURVEY BONE MINERAL DENSITY AND BODY COMPOSITION DATA COLLECTIONS

NHANES surveys have made significant contributions to defining the US national prevalence of osteoporosis as well as to osteoporosis epidemiology. Since 1999, osteoporosis data collection has become a continuous NHANES core survey component. Datasets collected are large and complex, and there is a substantial body of literature published in the peer-reviewed journals. A comprehensive treatment of NHANES osteoporosis datasets and results is well beyond the scope of the current article, and a summary of data collection campaigns and data highlights are reviewed herein. Data collection for osteoporosis commenced in NHANES I (1971–1975) with bone densities determined using a radiograph of the left hand and radiographic absorptiometry. This technique used direct exposure radiographs of the left hand alongside an aluminum alloy reference wedge digitized by a high-resolution camera, and showed comparability with other accepted methods of bone densitometry used at that time. Two measurements were obtained: the aluminum equivalency of the middle phalanx of the little finger and of the distal radius.[66–69] NHANES III (1988–1994) introduced the use of modern dual-energy x-ray absorptiometry (DEXA) measurement of bone mineral density into NHANES surveys, and this has since become the NHANES standard. NHANES III was also one of the first studies to use DEXA in a mobile setting and, significantly, it collected the first US nationally representative data on bone mineral density of the hip for men and women ages 20 years and older.[70] This study reported bone mineral density and bone mineral content at the femur neck, trochanter, intertrochanter, and for the total femur (the neck, and trochanteric and intertrochanteric regions). For women ages 50 years or older, osteoporosis prevalence (bone mineral density >2.5 standard deviations below reference values) varied by specific region ranging from an estimated 13% to 18%. Osteopenia (bone mineral density between 1.0 and 2.5 standard deviations below reference value) prevalences ranged from 37% to 50% across the 4 regions. The femur neck region had the highest estimated prevalence for both osteoporosis and osteopenia.

NHANES 1999 to 2004 performed whole body DEXA scans on survey participants age 8 years and older. The aim was to provide nationally representative DEXA for body composition measures, both to support national nutrition assessment and to complement NHANES obesity-related examination data (obesity-related anthropometry measures and bioelectric impedance data). The body composition data captured included estimates for the total body as well as for major body regions. These measures included total mass, fat mass, percentage fat, lean soft tissue (excluding bone mineral content), and fat-free mass (including bone mineral content).[71,72] Because valid data were obtained for 80% of eligible participants owing to exclusions for pregnancy, weight greater than 300 lbs, the presence of metal objects (implants or pacemakers), and truncal adiposity effects on scanning, invalid and missing data could not be treated as a random subset of the data. Therefore, a special multiply imputed dataset was created. Results for the body composition measures and an analysis of the relation of the DEXA-based estimates to traditional measures of adiposity have been published.[71,72] Subsequent NHANES survey cycles from 2005 onward performed DEXA scans for the proximal femur and posterior-anterior lumbar spine. Overall, summary US prevalence estimates for adults ages 50 years and older for the survey years 2005 to 2010 by World Health Organization criteria were 10.3% for osteoporosis and 43.9% for low bone mass. The US prevalences of osteoporosis and low bone mass in older women and men, respectively, were osteoporosis 51.4% versus 35.2% and low bone mass 51.4% versus 35.2%.[73] An analysis of temporal trends in hip osteoporosis and osteopenia between NHANES III and NHANES 2005 to 2006 as well as an analysis of prevalence trends over the periods 2005 to 2010 and 2013 to 2014 have been published elsewhere.[74,75] Also, using the NHANES 2013 to 2014 data, overall US spine fracture prevalence vertebral fracture assessment (lateral DEXA scan graded by semiquantitative measurement) was 5.4% and the prevalence did not significantly differ between men and women.[76] By age, the prevalence of spinal fractures was less than 5% in those less than 60 years, 11% in 70- to 79-year-old patients, and 18% in those 80 years and older. Fractures frequency was similar in both genders at most spinal levels except for an increase in T11 and T12 fractures among men.

OTHER RHEUMATIC DISEASES

Gout

As reviewed in the National Arthritis Data Workgroup report,[77] US national-level prevalence estimation for gout has primarily been based on interview questionnaire data from the US National Health Interview Survey (NHIS). As noted, this has acknowledged methodologic limitations; however, the NHIS has fielded the same gout questions consistently over time, and notably clear temporal trends are evident for increasing self-reported gout prevalence.[78] Historically, almost all NHANES surveys since the 1960s have had only limited gout-related data collection and a systematic approach has not been taken to data collection to support national gout prevalence estimation. Virtually all NHANES surveys have fielded a similar basic interview question for a self-reported prior medical diagnosis of gout. In addition, beginning with NHANES I in the 1970s, participant serum uric acid levels have been collected as a part of a standard biochemistry profile. Also, beginning with NHANES III, survey participant prescription drug data have been systematically collected that provided data on current urate-lowering therapy use. This ensemble of this data has, however, enabled a variety of useful analytical studies relating to gout and the potential health risks of hyperuricemia.[79–84]

The NHES I (1960–1962) fielded a single question for lifetime prevalence of doctor-diagnosed gout. This cycle was the only one in the NHANES survey to obtain radiographs of the foot, but unfortunately these films were not read for gouty changes. NHANES I in the 1970s collected a question for lifetime gout prevalence in the general household as well as questions for current gout status and the number of years since the participant first had gout. The NHANES I detailed health history supplement asked general-level questions about foot pain (currently on most days for 6 weeks, age at first occurrence, when last had it, ever had foot swelling painful to touch for 1 month, history of foot morning stiffness, and typical stiffness duration). The NHANES I physician's examination included the feet, but contained only a single categorical variable for the presence or absence of any foot abnormality. NHANES II (1976–1980) had the same data collection format as NHANES I, except that the question on current prevalence (still have) was not asked. NHANES III (1988–1994) had only limited gout data; there was a single question for lifetime prevalence of doctor-diagnosed gout and the number of years since the participant first had it. Notably, however, the NHANES III physician's examination included a selective examination of the right and left great toes, with tenderness to palpation, joint swelling, and pain on passive motion recorded. Current NHANES has had minimal gout data collection; no data were collected from 1999 to 2006, but a single interview question with modified wording to capture self-reported lifetime prevalence of medically diagnosed gout resumed for the 2007 to 2016 survey cycles.

Systemic Lupus Erythematosus

In the NHANES III (1988–1994) household interview, a single question was asked regarding a prior history of physician-diagnosed systemic lupus erythematosus (SLE). These data and NHANES III prescription drug data were used to estimate the US national prevalence of SLE in adults.[85] Two prevalence definitions were used: (a) self-reported physician diagnosis of SLE, and (b) self-reported physician diagnosis SLE plus and a current prescription for SLE medications (antimalarials, corticosteroids, or other immunosuppressive medications, including methotrexate, azathioprine, cyclosporine, or cyclophosphamide). In a sample of 20,000 adults 17 years of age and older, 40 stated that they had a history of a lupus diagnosis (32 women, 8 men) and 12 were currently being treated with index drugs. These small numbers preclude detailed data analysis; however, the overall self-reported lifetime prevalence of physician-diagnosed SLE was 0.2% and, among women, the prevalence of treated SLE was 0.1%. These estimates were in a similar range to those in a smaller previous SLE questionnaire survey study that used medical record review to verify self-reported diagnosis.[86]

US NATIONAL HEALTH AND NUTRITION EXAMINATION SURVEY DATA AND PUBLIC HEALTH ARTHRITIS PREVENTION SURVEILLANCE SYSTEMS

As seen, NHANES, in partnership with the National Institutes of Health and other federal agencies and guided by the National Arthritis Data Workgroup, successfully produced a wide body of health examination data that defines the US population prevalence for the principal rheumatic diseases. This compilation is the essential first step in public health risk assessment. However, to put those results to use on a national level to reduce the incidence of arthritis and to reduce the burden of existing disease, 2 additional steps need to be taken: establishing programs for the primary prevention and for the secondary prevention of disease, that is, reducing or eliminating causal factors to prevent arthritis occurrence, and programs for early diagnosis and treatment prevent disease complications, respectively. Population-level surveillance tracking over time needs to be established to ensure reductions in population disease incidence as well as adverse outcomes among those already affected. The NHANES surveys were specifically designed to provide national-level surveillance examination data and biomonitoring to support primary and secondary disease prevention programs, and NHANES has had success with major diseases such as hypertension and cardiovascular disease, among others. However, for the major arthritis-related disorders such as OA, RA, and gout, which collectively make arthritis rank among the most common disabling health conditions, a systematic program for NHANES national-level primary and secondary prevention surveillance was not designed and implemented. This is in contrast with the case for osteoporosis, where well-developed primary and secondary prevention guidelines exist and NHANES osteoporosis surveillance data have been incorporated into national-level *Healthy People* public health tracking efforts to prevent disease as well as to reduce overall disease burden.[87–89] A number of primary and secondary prevention guidelines currently exist for gout that could be harmonized.[90] Also, gout has clearly defined causes, natural history, and treatments, so systematic NHANES surveillance to track primary and secondary prevention efforts should be feasible. However, as reviewed, although there are important NHANES publications regarding hyperuricemia population distributions and its health risks as well as factors related to the secondary prevention of gout, the current limited NHANES gout data collection would need to be redesigned to fully support a national gout prevention program.

A perceived barrier to developing OA and RA primary prevention surveillance programs to reduce their incidence is that, despite there being an impressive body of scientific knowledge, there remains ongoing scientific uncertainty regarding ultimate causal mechanisms. However, public health intervention programs can in fact effectively be pursued in the absence of precise knowledge causal mechanisms if descriptive data can identify critical elements in a causal pathway for a disease outcome, for example, John Snow's classic demographic analysis of cholera distributions in 18th-century London. A number of scientific papers have reviewed possible OA and RA primary prevention targets, but a practical set of operationally feasible targets for OA and RA public health surveillance systems has not been defined.[91,92] The issue at hand is to identify a key set of risk factors or medical conditions that, if treated or eliminated, could substantially reduce subsequent OA or RA incidence. Ideally, surveillance targets thus defined should be practical for temporal trend tracking and be internationally harmonized. Existing NHANES arthritis publications have significantly contributed to the scientific discussion on OA and RA primary prevention surveillance targets, and additional analysis of the extensive NHANES arthritis datasets could likely provide more insights.

A key role of NHANES is to provide surveillance intelligence to track progress toward public health goals in improving outcomes in established disease. These goals include surveillance to track rates of early diagnosis and intervention, for treatment control to prevent secondary complications and target organ damage, and efforts to reduce disability and mortality rates. However, in general the secondary prevention of OA and RA has not been adequately or systematically addressed using NHANES data. RA has well-developed protocols for early diagnosis and intervention that are available. Existing NHANES data variables (medical history, prescription medication use, and others) could potentially provide an initial population-level perspective for RA and OA, including diagnosis rates, the prevalence of undiagnosed disease, treatment rates, functional status, target organ involvement, functional impairment, and mortality. Thus far, little if any secondary prevention-oriented analysis of the existing NHANES data has been accomplished; however, important analyses related to identifying primary prevention targets have been performed.

OA has the largest body of these studies and, in fact, NHANES cross-sectional research studies were some of the earliest population-based studies in this area. Radiologic OA data from NHES I and NHANES I were pivotal in helping to confirm on a population-level preventable risk factors for OA previously identified in previous smaller scale studies. These were biomechanical causes (prior traumatic joint injury, joint loading from the physical demands of work) and obesity. The NHANES data also helped show that, although there are shared risk factors for OA in different joint locations, there are also important joint-specific variations in risk factors. For example, with reference to potential public health OA surveillance target conditions, the NHANES I radiologic data showed that prior knee injury was a strong risk factor for unilateral knee OA with multivariate adjusted odds ratios of 16 and 11 for injury in the right and left knee, respectively; knee injury had a lesser but still significant association with bilateral knee OA (odds ratio, 3).[93] Also, in the NHANES I data, prior hip injury was a strong predictor of unilateral radiographic hip OA.[94] Developmental acetabular abnormalities of the hip have been identified as risk factors for development of OA in adulthood and, thus, could be another potential public health surveillance target; recent population-based studies indicate that these may be more common than previously assumed. The previously collected set of pelvic radiographs from NHANES I (1971–1975) could potentially be used to investigate population prevalences for major variants of this condition.[95,96] Clearly, the generation of this hypothesis (developmental abnormalities as a risk factor for hip OA) should spur additional research on why this happens and to whom it happens. The extraordinary amount of resources currently spent on hip replacements is a wake-up call for this needed effort.[97]

An analysis of NHANES I detailed occupational code data using US Department of Labor ratings for job physical strength demands and knee bending, demonstrated a 3-fold increase in radiologic knee OA in adults 55 years, especially for job-related knee bending, but also for work strength demands.[98] Although these detailed occupational data were collected in subsequent NHANES surveys with an enhanced capability to examine lifetime occupational risks and occupational ergonomic databases exist, this type of detailed biomechanical exposure study has not been performed using the NHANES II and III radiographic survey data.[99] However, NHANES studies with much lower sensitivity have shown associations between general job titles categories and radiographic OA. For example, NHES I in the 1960s showed significant showed associations with manual labor occupations for both hand and foot OA.[100] In NHANES III, both radiographic OA and symptomatic radiographic OA of the knee showed significantly increased prevalence among men who were manual laborers.[33] Subsequent to these NHANES studies, both knee and hip OA have been demonstrated in non-NHANES research to be clearly associated with occupation and biomechanical occupation risk factors.[101–103] The NCHS has published a useful review of NHANES and other NCHS survey occupational data collection methods.[104]

NHES I 1960s radiograph data provided the initial US population-based data indicating a connection between obesity and both foot and hand OA. In a concise but elegant descriptive study of NHES I anthropometry data, a significant association between OA in these weight-bearing and non–weight-bearing joints and total body weight was demonstrated. Analysis of NHES I anthropometric data also showed a significant association with body fat determined by skinfold measurement. Notably, body measures denoting the body and limb girths and breadths also had significant associations with OA as opposed to body or limb length measurements.[105] In weight-bearing joints, the NHANES I radiographic knee OA data[93,98] provided clear epidemiologic evidence for an association between obesity and knee OA, and this was subsequently confirmed for both radiologic and symptomatic radiologic knee OA in NHANES III data.[33,106] In the NHANES I radiologic data, significant increases in hip OA were not seen with obesity measures, but bilateral hip OA was more common among obese persons.[94] Subsequent longitudinal studies have shown that an association of obesity with knee OA is stronger than hip OA and confirmed an obesity association with bilateral hip OA.[91]

There are a limited number of NHANES studies addressing RA primary prevention targets. The 3-year NHANES III phase II dataset for adults 60 years and older that supports ACR RA Classification Criteria is the principal data resource but has not been used extensively. Dental public health surveillance examinations for the US population have been a core NHANES data collection component since the survey's inception. Periodontitis as a possible trigger for RA has been a topic of considerable interest.[107] The NHANES dental examination includes a periodontal assessment to provide population-based data on periodontitis health risks. Two NHANES III studies examined the association of periodontal disorders with RA. The first examined the association of clinical periodontal disease to RA.[108] Periodontitis was defined as at least 1 site exhibiting attachment loss with a probing depth of 4 mm or greater. Periodontitis was thus defined as well as tooth loss status. Those classified with RA had more missing teeth but less current tooth decay than those without RA. In a multivariate adjusted analysis, those with RA were more likely to be edentulous (odds ratio, 2.3) and to have periodontitis (odds ratio, 1.8) compared with non-RA subjects. In seropositive RA cases, there were stronger associations with poor dental health status. NHANES has also fielded a panel of serum antibodies to periodontal bacteria to determine whether a subset of antibodies to the wide variety of periodontal microorganism usually found can be useful serologic indicators of markers of periodontitis in public health surveillance.[109] An initial study has been published investigating possible associations between serum immunoglobulin G antibodies to 19 periodontal species and the prevalence of rheumatoid factor in adults ages 60 years and older using NHANES III data. The periodontal immunoglobulin G that was studied was unassociated with rheumatoid factor seropositivity, although the study sample size was reduced owing to exclusion of edentulous participants.[110] It should be noted that these studies were focused on periodontal factors as a risk factor, and although detailed they did not present a full analysis of all the NHANES dental health data collected. Also, general dental health status in RA cases could also be examined in NHES I, the oldest NHANES survey cycle.

THE RANGE OF US NATIONAL HEALTH AND NUTRITION EXAMINATION SURVEY STUDY CAPABILITIES

The characterization of NHANES as a cross-sectional survey has truth; however, this statement deserves comment. The major classes of epidemiologic models, cross-sectional studies, retrospective case referent studies, and prospective longitudinal studies are properly fielded in a coordinated fashion in any given research context and serve to provide independent confirmation of disease associations via different study designs. Traditionally, cross-sectional studies, because they are time and cost efficient and thus can more readily executed, have been the backbone of hypothesis generation and risk factor identification. Retrospective case-referent studies are also resource efficient and provide additional confirmation and clarification of risks, whereas prospective incidence studies, conducted over long durations and at greater expense, are used to directly measure incidence rates, confirm temporal sequences of causes and effects, and develop final models of disease causation. This paradigm comes with the additional overall caveat that the quality of any particular study design and its execution largely determines its research value; true population-based studies such as NHANES in which sampling and potential nonresponse biases are controlled in a planned manner are considered to have the highest quality.

Depending on exposure-outcome time scales and dose/dose rates, purely cross-sectional studies of disease and risk factor associations can closely approximate the results seen in retrospective and longitudinal study designs in a number of key situations, that is, (a) where the risk factor or exposure for a disease is a fixed attribute (eg, childhood developmental abnormality or a genetic disorder with high penetrance or a factor which is known to be constant over long time periods before the development of the disease in question), (b) where a 1-time exposure that conveys a high probability of an adverse health outcome (intraarticular knee fracture and subsequent OA), and (c) when the time period between exposure and a health outcome is very short. For example, similar associations will be seen in NHANES cross-sectional data, in retrospective and in longitudinal study data for long-standing hypertension or high cholesterol as risk factors for and heart disease; conversely, short-term ambient air pollution levels have shown clear associations with NHANES hematology and pulmonary function testing data.[111,112]

Also, NHANES data do have the capability to support retrospective epidemiologic investigations via its data linkages and its retrospective household interview modules (ie, weight history and smoking history data, disease duration history vs target organ outcomes, prescription drug duration of use vs potential adverse effects, and NHANES occupational history data, among others). Further, as a nationally representative cross-sectional survey, NHANES provides a platform for population-based longitudinal health outcome and mortality studies. As mentioned, in the 1960s an initial small-scale longitudinal study of children's growth and development was performed across the NHES II to NHES III survey cycles. Subsequently for the NHANES I survey conducted in 1971 to 1975, the NHANES I Epidemiologic Follow-Up Study (NHEFS) was fielded.[113,114] This study, sponsored jointly by NCHS and the National Institute on Aging, collected questionnaire data, which included elements of the arthritis Health Assessment Questionnaire,[115] limited physical examination measures, hospital and nursing home records, and death certificates. The initial follow-up took place in 1982 to 1984, with subsequent follow-up in 1986 to 1987 and 1992.[116–119] The NHEFS data are publicly available[120] as well as methodologic guidelines for analyzing this data.[121] A chief purpose the NHEFS was to validate in a general US population setting the usefulness of coronary heart disease risk factor models for predicting coronary heart disease outcomes that had been developed in major epidemiologic studies in the setting of the US population. Jointly with the National Heart Lung and Blood Institute, a Framingham model verification component was added to the NHEFS follow-up. The effect of baseline coronary heart disease risk factors on coronary heart disease mortality was compared between the Framingham seventh cohort examination and NHANES I 1971 to 1975 examination data as baselines. NHEFS mortality data using previously developed Framingham risk models were directly applicable to the United States white adult population. NHEFS data have been used extensively by arthritis researchers to look at pain associations, long-term impairment mortality outcomes in OA,[122–125] by osteoporosis researchers to assess long-term fracture and mortality risks,[126–128] as well as for general studies of risk factors for long-term physical disability[129–131] and, in addition, for analytical studies or uric acid associations with cardiovascular mortality.[80]

US NATIONAL HEALTH AND NUTRITION EXAMINATION SURVEY LONG-TERM MORTALITY AND DATA LINKAGE STUDIES

NHANES is housed in the NCHS, which fields a variety of US national health surveys (NHIS, the National Ambulatory Care Survey, and others) as well as the NCHS Division of Vital Statistics that tracks US national birth and death records. The Division of Vital Statistics provides the US National Death Index for researcher's use.[132] In addition, NHANES data as well as data from other NCHS surveys are linked to the US National Death Index. Public release NHANES participant mortality data files are available for selected major mortality categories. Owing to concerns about participant confidentiality, detailed mortality data are available only by arrangement with the NCHS Research Data Center (RDC).[133] Mortality follow-up data are also available for NHANES I and its Epidemiologic Follow Up Study, for the NHANES II and III surveys as well as for NHANES 1999 to 2004. NCHS mortality data have been and continue to be extensively used by a wide variety of researchers in different fields and, as mentioned, have been used by arthritis researchers. In addition to mortality data files, a number of other major health datasets are also available through the RDC for linkage with NHANES data. These can support longitudinal studies, for example, and Medicare and Medicaid Claims data, US Renal Data System, and US Department of Housing and Urban Development data.[134,135] Cross-sectional air pollution exposure studies using geographic linkage to national air monitoring data compared with NHANES examination and laboratory data have been conducted since NHANES II and since NHANES III data linkage studies have been performed using geocoded participant residence and air monitoring data.[136–139]

THE SCOPE AND AVAILABILITY OF US NATIONAL HEALTH AND NUTRITION EXAMINATION SURVEY DATA

US National Health and Nutrition Examination Survey General Survey Data Collection and Content

Although the distinction does not have a formal definition, NHANES data collections are usually spoken of as being "core," ongoing survey content as opposed to other data collection modules that may be fielded from time to time in different survey cycles. Core survey content relates to the main public health objectives of the survey, which include data collections, such as those for hypertension and cardiovascular disease, diabetes, anthropometry and obesity, and dental and oral health, and the basic NHANES household interview questionnaire are in the main fielded under the NCHS operational budget for basic survey operations. Also, as reviewed, arthritis data collection was a core component of in NHANES surveys from 1960 through 1994. National level nutrition-related data collection are jointly designed and sponsored by the NCHS and the US Department of Agriculture,[140] and the large panel of nutritional biochemistry studies including water- and fat-soluble vitamins, trace elements, isoflavones, lignans, acrylamide, and hemoglobin adducts, is analyzed by National Center for Environmental Health laboratories at the Centers for Disease Control and Prevention,[141] which also analyze NHANES environmental health biomarkers.[142] NHANES infectious disease serology studies are also analyzed in the Centers for Disease Control and Prevention's Atlanta laboratories. Biomarker and interview data collection relating to smoking and second hand smoke exposure are extensive.[143,144] In addition to this core, other federal agencies sponsor NHANES data collection modules, which may be in the survey continuously (the National Institute of Deafness and Communication Disorders audiometric testing), or periodically cycled in and out over a longer time frame (the National Heart, Lung, and Blood Institute respiratory health and spirometry module). A substantial number of data collection modules are funded on a one-time basis as for the 2009 to 10 IBP/SpA study and the 2003 to 2004 National Institutes of Health National Institute of Arthritis, Musculoskeletal and Skin Diseases–sponsored digital image dermatology examination components,[145] or only for a limited number of survey cycles, as was the case for and the NHANES 1999 to 2004 MPQ questionnaire for CWP. NHANES solicits open proposals for new survey modules on a biannual basis, with the proviso that proposals must come with funding attached, either through federal interagency agreement or for nongovernmental proposals, via an unrestricted grant from the Centers for Disease Control and Prevention Foundation.[146]

The NHANES data collection model differs significantly different from the typical detailed clinical examination: it is not an in-depth clinical examination; rather it is standardized, focused survey data collection. NHANES is a multipurpose health examination survey with simultaneous data collection components for many different health conditions. Public health assessment needs drive survey content selection and the amount of survey time allotted to each component. Typical fielded NHANES survey cycle components include a household interview questionnaire module, mobile examination center (MEC) examination module, and blood or urine studies. For example, the NHANES 2009 to 2010 IBP/SpA component had a household interview (overall, 2½ minutes; range, ½-5 minutes according to back pain status); a 3- to 4-minute arthritis body measures examination; and used standard phlebotomy specimens. Questionnaires and examinations must be time efficient, standardized, unambiguous, and readily intelligible to the general public and those with lower literacy (ie, an 8th-grade reading level).

An initial participant health interview is conducted in the home and may take from 20 minutes to 2 hours. Household interview questionnaire modules have time constraints to reduce overall respondent burden and a typical questionnaire module is 3 minutes or less. Skip patterns are extensively used in questionnaire administration to limit questions only to appropriate subgroups and to minimize total questionnaire administration time. Questionnaire content from well-validated instruments is preferred in NHANES, for example, the Rose Angina and American Thoracic Society-Division of Lung Disease Respiratory Health questionnaires, or the Health Assessment Questionnaire content added to the NHANES I Epidemiology Follow-Up Study. When validated questionnaire instruments are not available, questionnaire content is developed by benchmarking, cognitive testing, and pilot testing.

Standardized NHANES examinations are carried out in MEC. During each survey year, 3 separate MEC units are continually in service. At any given time, 2 MECS are collecting data at field locations while the third is either traveling or being prepared for operation at a new location. Participants come to a NHANES MEC where a total of 4 hours are available in each MEC morning, afternoon, or evening session for data collection. Interview and examination data collection must, therefore, be designed to be as time efficient as possible to minimize respondent burden and to allow a maximum of content to be collected and real-time intra-MEC computer scheduling is used to achieve this goal. Logistical time constraints include time to greet the participant, sign consent forms, change into examination gowns, and be escorted between examination rooms. Anthropometry body measures, phlebotomy, urine sample collection, blood pressure measurements, and the 24-hour dietary recall interview data collections are prioritized. MEC computer-assisted and audio-assisted interviews are also administered for topics requiring confidentiality (sexually transmitted disease history, drug use). Additional examination components are then performed, including the dental examination, DEXA, audiometry, and the any examination testing required for the specific survey cycle.

Typical data collection times required for examination components range from 5 minutes (urine sample) to 20 minutes or more (24-hour dietary recall interview). As a rule of thumb, a "long" examination component in the NHANES context is one that requires more than 10 minutes to complete. Passive examination data collection that does not require active participant instruction/performance or coaching (ie, examination components like blood pressure measurement, electrocardiographs, or radiographs) is preferred wherever possible because of higher data quality, less time requirements, and because longer components can cause bottlenecks in session examination component scheduling, leading to subsequent component nonresponse. However, participant effort examination components such as spirometry are performed typically in 12 minutes, a credit to the instructional and coaching skills of the MEC health technicians.

Supplemental US National Health and Nutrition Examination Survey Data Collection Capabilities

Currently as well as in past survey cycles, NHANES has fielded ancillary data collection modules alongside the main household interview and MEC examination. For example, to examine the subset of participants consenting to household interviews but considering themselves too impaired to travel to the MEC examination site, NHANES III and NHANES 1999 to 2000 both fielded home examinations to collect data for this subpopulation.[147] Also, NHANES home interviewer collection of environmental health-related samples is periodically done; for example, collections of wipe samples for lead in household dust as well as samples of household drinking water for volatile organic compounds.[148,149] Specific post-MEC examination follow-up questionnaire data have been collected by telephone interview as well as by mail. Further, NHANES participants have also shown high participation rates in additional post-MEC examination data collections such as the NHANES 2005 to 2006 household dust sample collection for dust allergens and endotoxin, the 24-hour urine sodium data collection study, as well as the previously mentioned ambulatory accelerometry studies.[150–152]

US NATIONAL HEALTH AND NUTRITION EXAMINATION SURVEY LABORATORY DATA

NHANES surveys routinely collect blood and urine samples, and genetic samples have been collected in certain survey cycles. The various NHANES survey components that have been fielded and laboratory analytes collected are summarized in 2 useful tables: one summarizing the earlier NHANES surveys and one for continuous NHANES 1999 to 2016.[153,154] Since NHANES I in the 1970s, a basic complete blood count and differential and a standard biochemistry profile have been collected on a full sample of all survey participants. The primary public health focus of NHANES hematology studies, however, is population biomonitoring to support national and international efforts to control rates of anemia among women of reproductive age and young children 0 to 5 years of age. Serum iron and iron indices, red blood cell folate levels, and serum ferritin have been most commonly measured; however, more recently, transferrin receptors are routinely measured in these specific survey subsamples. Reticulocyte counts and hemolysis indicators, however, have not been routinely measured in NHANES surveys. In some NHANES survey cycles vitamin B_6 and B_{12} levels have been obtained as well; however, hepcidin has not been measured. Full sample data for all ages are available for certain analytes; for example, serum iron and its indices are typically available in all NHANES survey cycles. Also, full-sample serum ferritin data are available for the NHANES II, HHANES, NHANES III, and NHANES 1999 to 2002 survey cycles. For arthritis researchers, this existing hematology data provides basic data relevant to detecting anemia generally as well as white cell and platelet cytopenias.

Typically, in NHANES survey cycles only 1 primary inflammatory marker has been fielded, and in a number of survey cycles none have been collected (NHES I-III NHANES II, HHANES, and NH2011–2014). C-Reactive protein was the acute phase reactant measured from NHANES III through NHANES 2009 to 2016. The erythrocyte sedimentation rate was measured only in the NHANES I survey. No interleukins have been studied in NHANES with the "exception" of leptin in NHANES III. Serum fibrinogen, however, was collected on a full sample of NHANES participants from 1988 through 2002. Serum ferritin was also collected in these same survey years and can be used as an indicator of more chronic systemic inflammation. As an additional note, the NHANES biochemistry profiles collected have not included creatine kinase levels, which can be an indication of muscle injury or primary destructive muscle disease. However, in 2011 total creatine kinase without isoenzymes was added to the NHANES Biochemistry profile. US population-level creatine kinase reference ranges have been published from the NHANES 2011 to 2014 data.[155] Serum troponin has not been measured in NHANES.

Autoimmune serology has been performed in a number of NHANES survey cycles. As mentioned, rheumatoid factor was measured in both NHES I and NHANES III. NHANES III also collected data for the 2 principal thyroid autoantibodies, antithyroglobulin and antithyroperoxidase as a part of its thyroid serology panel.[156] Antithyroglobulin and antithyroperoxidase were again measured in a one-third subsample of survey participants in NHANES 2003 to 2004 and on a full sample of participants in 2007 to 2012. NHANES stored surplus sera and urine samples from its surveys and this was retrospectively used to measure autoantibodies. Two such studies have been accomplished, the first was an National Institute of Environmental Health Sciences–sponsored study of antinuclear antibodies and specific autoantibodies by immunoprecipitation using the NHANES 1999 to 2004 Environmental Health Dioxins one-third subsample data[157] and the second was a study of celiac disease-related autoantibodies to tissue transglutaminase (immunoglobulin A antitransglutaminase) and endomysial antigens (immunoglobulin A antiendomysial antigens) in NHANES III, NHANES 1999 to 2004, and 2009 to 2010.[158] Finally, in NHANES III a subsample case-referent study of 65-kDa isoform of glutamic acid decarboxylase antibody has been performed for participants 40 years of age and older.[159]

US NATIONAL HEALTH AND NUTRITION EXAMINATION SURVEY STORED BIOSPECIMENS PROGRAM

The US Centers for Disease Control and Prevention maintains biorepositories for the collection, processing, and storing of NHANES biospecimens, including participants' blood (serum or plasma), urine, and DNA samples. These samples can be used to analyze specimens for new analytes not included in previous NHANES data releases and are a national resource for assessment of new emerging health conditions. For example, when hantavirus and the hepatitis C virus were initially identified, NHANES stored sera and health examination were pivotal in providing a US national risk assessment. These specimens are in regular use by researchers and with the exception of DNA samples; after data processing, the results for the analytes studied are added to the NHANES public release data files for general use, as was the case for the US antinuclear autoantibodies study mentioned. Currently available stored specimens include samples from NHANES III and current NHANES 1999 to 2016; however, specimens from earlier NHANES survey cycles have been exhausted. The scope and procedures for accessing specimens is summarized in an NCHS documentation report.[160] Other examination records, such as the original sets of radiographs for

NHANES I through NHANES III are stored in the US Federal Archives. Blood collection for the extraction of DNA was first performed from consenting participants in NHANES III phase II and then in NHANES 1999 to 2002, 2007 to 2008, 2009 to 2010, and 2011 to 2012. Data from genetic studies performed is placed in a restricted genetic repository for linkage studies with NHANES public use and restricted datasets and is accessible through the NCHS RDC.[161] The majority of genetic data in the repository are single nucleotide polymorphisms.

US NATIONAL HEALTH AND NUTRITION EXAMINATION SURVEY PRESCRIPTION AND NONPRESCRIPTION MEDICATION DATA

In the early NHANES arthritis studies, selected nonprescription and prescription medication data were collected by questionnaire. NHANES III (1988–1994) fielded the first comprehensive data collection for all participant prescription medications that has remained a standard in current NHANES 1999 to 2016.[162,163] These data have proved to be a very useful resource for researchers and are widely used in publications using NHANES data. Data collection took place in the household interview by professional interviewers. Participants are asked to bring all bottles or tubes of medications used in the previous 30 days and the interviewer reviews these and records the medication information. Data recording incudes the medication name, the duration of use, and the self-reported reason for medication use, but not dosage. If the respondent has previously reported being diagnosed with key target survey diseases such as hypertension or diabetes and no medications for these diseases are noted, they are prompted for further information. This information is coded electronically in current NHANES using the Multum™ database, which provides generic drug identification codes for medication ingredients and drug class classification data that is publicly released. The scope of prescription data collection is limited to drugs taken at home; medications administered in doctor's offices, clinics or hospitals is not included. These prescription drug data have a wide variety of potential uses in arthritis and musculoskeletal disease research. As mentioned, the NHANES III prescription drug data was used in published analytical case definitions for RA and SLE. Other recent papers have defined the general US population prevalence of chronic steroid use as well as steroid effects on serum lipid values[164,165] and the US prevalence of skeletal muscle relaxant use.[166] Also, 2 papers have examined the prevalence of musculoskeletal pain and statin use using the NHANES 1999 to 2002 MPQ pain questionnaire and prescription medication data.[167,168]

NHANES has collected less nonprescription over-the-counter medication data. However, some significant data collections do exist in this area, which include the NHANES dietary supplements data, antacid use data, and low-dose preventive aspirin use.[169–171] For example, in NHANES 2005 to 2008, data for adults taking prescription medications, the prevalence of concomitant dietary supplement use (including vitamin preparations), was 53% among those with arthritis versus 14% among other US adults on a prescription drug.[172] Current dietary supplements use in the US among persons with arthritis has been described using these data.[173] The early arthritis survey cycles including NHES I and NHANES I and II, as well as NHANES 2009 to 2010 did collect some amount data on over-the-counter analgesic use, as well as information on self-reported analgesic efficacy in participants with musculoskeletal pain. Notably, a comprehensive effort to survey the detailed prevalence of the use of both prescription and nonprescription analgesics use was conducted in NHANES 1999 to 2004, which is a potentially important data resource for arthritis-related research.[174,175] A main public health concern prompting this effort was to obtain accurate US population-level data to assess risks of analgesic nephropathy, which were not evident in the data[176]; however, evidence was found for inappropriately high rates of over-the-counter medication nonsteroidal antiinflammatory drug use among persons with mild as well as moderate and advanced degrees of renal impairment.[177]

US NATIONAL HEALTH AND NUTRITION EXAMINATION SURVEY DATA FOR PHYSICAL ACTIVITY, FUNCTIONAL LIMITATIONS, AND SOCIAL SUPPORT

Historically, most NHANES survey cycles have collected some degree of data on participant's levels of physical activity, short-term and long-term functional limitations, and impairments and disabilities. NHANES III (1988–1994) and current NHANES 1999 to 2016 have had the most extensive data collection in these areas. Self-reported physical activity was captured in the exercise module in the NHANES III and in the physical activity questionnaire module in the household interview in NHANES 1999 to 2016.[178,179] NHANES has also collected examination data on physical capacity. In NHANES 1999 to 2004, fitness levels of participants ages 20 to 49 years were assessed by submaximal treadmill testing,[180] and in NHANES 2008 to 2016 ambulatory physical activity monitoring was done using accelerometers over a 7-day time span.[180,181] NHANES accelerometry data have been used to assess daily physical activity levels in subsamples of adults with musculoskeletal pain and mobility limitations to determine whether accelerometry profiles accompany pain at different sites of the body.[182] Physical activity and exercise capacity among children has been a special NHANES focus; in NHES III in the 1960s, treadmill exercise testing was done in children ages 12–17 years, and a comprehensive National Survey of Youth Fitness was performed in 2011 to 2012.[183,184]

The NHANES physical functioning questionnaire is the primary instrument that collects data on functional limitations.[185] The physical functioning questionnaire contains variables to define activities of daily living, instrumental activities of daily living, and basic functional activities. The physical functioning questionnaire can be used to construct other impairment-related metrics as well. The physical functioning questionnaire also contains disability outcome variables and self-reported data on the general categories of disease that have caused impairments, including arthritis. The NHANES social support questionnaire module provides interview data on emotional, material, and network support (ie, the number of members in a network).[186–188] In addition, NHANES III and NHANES 1999 to 2004 both performed physical examination testing for functional capacity. NHANES III fielded 3 physical performance tests: an 8-foot timed walk, 5 timed chair stands test, and a key-in-lock test of manual dexterity.[189] As noted, these tests have been used to assess functional status in NHANES III participants with radiographic OA of the knee.[33] NHANES 1999 to 2004 also fielded the 20-foot timed walk test and in 1999 to 2002, examination isokinetic testing of knee extensor muscle strength was performed in participants ages 50 years or older.[190] This test has been used, for example, to assess lower extremity muscle strength among diabetics and in those taking prescription statins.[191,192]

US NATIONAL HEALTH AND NUTRITION EXAMINATION SURVEY METHODOLOGY STUDIES

A principal function of NHANES is to provide national-level reference ranges for health examination tests and laboratory analytes. This was a primary goal from the inception of the NHANES survey and continues to be a major goal. Examples of examination-based standard reference include reference ranges for pulse and blood pressure hearing testing and age-related hearing loss (presbycusis) developed from the 1960s NHES I audiometric data, which continue to be a standard[193–195]; the widely used NHANES standard pediatric growth charts for children are derived from children's anthropometry data; reference ranges for spirometry testing from NHANES III, as well as the recent SPA arthritis body measures study are also standards in widespread use.[55,196–198] In NHANES radiology studies, DEXA scan data have provided national-level age, sex and race/ethnicity specific reference range data for bone mineral density and bone mineral content.[199,200] NHANES musculoskeletal radiology image dataset methodology studies include the NHANES III hand and wrist radiograph image study to model effective levels of digitization for the set of images and digital methodology studies for content retrieval and vertebral segmentation using the publicly available NHANES II cervical and lumbar spinal film images[34,201–204] In a similar fashion, NHANES have provided national reference standards for blood, urine, and other biological sample analytes. Examples include serum lipids and cholesterol, serum vitamin levels including folate and vitamin D, and most recently NHANES samples have been analyzed by the National Center for Environmental Health laboratories to provide for the first time an unprecedented comprehensive set of national level reference values for environmental health–related analytes, including heavy metals (lead, mercury, cadmium, arsenic, and others), dioxins, polychlorinated biphenyls and persistent organic pollutants, pesticides and fungicides, and others.[141,142] Also of methodologic relevance are the second-day examinations performed in NHANES III and NHANES 1999 to 2002. These repeat examinations were performed on a nonrandom sample of participants who had already completed the standard NHANES examination and were reexamined an average of 2 weeks after their initial examination, providing data on the short-term temporal biological variation of NHANES examination and laboratory data.[147] Peer-reviewed journal articles have also addressed methodologic analysis of NHANES data.[205–207]

US NATIONAL HEALTH AND NUTRITION EXAMINATION SURVEY ONLINE DATA AND PUBLICATIONS

The main data site for researchers is the NHANES Questionnaires, Datasets, and Related Documentation webpage.[208] This contains questionnaire, health examination, laboratory, and imaging data for all NHANES surveys from 1960 to the present. Researchers can used the 2 previously mentioned data overview matrices to locate survey cycles with specific datasets of interest from 1971 to 2006.[153,154] The NHANES data website also provides a search engine to identify specific variables in NHANES 1999 to 2016. The continuous NHANES 1999 and onward datasets are formatted similarly; in each survey cycle dataset, a data documentation PDF provides an introduction to the data, technical notes, and a code book listing each variable and its permissible values and frequencies; the data are provided as a SAS transport data file. Datasets are available in 5 categories: demographic, dietary data, examination data, laboratory data, and questionnaire data (radiographic and imaging studies are considered examination datasets). Separate links are also provided for copies of the questionnaire instruments and the laboratory and examination procedure manuals. To create the typical arthritis dataset, data files for the questionnaire, examination, and laboratory datasets need to be downloaded and merged. Earlier NHANES survey data from 1960 to 1994 were typically processed by mainframe computers and are publicly released as "flat files" (ie, row and column data format). NHANES provides SAS programming code to read the files and assemble them as a formatted, labeled SAS dataset. In the earliest NHANES surveys, separate topic area datasets (ie, arthritis, diabetes, etc) were released that included all the relevant questionnaire, examination, and laboratory data.

NHANES provides detailed online tutorials with explanation of the NHANES survey and procedures for analyzing NHANES data.[209] These tutorials include worked examples for data downloading, dataset assembly, data quality evaluation, and recommended statistical procedures for analysis. Program code for these purposes is provided for major software packages including SUDAAN, SAS, and STATA. The introductory base tutorial is for continuous NHANES 1999 and onward, which should be completed before using tutorials for earlier NHANES surveys, such as NHANES I, II, or III. In addition, NHANES provides special topic tutorials including the NHANES dietary tutorial, the NHANES environmental chemical data tutorial, the physical activity and cardiovascular fitness data tutorial, and the NHANES–Centers for Medicare and Medicaid Services linked data tutorial.

A considerable amount of technical documentation on the NHANES surveys and analysis of NHANES data is contained in NCHS publications. These are referenced in Medline, but their significance is often overlooked. The NCHS vital and health statistics publications have several series: series 1, Programs and Collection Procedures Plan and Operations Reports, contains the primary documentation reports for the NHANES and other surveys and, in older surveys, includes copies of the original data collection instruments; Series 2, Data Evaluation and Methods Research, contains methodology studies; and Series 11, Data from NHES, NHANES and Hispanic Health and Nutrition Survey, contains reports on the results of NHANES data analysis in key topic areas. Series 11 has been a primary venue for publishing NHANES data, especially in the early survey years, and currently has 253 reports.[210] The NHCS's Advance Data from Vital and Health Statistics also publishes many important analytical reports and in 2008 was renamed the National Health Statistics Reports.

US NATIONAL HEALTH AND NUTRITION EXAMINATION SURVEY DESIGN, FIELD OPERATIONS, AND DATA PRODUCTS

This section provides a general overview of the NHANES survey design, its sampling frame, and data collection aims. Although NHANES obtains nationally representative samples of health examination and laboratory data, data collection is not based on a simple random sample of the US population.[211] Rather, the NHANES survey uses a complex, multistage, demographically based survey design that requires special statistical analysis.[212] This demographic sampling strategy may not be familiar to medical researchers; however, it has numerous advantages. It ensures an overall nationally representative sample will be achieved while at the same time it enables adequate study sample sizes to be collected for key US subpopulations, such as minorities, those with low income, young children, and older adults. The demographic sampling strategy is also key to reducing overall sample sizes to an operationally feasible level for data collection. Because demographic sampling is based on a combination of probability sampling, cluster sampling, and stratified sampling, in NHANES the public release data files include survey design variables for strata and primary sampling units (PSU) as well as individual participant sample weights, which reflect the estimated proportion of the US population represented by an individual sample person. Statistical analysis of NHANES data must incorporate these design variables and sample weights, and software routines for complex survey analysis for this purpose; they are available in most current statistical packages.

The sampling frame for NHANES is the US resident civilian population currently residing in the 50 states and the District of Columbia that is not institutionalized. It excludes persons in hospitals, nursing homes, those in custody, active duty military personnel, and US citizens living overseas. Other NCHS surveys such as the National Hospital Care Survey and The National Survey of Long-Term Care Providers provide data on institutionalized populations.[213] NHANES uses a 4-stage sampling strategy to assemble a nationally representative sample. In the first stage, a sample of PSUs is selected from a frame of all US counties with selection probabilities proportionate population size. The second stage selects local area segments, that is, census blocks or combinations of blocks. In the third stage, based on a field listing of all dwelling units in each segment, a sample of dwelling units (households) is chosen. Subsampling rates here are designed to produce a national, approximately equal probability sample of households. The fourth stage is the actual selection of individual persons within households. A listing is made of all eligible members within a household and a subsample of individuals is selected based on the primary NHANES subsample domains: sex, age, race and Hispanic origin, income levels, and any special subsample requirements. There are differences across the set of NHANES surveys with respect to sample and especially subsampling design. The original NHES surveys (I, II, and II) did not use subsampling, NHANES I, NHANES II, and HHANES did not include persons aged 75 years and older, and oversampling of Hispanic or black persons did not occur until NHANES III. Specific continuous NHANES 1999 to 2016 survey cycles have oversampled pregnant women, Mexican Americans and then all Hispanic persons, adolescents, elderly persons, and most recently Asian Americans. In current NHANES, sampling design targets for a single survey year are 360 segments within 15 PSUs, approximately 12,400 households within segments, 6525 selected and 5000 examined sample persons. At each of the 15 field locations, an average of 450 participants are selected with an expected yield of 333 examined per location.[211]

ANALYTICAL PERSPECTIVES FOR US NATIONAL HEALTH AND NUTRITION EXAMINATION SURVEY DATA USE

NHANES publishes analytical guidelines for its survey cycles and these provide readable, practical overviews of issues in study design and analysis of data for the different survey cycles.[214] As mentioned, NHANES also has a step-by-step online tutorial that provides detailed guidance on NHANES survey design and data analysis. The following general points from those documents are particularly pertinent to NHANES arthritis data analysis. The complex demographic NHANES survey design was fielded to produce reliable data for high-frequency medical conditions such as heart disease, diabetes, and obesity. Central to survey planning is an overall objective of producing reliable prevalence estimates for medical conditions having a 10% population prevalence with a 30% relative standard error. For the researcher, it is useful to put this into perspective with respect to NHANES sample sizes, that is, the number of survey cycles that need to be combined to produce reliable statistical estimates. A single-year study can be performed with data from NHANES 1999 and onward because the sample design allows for the production of yearly aggregate-level national estimates. However, because of limited sample size, annual estimates can only be produced for the nation as a whole for very broad age categories, for gender, and for 3 major race ethnicity subdomains. Also large, potentially unstable variance estimates occur because singe year estimates are based on a small number of PSUs. The NHANES 2009 to 10 HLA-B27 prevalence study is an example where resources were sufficient to field only a 1-year study. NHANES data at the 1-year level are available only through the NCHS RDC because of the possibility of disclosure of a sample person's identity.

From this discussion, it can be seen that much larger study sample sizes are clearly preferred for routine analysis. This is seen clearly in the design of older NHANES studies that were publicly released as 4- to 6-year datasets. The current recommendation is that a single NHANES survey cycle representing 2 years of data is the *minimum* needed for analysis. To improve the statistical reliability and stability of estimates, analysts are advised to use combinations of 2-year cycles (ie, 4-year data or preferably 6-year data). Combining data from multiple 2-year survey cycles is especially necessary for the analysis of rare conditions, and reliable analysis in detailed demographic subdomains. The example of the NHANES III phase II ACR RA prevalence study shows that a 3-year dataset can effectively estimate overall US prevalences in the 2% range. For many types of arthritis, US population prevalences may be lower than this; however, a prevalence of 1% or even 0.5% are of potential public health significance because these small percentages correspond with hundreds of thousands or even 1 million or more cases nationally for diseases with significant adverse health outcomes. Also, the collective burden of such low prevalence disorders in the general population may well equal or exceed that of higher prevalence disorders. Some NCHS research has been done to address the issue of reliable statistical estimation for low prevalence conditions.[215] The innovative methodology developed NHANES's sister survey, the National Ambulatory Care Survey, also can potentially provide estimates of the prevalence of less commonly encountered rheumatologic conditions.[216,217]

The NHANES III Analytical Guidelines Appendix B[218] provides a general quality control algorithm for assessing reliability of prevalences and, as demonstrated in the NHANES online tutorial, this procedure should in fact be performed in all studies regardless of prevalence magnitudes. It should be recalled here that, because NHANES is a complex survey and not a random sample, significance testing for prevalences is performed with *t* tests according to the observed degrees of freedom in the particular sample. The recommended procedure is to produce a spreadsheet containing all study prevalence estimates, with columns for total sample size, number of cases, percent prevalence, standard errors, 95% confidence intervals, degrees of freedom, design effects, and relative standard errors. At a minimum, individual prevalence estimates based on less than 12 degrees of freedom or with a relative standard error of greater than 30% should be flagged as potentially statistically reliable. Also, a check of the average design effect across the major demographic variables should be made. Additional general NCHS guidelines on the reliability of prevalence estimation and its confidence interval estimation have also been recently published.[219]

NHANES sample weights and design variables (strata, PSU) should be used in all analyses. Strata and PSU variables must be included in data analysis because, as a complex survey, overall net study variances are typically increased over those seen in simple random sampling.[212,220] This ratio of variances between the 2 types of sampling is called the design effect, that is, complex survey sample variances are characteristically inflated compared with those under simple random sampling and this must be accounted for in published estimates. Also, in a demographically based survey, sample weights must be used. These weights account for differential selection probabilities of demographic subgroups in the survey design (age, gender, race/ethnicity, income, pregnancy status, etc). To help estimate a nationally representative sample, however, they also have other key functions; they are designed to control for selective nonresponse bias, include adjustments to compensate for inadequacies in the sampling frame, include adjustments to account for specific location characteristics known with certainty, and include a post-stratification step in weighting where known population totals compensate for undercoverage or overcoverage of certain demographic groups and for any residual differential nonresponse among these groups.[211]

The sum of NHANES data file sample weights can be considered as approximations of the absolute numbers of persons in the United States; however, they should not be used to estimate the numbers of persons in the United States affected by a medical condition. Rather, the statistically estimated prevalence of a condition should be multiplied by the official US Census Current Population Survey population counts for the demographic groups analyzed. Current Population Survey tables for the different NHANES survey are provided for this purpose on the NHANES website.[1] Generally, it is best to present estimates for the absolute number of persons affected by the condition sparingly for the main points in an analysis, as long detailed lists of population counts can detract from public health messaging.

ANALYZING NHANES ARTHRITIS-RELATED DATA: ISSUES AND OPPORTUNITIES

Using Self-Reported Arthritis Variables

This article emphasizes NHANES studies using recognized disease classification criteria and case definitions primarily based on NHANES examination or radiologic studies. This method is the recommended one for analyzing the NHANES arthritis related data; however, a number of studies have used only the self-reported NHANES medical conditions questionnaire arthritis history question variable for the study case definition of OA or RA. The medical conditions questionnaire arthritis questions (past physician diagnosis of arthritis generally; or of RA or OA) are interview questions fielded generally in federal health questionnaire surveys such as the NCHS's NHIS, with the primary intent of having a single overall indicator variable to track the prevalence of diagnosed arthritis over time.[221,222] Typically, the data are presented briefly in the introduction section of public health reports to frame the general scope of arthritis prevalence in the United States, for example, the National Arthritis Data Workgroup arthritis data needs assessment reports.[9–12] However, currently, self-reported arthritis and other arthritis-related interview questions are the primary data used in nationwide public health goals tracking, for example, in *Healthy People 2020* and the Centers for Disease Control and Prevention Surveillance Reports.[87,223,224] An additional use of the general self-reported arthritis variables is to provide NHANES data analysts with a summary arthritis adjustment variable for multivariate analyses to examine the effects of confounding and effect modification. The NCHS has done a number of methodology studies on these types of questionnaire variables that show that although they do not have extremely high sensitivity and specificity for the target diseases in question, they do have sufficient sensitivity and specificity to be used for these general level surveillance purposes when fielded in large-scale survey studies such as the NHIS.[225–228]

The issue of the validity of self-reports of specific type of arthritis (RA, OA) has been studied for many years with variable results and in the end the validity of this type of data may depend on the particular study population and context. In the NHANES context, the relation between the medical conditions questionnaire self-reported RA versus the 1987 ACR RA criteria was examined using NHANES III data, and a low sensitivity of self-reported RA for examination based RA was seen.[37] Most sample persons classified by ACR criteria as having RA gave a history of a prior arthritis diagnosis; however, they were unaware of the specific type of arthritis. Thus, self-reported RA is not desirable for use in NHANES prevalence studies in the age group. The issue of developing validated case definition module questionnaire instruments for arthritis surveillance is an important one but somewhat neglected as a public health goal. The existing NHANES arthritis questionnaire, examination, and laboratory data represent an opportunity for modeling in this regard. Although many feel questionnaire data to have low validity, this is not the case with well-validated questionnaire instruments. Further, some arthritis-related data can only be collected by self-report, for example, pain experience. Also, more detailed and nuanced analytical data modeling can significantly improve the validity of self-reported data, for example, the recent NCHS methodology studies for medical conditions questions and body measures metrics such as body mass index.[229,230]

NHANES: Identifying Unpublished NHANES Survey Arthritis Data

As outlined, NHANES data collection content has changed significantly over time. This is true both within the NHANES core modules, but especially so for the remainder of NHANES survey content, which has changed significantly over time as examination components come and go. The result is an impressive body of data collected over a 50-year period of data collection; however, the individual researcher focusing on a specific topic, NHANES data collections, presents something of a mosaic of studies performed for different purposes, at different times and targeted at different subgroups of the US population. The challenge is to identify sufficient data resources for the particular research problem at hand. In some case, NHANES data collection will be insufficient to support a particular research aim; nevertheless, in many instances data may exist but be overlooked. Therefore, a significant general issue in publications using NHANES data is that investigators typically use only a very limited set of variables from 1 or 2 NHANES datasets for analysis, whereas in fact much more extensive data are available. The focused review here will hopefully decrease that possibility for arthritis researchers. It should be remembered that NHANES datasets contain extensive demographic, questionnaire, examination, and laboratory analyte variables, as well as other information. In planning research, investigators should review available data in each of these data collection areas. Also, it is important to review the detailed NHANES data collection procedure manuals and laboratory methods manuals to understand how the NHANES data were actually collected and processed, and how this compares with other published studies.

Many journals aim to selectively publish only newly collected data, and the NHANES data website has a monthly update of new NHANES data modules that have been publicly released. Because NHANES arthritis data collection has been minimal in recent years, researchers may feel some reluctance to spend time analyzing the "old" NHANES arthritis data described herein, particularly because, as seen, so many important publications on the NHANES arthritis data have been authored by prominent rheumatologists and epidemiologists. However, NHANES data are unique in that there are no other nationally representative health examination based surveys in the United States. Also, the scope of the NHANES arthritis data collection is extensive and many, if not most, of the basic analytical studies that could have been and should be pursued have not been published. This is in fact generally the case for most NHANES datasets. This phenomenon of underpublished data could legitimately be called the "NHANES disease." Although its causes are uncertain, it is often the case that for a newly released NHANES dataset, either a single journal article, or a very limited number of articles are published in highly respected journals. This may give the impression that the dataset in question has been "published" despite the fact that authors often characterize their work as preliminary. However, recently analyzed NHANES data from prior NHANES has clearly provided pivotal population-based disease risk assessments. A notable recent example relevant to obesity research is the recent digitalization and rereading of the NHANES III gallbladder ultrasound tapes to provide the first national-level prevalence data for and analytical studies of hepatic steatosis, confirming the genetic association hepatic steatosis with PNPLA3, GCKR, and PPP1R3B.[231,232]

A clear arthritis-related example of an underpublished dataset is the publicly available NHANES III ACR-RA data. This is a useful 3-year dataset, but not large by NHANES standards. Current publications include basic RA prevalence estimates and several analytical papers relating to RA risk factors.[37,108,110,233] However, the basic NHANES III RA prevalence article was primarily a methodology-oriented study and a more detailed analysis of NHANES demographics and occupational history variables was not presented. Current publications on the RA dataset do not include a detailed analysis of public health and clinical surveillance parameters; that is, population prevalences of undiagnosed and diagnosed disease, disease durations, RA case stage distribution estimates, and RA treatment and control rates. Questionnaire and physical examination based descriptive data for hand and knee joint involvement distributions were not published, nor were NHANES III examination and questionnaire data relating to functional limitations or social support considered. Other NHANES data that remain unpublished of potential relevance to RA are data for inflammatory markers (C-reactive protein, ferritin fibrinogen), distributions of RA target organ involvement (NHANES renal function data), and hematologic indices (normochromic normocytic anemia, other cell counts). In addition, relevant to current hypotheses of lung inflammation as a potential trigger for RA, a specific focus of NHANES III data collections was population assessment of respiratory health and chronic obstructive lung disease. Pulmonary function testing, respiratory symptom, and history questionnaire data were collected and have been extensively analyzed to support that goal, but not analyzed with respect to RA. Further, NHANES data collections can also support RA target organ and comorbidity studies. For example, a NHANES III ACR-RA study did not show a clear association between RA and diabetes.[233] Notably, however, a more recent NHANES III analysis of stored biospecimens showed a higher risks of diabetes-related autoantibodies in non-Hispanic white and black adult diabetics as compared with adults without diabetes (6% vs 2% and 4% vs 1%, respectively).[159] The NHANES III adult data file also contains autoimmune serology results for thyroid disorders and celiac disease. Finally, no longitudinal data linkage studies have been performed for the NHANES III RA cohort (ie, mortality data follow-up; Medicare/Medicaid data), although the incidence of RA among periodontal disease has been analyzed using NHANES I Follow-Up Epidemiology Study data.[234] Smoking is increasingly considered a major RA risk factor, as well as a risk factor for periodontitis.[235] In support of US public health initiatives, NHANES datasets have detailed smoking data including smoking history, specific types of current products used, as well as cotinine and urinary metabolite biomonitoring data to classify smokers as well as those with second hand smoke exposure. These smoking data have not been analyzed in any detail for RA.

Also remarkable with respect to the NHANES III RA data is that the US population distribution of rheumatoid factor for adults 60 years of age and older and its correlates and epidemiologic associations from the dataset remain unpublished. The NHANES III rheumatoid factor data are potentially significant; recent population-based longitudinal studies have demonstrated increased risks developing of RA in persons seropositive for rheumatoid factor, especially those with high titers,[236,237] outcomes that could be potentially examined via NHANES data linkage studies. Also, recently NHANES III stored biospecimens have been analyzed for monoclonal gammopathy of undetermined significance and these data are now publicly available.[238] Also, temporal biological variation data are available for rheumatoid factor in the NHANES III second-day examination files.[147] The value of NHANES III RA-related dataset has potential to be significantly upgraded to support modern RA case classification criteria by reading the existing set of NHANES III hand-wrist and knee radiographs for RA changes. Also, adding anticitrullinated peptide antibody data using NHANES biospecimen program stored sera is important, because anticitrullinated peptide antibody data are being used to define patients at risk for RA, and the general population distribution of this important autoantibody and associations with numerous NHANES variables can be examined directly.

Some Methodologic Issues in the US National Health and Nutrition Examination Survey Arthritis Data

Two additional and interrelated methodologic issues in the NHANES setting and in arthritis epidemiology studies generally are (a) the low prevalence of some clinically important rheumatic diseases and (b) the need to develop valid disease classification criteria for population-level public health surveillance. First, as seen for RA, with the current NHANES sampling design, a larger 6-year or even an 8-year dataset would be desirable to support epidemiologic analyses. Also, having classification criteria that include the entire RA disease spectrum (ie, preclinical and early disease as well as definite disease), is important for population-based studies. In the NHANES III RA data, the ACR case classification criteria used apply only to well-established disease and the study could not include radiologic data, and both of these factors served to decrease the observed estimated RA prevalences. Further, in RA as well as for other types of arthritis such as SpA, early diagnosis and treatment of mild disease to prevent progression is a key goal. For many disorders, the prevalences of a preclinical prodromal state and of early milder disease is often (but not necessarily) higher. Including this more complete disease spectrum with the additional cases NHANES data could significantly increase prevalences and thereby enhance NHANES RA study capabilities.

Second, important issues relating to disease classification and misclassification have arisen out of NHANES arthritis studies. These issues are key for developing arthritis public health surveillance monitoring, because optimal classification of arthritis cases is important for precision in arthritis prevalence estimates. One of the most significant of these issues is the definition of arthritis-related pain and especially discordances between pain reports and radiographic findings. This finding has been clearly seen in NHANES I knee OA radiology studies as well in the NHANES I sacroiliac joint disease data. In this respect, the NHANES I knee OA data have been the subject of important analyses.[239] A significant percentage of NHANES I cases with significant radiographic knee OA findings did not report joint-related pain by study criteria, whereas participants with no radiologic findings reported some prevalence of joint pain. Subsequent reviews of the early NHANES data and other subsequent major studies (reviewed in[240]) suggest multiple factors may help to explain these results, including questionnaire screening only at a high pain level (pain present on most days for 3 months in the NHANES data); variability in radiograph readings; more positive radiographic findings usually seen with multiple radiograph views of a joint; fewer positive radiographs seen non–weight-bearing knee films (as in NHANES III), which precludes assessment of early OA changes; therapeutic effects of drug treatment on pain report frequencies; patient reduction in physical activity or use of assistive devices to reduce or eliminate pain; and the presence of concomitant non-OA origin knee pain as well as other causes.[241,242] Further, the NHANES sample does not include disabled, institutionalized persons, and selective arthritis-related mortality in populations could also play a role. Using more modern imaging techniques such as MRI would detect a higher percentage of OA cases (or pathology studies even higher). Finally, as an additional note, both the NHANES I and the NHANES III knee radiographs were read for chondrocalcinosis, which could potentially be associated with increased pain reporting. These data are publicly available but apparently thus far not analyzed. Additional analysis of the NHANES knee OA and SI joint data seems to be needed, especially because the later NHANES III knee OA data have not yet been systematically analyzed in this regard, and an analysis of the relation of symptoms to radiographic findings should be broadened to include joint stiffness and NHANES functional limitations data. This type of analysis could potentially be usefully supplemented with new biomarker data. For the researcher, a useful inventory and review of pain data collections in NCHS surveys through the 1990s, including summaries of the NHANES data collections in this area, has been published.[243]

A related issue in defining a complete disease spectrum for arthritis surveillance studies is the question of "asymptomatic" disease. Although arthritis pain is of central importance in arthritis and a principal factor prompting patients to seek medical care, it is possible that the NHANES population-based survey data results cited previously may in part be pointing to a subpopulation of arthritis cases potentially presenting with minimal levels of pain or no pain at all, although they may otherwise experience functional limitations and adverse clinical outcomes characteristic of the arthritis syndrome in question. Many people may well ignore back pain or stiffness, which is considered to be a commonly occurring problem, but it is very hard to ignore knee pain or hand swelling because of the functional limitations imposed. Classical RA is usually thought to always be accompanied by significant joint pain; however, for ankylosing spondylitis, psoriasis-related axial arthritis, and SpA in inflammatory bowel disease, it is evident that a percentage of cases with definite and even advanced radiologic disease presents without a significant pain history, and these patients may have substantial functional impairments.[244–247] Reanalysis of the relevant NHANES data here could further research in this area, in this instance potentially giving more diagnostic weight to a combination of radiologic findings, target organ impairment, and functional status measures.

An additional important analytical issue relates to the NHANES I and NHANES III survey knee radiographs, both of which were read for OA using the Kellgren-Lawrence reference atlas standard. This is important because accurate tracking of arthritis trends over time is a major public health surveillance goal. The overall prevalence of radiographic knee KOA in NHANES I adults 60 years or older was 9%, whereas in NHANES III it was 30%. This finding has raised questions as to whether the radiographs from the earlier survey period may have been underread, or conversely whether the NHANES III films were overread. However, because obesity is a major known risk factor for knee OA, the well-documented marked increase in obesity over the time period between NHANES I and III might well explain a difference in the prevalence of radiographic knee OA. These questions could be clarified by further analytical research on these datasets.

Rheumatologic Approaches to Public Health Surveillance of Chronic Axial Pain

Rheumatology has demonstrated expertise in developing well-defined disease classification criteria. These criteria are developed jointly by rheumatologists, biostatisticians, and epidemiologists, and have had proven usefulness in international epidemiology studies of the prevalence, scope, and impact of specific disorders such as RA, OA, gout, SLE, and other syndromes. They are pivotal in standardizing clinical trials to evaluate therapies. The criteria typically have undergone a number of iterations as knowledge has advanced. Classification criteria suitable for public health surveillance for diseases such as RA, SLE, and OA are, thus, available and have been usefully applied in the NHANES data. Potentially, rheumatologic expertise in developing classification criteria could be usefully applied to help identify and define additional and specific public health surveillance monitoring targets, especially for musculoskeletal conditions that remain as significant unresolved outstanding issues for the general population. A useful example is chronic axial pain (ie, chronic neck; upper, mid, lower back; or buttock pain) that, as reviewed herein, has a US population prevalence approaching 20% of adults. Specific causes of axial pain are not often attained with any diagnostic certainty and effective, specifically targeted therapy is typically not available, which make primary and secondary prevention efforts for chronic neck and back pain problematic. Although important research advances have been made, there is no clear evidence that, at a patient level, there is any significant progress. Rheumatology does not have ownership of this general public health issue; however, chronic axial pain does intersect with rheumatologic disorders in many specific instances. Defining these additional rheumatic conditions clearly, providing clear screening guidelines for medical practitioners to use, and placing these under direct public health surveillance could potentially be a major contribution to public health efforts to reduce the population burden of chronic axial pain. The rheumatologic subgroup of patients with chronic axial pain otherwise would continue to routinely present to a variety of practitioners with varying clinical skills,[248] and thus by default would largely remain under the umbrella category chronic back pain (ie, undiagnosed).

IBP associated with ankylosing spondylitis and SpA is a specific case in point. For example, rheumatologic IBP case classification criteria were designed in the first instance by Calin and colleagues[46] as a general population screening instrument. The NHANES 2009 to 2010 IBP/SpA survey was the first large-scale, population-based effort to field IBP screening criteria and to directly estimate its prevalence in relation to the frequency of overall chronic neck and back pain. The results were similar for each of the 4 IBP criteria studied. For example, in the NHANES 2009 to 2010 US general population sample of 5013 sample persons, 980 or 19.2% of all US adults, had chronic axial pain of all types. Of these 980 persons, 274 (29%) initially screened positive for IBP by ESSG criteria. When ESSG SpA criteria are applied to the total chronic axial pain sample (IBP being a mandatory ESSG SpA feature), 70 persons, equivalent to an estimated 7% of the US chronic back pain population, met ESSG criteria for SpA. This number is likely a lower bound estimate of the true prevalence of IBP in patients with chronic axial pain, because many true IBP cases may never develop SpA. However, the example suggests that a finite and important percentage of chronic axial pain cases may have IBP. This finding highlights a specific situation where, potentially, a specific diagnosis can be given to a subset of chronic axial pain cases and disease-specific diagnostic testing (MRI or HLA-B27 testing, for example) and therapy offered. From a public health viewpoint, this enables population-based disease surveillance and control for a clearly defined target; that is, early diagnosis and treatment efforts aimed at secondary prevention of disease complications as well as more specifically focused primary prevention research. The NHANES IBP data clearly need further analysis and comparison with ongoing IBP research elsewhere. Additional general tasks necessary to fully develop IBP surveillance criteria will include the evaluation of the newer Assessment of Spondyloarthritis International Society IBP classification criteria in population-level studies as well as developing formal exclusion criteria. For instance, the published literature includes a variety of possible IBP mimics with an axial pain component, such as sarcoidosis, spinal and perispinal inflammatory conditions (vertebral osteomyelitis, inflammatory infected aortic aneurysm in older adults), Paget's disease, drug-induced disease (isotretinoin), and chronic infected pilonidal cyst (author's case).[249–253] Common diseases with retroperitoneal involvement and back pain, for instance, conditions like endometriosis, could also potentially be IBP mimics.[254]

From a public health perspective, a fundamental problem impeding progress in decreasing the incidence of or controlling chronic axial pain is an epidemiologic one, namely, its underlying diagnostic heterogeneity. As it currently stands, chronic back pain remains largely an undiagnosed disease. Chronic back pain is essentially an umbrella term for a number of clinically distinct entities, potentially 10 or more important ones, and their root causes and therapeutic approaches may differ greatly. Attempting to deal with such an inherently heterogeneous aggregate case definition sets a very high bar for finding effective therapies and for public health intervention programs. However, this is in fact a common epidemiologic problem in many chronic disorders, for example, the underlying heterogeneity in asthma and autism studies that impedes progress and can potentially bias clinical trial results toward the null. A general strategy to counter disease classification heterogeneity is to seek opportunities to define disease subsets that have specifically defined etiology and, ideally, a specific therapy as well. For example, if 1 or more chronic axial pain subsets can be identified and removed from the general umbrella axial pain category, the residual category of chronic back pain becomes more homogeneous and tractable, and more amenable to clinical and epidemiologic investigation. For instance, the ability to identify just 2 additional etiology-specific axial pain target conditions with US population prevalence similar to IBP could, together with IBP, potentially remove almost 20% of currently defined patients out of the nonspecific axial pain case definition. With the advent of advanced imaging studies available on a widespread scale, the use of these case ascertainment criteria as discussed would allow for an efficient use of an expensive diagnostic modality.

The NHANES back pain datasets are detailed and extensive and offer an unbiased population-based data platform for exploratory scoping studies, hypotheses development, as well as analytical studies. Although a small number of articles on basic prevalence have been published, these data collections are otherwise largely unanalyzed. There are several possible approaches for identifying additional etiology-specific rheumatologic subsets in the NHANES data: that is, rheumatologic syndromes with chronic axial involvement as a principal component. For example, diffuse idiopathic skeletal hyperostosis most typically affects the cervical and upper thoracic spine, but may also occur in the lumbar spine. The prevalence and distribution of radiographic diffuse idiopathic skeletal hyperostosis and its association with axial symptoms has been examined in some studies but not others[255,256] but remains to be explored on a population level. Further its potential role in producing chronic axial pain could be evaluated in the large-scale, nationally representative set of online NHANES II cervical and lumbar spine radiographs, arthritis questionnaires, and other NHANES II data. Acute and chronic reactive arthritis secondary to enteric and genitourinary infection, a disorder in the SpA family, most typically presents with peripheral arthritis, but its spectrum does include axial involvement. This disorder is diagnosable, with specific treatment protocols. Reactive arthritis was not included in the 2009 to 2010 IBP/SpA data collection, but has the potential to be studied in NHANES, especially because of the NHANES emphasis on the control of infectious disease-related morbidity. NHANES has the capability for examining serology for enteric and other arthritogenic pathogens as a part of its infectious disease surveillance programs, and has performed serologic surveys of rubella, chlamydia, cryptosporidium, toxocara, hepatitis B, and hepatitis C. Beyond this, the NHANES 1999 to 2004 data MPQ CWP dataset has not been screened for candidate axial pain disorders. The detailed body pain diagram data support site-specific analysis of distributions of axial and peripheral joint involvement. Potential CWP associations with the range of specific NHANES medical conditions and the NHANES laboratory data could usefully be examined.

Apart from rheumatologic syndromes, the possibility of chronic axial pain associated with the principal high prevalence chronic diseases targeted in the NHANES survey design should be examined. Sample sizes here are large, because these are the primary foci of NHANES data collection. The current index of suspicion that these medical conditions may cause chronic axial pain disorders is not high; however, the possibility has not been evaluated formally using large, nationally representative NHANES datasets. Osteoporosis is not typically thought to be associated with axial pain, except for vertebral fractures. As noted, the US osteoporosis-related vertebral fracture prevalence is published.[76] However, the NHANES osteoporosis data have not otherwise been analyzed with respect to the possibility of chronic axial pain. If there proved to be either a higher or a lower prevalence of chronic axial pain in osteoporosis cases than in the general population, this finding could be significant. Diabetes and obesity are also chief high-prevalence disorders studied in NHANES and, although there has been 1 preliminary report regarding diabetes and back pain,[257] these datasets have not been evaluated in detail with respect to the possibility of either chronic axial disease or even peripheral arthritis syndromes. Finally, the set of NHANES II radiographs could also be used for their originally intended purpose: to examine associations between spinal OA, lumbar disc degeneration, and their degree of axial pain and functional impairment. Results of a recent systematic review and metaanalysis of associations between lumbar spine radiographic features and low back pain suggest that evaluating these data to identify axial pain public health surveillance targets is important.[258]

SUMMARY

It is important to understand how NHANES data compare with the standard case of clinical research data collection. NHANES arthritis data collections typify the demographic survey approach to describing rheumatic disorders. NHANES does not perform detailed clinical examinations but rather executes planned, high-quality, protocol-driven active data collection designed to assess arthritis prevalence, risk factors, and outcomes. Furthermore, the NHANES sample target is the ambulatory, noninstitutionalized US population. This is in fact the bulk of the population; however, it may not provide a representative sample of the sickest cases, which is the subject of so many clinical and epidemiology studies. In terms of disease spectrum, NHANES data can potentially effectively capture population-based samples of preclinical, mild, and moderate cases of a specific disease as well as some proportion of more severe cases. NHANES also has the specific advantage of being able to study representative samples of undiagnosed disease cases not presenting to medical practitioners. NHANES data are, therefore, highly relevant to current clinical research agendas to identify prodromal disease states with precision and to effectively make early diagnosis and treatment to prevent disease complications, a shared goal with public health arthritis prevention programs.

Finally, it should also be recognized that the NHANES coverage of arthritis syndromes is incomplete in some respects. Significantly, NHANES arthritis surveys have not collected data on either Sjogren's syndrome or polymyalgia rheumatica, which primarily affect older adults. These were identified as National Arthritis Workgroup priorities for NHANES, but thus far have not been studied.[12] Also remarkable it is that NHANES, with its emphasis on infectious disease surveillance, has not performed Lyme disease or parvovirus B19 serology in any arthritis data collections, even though the former is a public health focus.[259] Nevertheless, the body of NHANES arthritis data and publications remains substantial, and still offers significant opportunities for productive research to improve the nation's health.

REFERENCES

1. National Health & Nutrition Examination Survey. NHANES response rates and population totals. Available at: https://www.cdc.gov/nchs/nhanes/response_rates_cps.htm. Accessed November 1, 2017.
2. Oliver SE, Unger ER, Lewis R. Prevalence of human papillomavirus among females after vaccine introduction-National Health and Nutrition Examination Survey, United States, 2003–2014. JID 2017;216:594–603.
3. Pirkle JL, Flegal KM, Bernert JT, et al. Exposure of the US population to environmental tobacco smoke: the Third National Health and Nutrition Examination Survey, 1988 to 1991. JAMA 1996;275:1233–40.
4. US Centers for Disease Control and Prevention (CDC). Disparities in secondhand smoke exposure - United States, 1988-1994 and 1999-2004. MMWR Morb Mortal Wkly Rep 2008;57:744–7.
5. Homa DM, Neff LJ, King BA, et al. Vital signs: disparities in nonsmokers' exposure to secondhand smoke-United States, 1999–2012. MMWR 2015;64:103–8.
6. Pirkle JL, Brody DJ, Gunter EW, et al. The decline in blood lead levels in the United States: The National Health and Nutrition Examination Surveys (NHANES). JAMA 1994;272:284–91.
7. US Centers for Disease Control and Prevention (CDC). Vital Signs: prevalence, treatment and control of hypertension-United States, 1999-2002 and 2005-2008. MMWR Morb Mortal Wkly Rep 2011;60:103–8.
8. Roberts J. Information on arthritis and other musculoskeletal disorders from the interview and examination survey programs of the National Center for Health Statistics. In: Lawrence RC, Shulman LE, editors. Epidemiology of the rheumatic diseases. Proceedings of the fourth international Conference national Institutes of health. New York: Gower Medical Publishing Limited; 1984. p. 341–8.
9. Lawrence RC, Hochberg MC, Kelsey JL, et al. Estimates of the prevalence of selected arthritic and musculoskeletal diseases in the United States. J Rheumatol 1989;16:427–41.
10. Sokka T, Krishnan E. National databases and rheumatology research II: the National Health and Nutrition Examination Surveys. Rheum Dis Clin North Am 2004; 30:869–78.
11. Helmick CG, Felson DT, Lawrence RC, et al. Estimates of the prevalence of arthritis and other rheumatic conditions in the United States. Arthritis Rheum 2008;58:15–25.
12. Lawrence RC, Felson DT, Helmick CG. Estimates of the prevalence of arthritis and other rheumatic conditions in the United States, Part II. Arthritis Rheum 2008;58:26–35.
13. Engel A, Burch TA. Chronic arthritis in the United States Health Examination Survey. Arthritis Rheum 1967;10:61–2.
14. Kellgren JH, Lawrence JS. Radiological assessment of osteoarthritis. Ann Rheum Dis 1957;16:494–502.

15. Ropes M, Bennett GA, Cobb S, et al. Revision of diagnostic criteria for Rheumatoid Arthritis. Bull Rheum Dis 1958;9:175–6.
16. Engel A, Burch T. A osteoarthritis in adults by selected demographic characteristics: United States, 1960-1962. Vital Health Stat 11 1966;20:1–33.
17. Roberts J, Burch TA. Prevalence of osteoarthritis in adults by age, sex, race and geographic area: United States, 1960-1962. Vital Health Stat 11 1966;5:1–34.
18. Engel A, Roberts J, Burch TA. Rheumatoid Arthritis in Adults: United States, 1960-1962. Vital Health Stat 11 1966;17:1–50.
19. Engel A. Rheumatoid arthritis in U.S. adults 1960-1962. In: Bennett PH, Wood PHN, editors. Population studies of the rheumatic diseases. International Congress Series No. 148. Amsterdam: Excerpta Medica Foundation; 1968. p. 83–9.
20. Miller HW. Plan and operation of the health and nutrition examination survey: United States–1971–1973. Part A, development, plan and operation. Vital Health Stat 1 1973;10a:1–53.
21. Miller HW. Plan and operation of the health and nutrition examination survey: United States– 1971–1973. Part B, Data Collection forms of the Survey. Vital Health Stat 1 1973;10b:1–82.
22. Engel A, Murphy RS, Mauer K, et al. Plan and operation of the HANES I (Health & Nutrition Examination Survey) augmentation survey of adults 25–74 years. United States, 1974–75. National Center for Health Statistics. Vital Health Stat 1 1978;14:1–116.
23. Maurer K. Basic data on arthritis of knee, hip and sacroiliac joints in adults ages 25-74 years: United States, 1971-1975. Vital Health Stat 11 1979;213:1–31.
24. Cunningham LS, Kelsey JL. Epidemiology of musculoskeletal impairments and associated disability. Am J Public Health 1984;74:574–9.
25. Grubber JM, Callahan LF, Helmick CG, et al. Prevalence of radiographic hip and knee osteoarthritis by place of residence. J Rheumatol 1998;25:959–63.
26. Espino DV, Burge SK, Moreno CA. The prevalence of selected chronic diseases among the Mexican-American elderly: data from the 1982-1984 Hispanic Health and Nutrition Examination Survey. J Am Board Fam Pract 1991;4:217–22.
27. McDowell A, Engel A, Massey JT, et al. Plan and operation of the Second National Health and Nutrition Examination Survey, 1976–1980, programs and procedures. Vital Health Stat 1 1981;15:1–144.
28. Lawrence RC. New research opportunities associated with national data sets. J Rheumatol 1985;12:1035–7.
29. National Library of Medicine. NHANES II X-ray Images. Available at: https://ceb.nlm.nih.gov/proj/ftp/ftp.php. Accessed November 14, 2017.
30. Pouletaut P, Dalqamoni H, Marin F, et al. Influence of age, gender and weight on spinal osteoarthritis in the elderly: an analysis of morphometric changes using X-ray images. IRBM 2010;31:141–7.
31. Plan and operation of the Third National Health and Nutrition Examination Survey, 1988-94. Vital Health Stat 1 1994;(32):1–407.
32. National Center for Health Statistics. The Third National Health and Nutrition Examination Survey (NHANES III), 1988–94, series 11, no. 11A (Knee Osteoarthritis X-ray Data and Documentation) Data Release (updated October 2001). Available at: http://www.cdc.gov/nchs/about/major/nhanes/nh3data.htm. Accessed October 26, 2017.
33. Dillon CF, Rasch EK, Gu Q, et al. Prevalence of knee osteoarthritis in the United States: arthritis data from the Third National Health and Nutrition Examination Survey 1991-1994. J Rheum 2006;33:2271–9.

34. Ostchega Y, Long LR, Goh GH, et al. Establishing the level of digitization for wrist and hand radiographs for the third National Health and Nutrition Examination Survey. J Digit Imaging 1998;11:116–20.
35. Altman R, Alarcon G, Appelrouth D, et al. The American College of Rheumatology Criteria for the classification and reporting of osteoarthritis of the hand. Arthritis Rheum 1990;33:1601–10.
36. Dillon CF, Hirsch R, Rasch EK, et al. Symptomatic hand osteoarthritis in the United States: prevalence and functional impairment estimates from the third U.S. National Health and Nutrition Examination Survey (1991-1994). Am J Phys Med Rehabil 2007;86:12–21.
37. Rasch EK, Hirsch R, Paulose-Ram R, et al. Prevalence of rheumatoid arthritis in persons 60 years of age and older in the United States: effect of different methods of case classification. Arthritis Rheum 2003;48:917–26.
38. Arnett FC, Edworthy SM, Bloch DA, et al. The American Rheumatism Association 1987 revised criteria for the classification of rheumatoid arthritis. Arthritis Rheum 1988;31:315–24.
39. Zipf G, Chiappa M, Porter KS, et al. National Health and Nutrition Examination Survey: plan and operations, 1999–2010. National Center for Health Statistics. Vital Health Stat 1 2013;56:1–37.
40. National Health and Nutrition Examination Survey. Miscellaneous Pain Questionnaire. Available at: https://wwwn.cdc.gov/Nchs/Nhanes/1999-2000/MPQ.htm. Accessed November 14, 2017.
41. Margolis RB, Tait RC, Krause SJ. A rating system for use with patient pain drawings. Pain 1986;24:57–65.
42. Wolfe F, Smythe HA, Yunus MB, et al. The American College of Rheumatology 1990 criteria for the classification of fibromyalgia. Report of the multicenter criteria committee. Arthritis Rheum 1990;33:160–72.
43. Hardt J, Jacobsen C, Goldberg J, et al. Prevalence of chronic pain in a representative sample in the United States. Pain Med 2008;9:803–12.
44. National Health and Nutrition Examination Survey. Arthritis Questionnaire (ARQ_F). Available at: https://wwwn.cdc.gov/Nchs/Nhanes/2009-2010/ARQ_F.htm. Accessed November 14, 2017.
45. Dillon CF, Hirsch R. The United States National Health and Nutrition Examination Survey and the epidemiology of ankylosing spondylitis. Am J Med Sci 2011;341:281–3.
46. Calin A, Porta J, Fries JF, et al. Clinical history as a screening test for ankylosing spondylitis. JAMA 1977;237:2613–4.
47. Dougados M, van der Linden S, Juhlin R, et al. The European Spondylarthropathy Study Group preliminary criteria for the classification of spondylarthropathy. Arthritis Rheum 1991;34:1218–27.
48. Rudwaleit M, Metter A, Listing J, et al. Inflammatory back pain in ankylosing spondylitis: a reassessment of the clinical history for application as classification and diagnostic criteria. Arthritis Rheum 2006;54:569–78.
49. Sieper J, Rudwaleit M, Baraliakos X, et al. The Assessment of SpondyloArthritis International Society (ASAS) handbook: a guide to assess spondyloarthritis. Ann Rheum Dis 2009;68(Suppl 2):ii1–44.
50. Weisman MH, Witter JP, Reveille JD. The prevalence of inflammatory back pain: population-based estimates from the US National Health and Nutrition Examination Survey, 2009-10. Ann Rheum Dis 2013;72:369–73.
51. Weisman MH. Inflammatory back pain The United States perspective. Rheum Dis Clin N Am 2012;38:501–12.

52. Reveille J, Weisman MH. The epidemiology of back pain, axial spondyloarthritis and HLA-B27 in the United States. Am J Med Sci 2013;345:43–436.
53. Amor B, Dougados M, Mijiyawa M. Criteria of the classification of spondylarthropathies. Rev Rhum Mal Osteoartic 1990;57:85–9.
54. Reveille JD, Witter JP, Weisman MH. Prevalence of axial spondylarthritis in the United States: estimates from a cross-sectional survey. Arthritis Care Res (Hoboken) 2012;64:905–10.
55. Assassi S, Weisman MH, Lee M, et al. New population-based reference values for spinal mobility measures based on the 2009-2010 National Health and Nutrition Examination Survey. Arthritis Rheumatol 2014;66:2628–37.
56. Reveille JD, Hirsch R, Dillon CF, et al. The prevalence of HLA-B27 in the US: data from the US National Health and Nutrition Examination Survey, 2009. Arthritis Rheum 2012;64:1407–11.
57. Walsh JA, Zhou X, Clegg DO, et al. Mortality in American veterans with the HLA-B27 gene. J Rheumatol 2015;42:638–44.
58. Haroon N. Does a positive HLA-B27 test increase your risk of mortality? J Rheumatol 2015;42:559–60.
59. Gran JT, Husby G. Ankylosing spondylitis in women. Semin Arthritis Rheum 1990;19:303–12.
60. Boyer GS, Templin DW, Bowler A, et al. A comparison of patients with spondyloarthropathy seen in specialty clinics with those identified in a communitywide epidemiologic study. Has the classic case misled us? Arch Intern Med 1997;157:2111–7.
61. Deyo RA, Tsui-Wu YJ. Descriptive epidemiology of low-back pain and its related medical care in the United States. Spine 1987;12:264–8.
62. Andersen RE, Crespo CJ, Bartlett SJ. Relationship between body weight gain and significant knee, hip, and back pain in older Americans. Obes Res 2003;11:1159–62.
63. Altman RD, Bloch DA, Hochberg MC, et al. Prevalence of pelvic Paget's disease of bone in the United States. J Bone Miner Res 2000;15:461–5.
64. National Center for Health Statistics. Public Use Data Tape Documentation. Chest-X-Ray, Pulmonary Diffusion, and Tuberculin Test Results Ages 26-74. Tape Number 4251. National Health and Nutrition Examination Survey, 1971-1975. 162 pp. Available at: https://www.cdc.gov/nchs/data/nhanes/nhanesi/4251.pdf. Accessed November 1, 2017.
65. Carter OD, Haynes SG. Prevalence rates for scoliosis in US adults: results from the first National Health and Nutrition Examination Survey. Int J Epidemiol 1987;16:537–44.
66. Vose GP. Estimation of changes in radiographic densitometry. Radiology 1969;93:841–4.
67. CompuMed Inc. OsteoGram radiographic absorptiometry of NHANES I radiographs. Manhattan Beach (CA): CompuMed Inc; 1994.
68. Yang SO, Hagiwara S, Engelke K, et al. Radiographic absorptiometry for bone mineral measurement of the phalanges: precision and accuracy study. Radiology 1994;192:857–9.
69. Cosman F, Herrington B, Himmelstein S, et al. Radiographic absorptiometry: a simple method for determination of bone mass. Osteoporos Int 1991;2:34–8.
70. Looker AC, Orwoll ES, Johnston CC Jr, et al. Prevalence of low femoral bone density in older U.S. adults from NHANES III. J Bone Miner Res 1997;12(11):1761–8.

71. Borrud LG, Flegal KM, Looker AC, et al. Body composition data for individuals 8 years of age and older: U.S. population, 1999–2004. National Center for Health Statistics. Vital Health Stat 11 2010;250:1–87.
72. Flegal KM, Shepherd JA, Looker AC, et al. Comparisons of percentage body fat, body mass index, waist circumference, and waist-stature ratio in adults. Am J Clin Nutr 2009;89:500–8.
73. Wright NC, Looker AC, Saag KG, et al. The recent prevalence of osteoporosis and low bone mass in the united states based on bone mineral density at the femoral neck or lumbar spine. J Bone Miner Res 2014;29:2520–6.
74. Looker AC, Melton LJ III, Harris TB, et al. Prevalence and trends in low femur bone density among older US adults: NHANES 2005–2006 compared with NHANES III. J Bone Miner Res 2010;5:64–71.
75. Looker AC, Isfahani S, Fan B, et al. Trends in osteoporosis and low bone mass in older US adults, 2005–2006 through 2013–2014. Osteoporos Int 2017;28: 1979–88.
76. Cosman F, Krege JH, Looker AC, et al. Spine fracture prevalence in a nationally representative sample of US women and men aged ≥40 years: results from the National Health and Nutrition Examination Survey (NHANES) 2013-2014. Osteoporos Int 2017;28:1857–66.
77. Lawrence RC, Helmick CG, Arnett FC, et al. Estimates of the prevalence of arthritis and selected musculoskeletal disorders in the United States. Arthritis Rheum 1998;41:778–99.
78. Zhu Y, Pandya BJ, Choi HK. Prevalence of gout and hyperuricemia in the US general population: the National Health and Nutrition Examination Survey 2007-2008. Arthritis Rheum 2011;63:3136–41.
79. Choi WJ, Ford ES, Curhan G, et al. The independent association of serum retinol and β-carotene levels with hyperuricemia – a national population study. Arthritis Care Res (Hoboken) 2012;64:389–96.
80. Fang J, Alderman MH. Serum uric acid and cardiovascular mortality the NHANES I Epidemiologic Follow-Up Study, 1971–1992, National Health and Nutrition Examination Survey. JAMA 2000;283:2404–10.
81. Odden MC, Amadu AR, Smit E. Uric acid levels, kidney function, and cardiovascular mortality in US adults: National Health and Nutrition Examination Survey (NHANES) 1988–1994 and 1999–2002. Am J Kidney Dis 2014;64:550–7.
82. Kramer HM, Curhan G. The association between gout and nephrolithiasis: the National Health and Nutrition Examination Survey III, 1988-1994. Am J Kidney Dis 2002;40(1):37–42.
83. Juraschek SP, Kovell LC, Miller ER, et al. Gout, urate lowering therapy and uric acid levels among US adults. Arthritis Care Res (Hoboken) 2015;67:588–92.
84. Juraschek SP, Kovellc LC, Miller ER. Association of kidney disease with prevalent gout in the United States in 1988–1994 and 2007–2010. Semin Arthritis Rheum 2013;42:551–61.
85. Ward MM. Prevalence of physician-diagnosed systemic lupus erythematosus in the United States: results from the third national health and nutrition examination survey. J Womens Health (Larchmt) 2004;13:713–8.
86. Hochberg MC, Perlmutter DL, Medsger TA, et al. Prevalence of self-reported physician-diagnosed systemic lupus erythematosus in the USA. Lupus 1995; 4:454–6.
87. National Center for Health Statistics. Healthy people 2020 midcourse review. Chapter 3: Arthritis, osteoporosis, and chronic back conditions (AOCBC).

Hyattsville (MD): 2016. Available at: https://www.cdc.gov/nchs/data/hpdata2020/HP2020MCR-C03-AOCBC.pdf. Accessed November 1, 2017.
88. Donaldson MG, Cawthon PM, Lui LY, et al. Estimates of the proportion of older white men who would be recommended for pharmacologic treatment by the new US National osteoporosis foundation guidelines. J Bone Miner Res 2010; 25:1506–11.
89. Dawson-Hughes B, Looker AC, Tosteson NA, et al. The potential impact of the National Osteoporosis Foundation guidance on treatment eligibility in the USA: an update in NHANES 2005–2008. Osteoporos Int 2012;23:811–20.
90. Dalbeth N, Bardin T, Doherty M, et al. Discordant American College of Physicians and international rheumatology guidelines for gout management: consensus statement of the Gout, Hyperuricemia and Crystal-Associated Disease Network (CAN). Nat Rev Rheumatol 2017;13:561–8.
91. Felson DT, Lawrence RC, Dieppe PA, et al. Osteoarthritis: new insights. Part 1: the disease and its risk factors. Ann Intern Med 2000;133:635–46.
92. Callahan LF, Jordan JM. Arthritis and its impact: challenges and opportunities for treatment, public health, and public policy. N C Med J 2007;68:415–21.
93. Davis MA, Ettinger WH, Neuhaus JM. The association of knee injury and obesity with unilateral and bilateral osteoarthritis of the knee. Am J Epidemiol 1989;130: 278–88.
94. Tepper S, Hochberg MC. Factors associated with hip osteoarthritis: data from the First National Health and Nutrition Examination Survey (NHANES-I). Am J Epidemiol 1993;137:1081–8.
95. Raveendran R, Stiller JL, Alvarez C, et al. Population-based prevalence of multiple radiographically-defined hip morphologies: the Johnston County Osteoarthritis Project. Osteoarthritis Cartilage 2018;26(1):54–61.
96. Nelson AE, Stiller JL, Shi XA, et al. Measures of hip morphology are related to development of worsening radiographic hip osteoarthritis over 6 to 13 year follow-up: the Johnston County Osteoarthritis Project. Osteoarthritis Cartilage 2016;24:443e450.
97. Delanois RE, Mistry JB, Gwam CU, et al. Current epidemiology of revision total knee arthroplasty in the United States. J Arthroplasty 2017;32:2663–8.
98. Anderson JJ, Felson DT. Factors associated with osteoarthritis of the knee in the first national Health and Nutrition Examination Survey (HANES I). Evidence for an association with overweight, race, and physical demands of work. Am J Epidemiol 1988;128:179–89.
99. Dembe AE, Yao X, Wickizer TM. Using O*NET to estimate the association between work exposures and chronic diseases. Am J Ind Med 2014;57:1022–31.
100. Gordon T. Osteoarthrosis in US Adults. In: Bennett PH, Wood PHN, editors. Population studies of the rheumatic diseases. International Congress Series No. 148. Amsterdam: Excerpta Medica Foundation; 1968. p. 391–7.
101. Dulay GS, Cooper C, Dennison EM. Knee pain, knee injury, knee osteoarthritis & work. Best Pract Res Clin Rheumatol 2015;29:454–61.
102. Ezzat AM, Cibere J, Koehoorn M, et al. Association between cumulative joint loading from occupational activities and knee osteoarthritis. Arthritis Care Res (Hoboken) 2013;65:1634–42.
103. Harris EC, Coggon D. Hip osteoarthritis and work. Best Pract Res Clin Rheumatol 2015;29:462–82.
104. Wagener DK. Bibliographies and data sources no. 2: occupation and health data guide. Hyattsville (MD): National Center for Health Statistics; 1993.

DHHS Publication No. [PHS) 93-130S; Available at: https://www.cdc.gov/nchs/data/misc/bds_02.pdf. Accessed November 1, 2017.

105. Engel A. Osteoarthritis and body measurements. Vital Health Stat 11 1968;29: 1–45.
106. Mark AE. Separate and combined influence of body mass index and waist circumference on arthritis and knee osteoarthritis. Int J Obes 2006;30:1223–8.
107. Potempa J, Mydel P, Koziel J. The case for periodontitis in the pathogenesis of rheumatoid arthritis. Nat Rev Rheumatol 2017;13:606–20.
108. de Pablo P, Dietrich T, McAlindon TE. Association of periodontal disease and tooth loss with rheumatoid arthritis in the US population. J Rheumatol 2008;35:70–6.
109. Dye BA, Herrera-Abreu M, Lerche-Sehm J, et al. Serum antibodies to periodontal bacteria as diagnostic markers of periodontitis. J Periodontol 2009;80: 634–47.
110. Goh CE, Kopp J, Papapanou PN, et al. Association between serum antibodies to periodontal bacteria and rheumatoid factor in NHANES III. Arthritis Rheumatol 2016;68:2384–93.
111. Schwartz J. Air pollution and blood markers of cardiovascular risk. Environ Health Perspect 2001;109(Suppl 3):405–9.
112. Schwartz J. Lung function and chronic exposure to air pollution: a cross-sectional analysis of NHANES II. Environ Res 1989;50:309–21.
113. Cox CS, Rothwell ST, Madans JH, et al. Plan and operation of the NHANES I Epidemiologic Follow-Up Study, 1987. Vital Health Stat 1 1992;(27):1–190.
114. Cox CS, Mussolino ME, Rothwell ST, et al. Plan and operation of the NHANES I Epidemiologic Follow-Up Study, 1992. Vital Health Stat 1 1997;(35):1–231.
115. Bruce B, Fries JF. The Stanford Health Assessment Questionnaire: a review of its history, issues, progress, and documentation. J Rheumatol 2003;30:167–78.
116. Cornoni-Huntley J, Barbano HE, Brody JA, et al. National Health and Nutrition Examination I-epidemiologic follow-up survey. Public Health Rep 1983;8: 245–51.
117. Cornoni-Huntley JC, Huntley RR, Feldman JJ, editors. Health status and well-being of the elderly: National Health and Nutrition Examination Survey - I epidemiologic follow-up study. 1st Edition. Oxford (United Kingdom): Oxford University Press; 1990. p. 320.
118. Cohen BB, Barbano HE, Cox CS, et al. Plan and operation of the NHANES I Epidemiologic Follow-Up Study: 1982–84. Vital Health Stat 1 1987;(22):1–142.
119. Finucane FF, Freid VM, Madans JH, et al. Plan and operation of the NHANES I Epidemiologic Follow-Up Study, 1986. Vital Health Stat 1 1990;(25):1–154.
120. US National Center for Health Statistics. NCHS Research Data Center. Available at: https://www.cdc.gov/rdc/index.htm. Accessed October 21, 2017.
121. Ingram DD. Statistical issues in analyzing the NHANES I Epidemiologic Follow-Up Study. Vital Health Stat 2 1994;121:1–30.
122. Hochberg MC, Lawrence RC, Everett DF, et al. Epidemiologic associations of pain in osteoarthritis of the knee: data from the National Health and Nutrition Examination Survey and the National Health and Nutrition Examination-I Epidemiologic Follow-up Survey. Semin Arthritis Rheum 1989;18(4 Suppl 2):4–9.
123. Davis MA, Ettinger WH, Neuhaus JM, et al. Knee osteoarthritis and physical functioning: evidence from the NHANES I Epidemiologic Follow-Up Study. J Rheumatol 1991;18:591–8.

124. Ettinger WH, Davis MA, Neuhaus JM, et al. Long-term physical functioning in persons with knee osteoarthritis from NHANES. I: effects of comorbid medical conditions. J Clin Epidemiol 1994;47:809–15.
125. Leigh JP, Fries JF. Arthritis and mortality in the epidemiological follow-up to the National Health and Nutrition Examination Survey I. Bull N Y Acad Med 1994;71: 69–86.
126. Looker AC, Harris TB, Madans JH, et al. Dietary calcium and hip fracture risk: the NHANES I Epidemiologic Follow-Up Study. Osteoporos Int 1993;3:177–84.
127. Mussolino ME, Looker AC, Madans JH, et al. Risk factors for hip fracture in white men: the NHANES I Epidemiologic Follow-Up Study. J Bone Miner Res 1998;13: 918–24.
128. Langlois JA, Mussolino ME, Visser M, et al. Weight loss from maximum body weight among middle-aged and older white women and the risk of hip fracture: the NHANES I Epidemiologic Follow-Up Study. Osteoporos Int 2001;12(9): 763–8.
129. Launer LJ, Harris T, Rumpel C, et al. Body mass index, weight change, and risk of mobility disability in middle-aged and older women, the epidemiologic follow-up study of NHANES I. JAMA 1994;271:1093–8.
130. Idler EL, Russell LB, Davis D. Survival, functional limitations, and self-rated health in the NHANES I Epidemiologic Follow-Up Study, 1992. First National Health and Nutrition Examination Survey. Am J Epidemiol 2000;152:874–83.
131. Hubert HB, Bloch DA, Fries JF. Risk factors for physical disability in an aging cohort: the NHANES I Epidemiologic Follow-Up Study. J Rheumatol 1993; 20(3):480–8.
132. National Center for Health Statistics. NCHS Data Linked to NDI Mortality Files. Available at: https://www.cdc.gov/nchs/data-linkage/mortality.htm. Accessed November 14, 2017.
133. National Center for Health Statistics. Research Data Center. Available at: https://www.cdc.gov/rdc/. Accessed November 14, 2017.
134. Golden C, Driscoll AK, Simon AE, et al. Linkage of NCHS population health surveys to administrative records from Social Security Administration and Centers for Medicare & Medicaid Services. Vital Health Stat 1 2015;58:1–53.
135. Lloyd PC, Helms VE, Simon AE, et al. Linkage of 1999–2012 National Health Interview Survey and National Health and Nutrition Examination Survey data to U.S. Department of Housing and Urban Development administrative records. Vital Health Stat 1 2017;(60):1–40.
136. Kravets N, Parker JD. Linkage of the third National Health and Nutrition Examination Survey to air quality data. Vital Health Stat 2 2008;(149):1–16.
137. Parker JD, Kravets N, Nachman K, et al. Linkage of the 1999-2008 National Health and Nutrition Examination Surveys to traffic indicators from the National Highway Planning Network. Natl Health Stat Rep 2012;45:1–16.
138. Chen JC, Schwartz J. Neurobehavioral effects of ambient air pollution on cognitive performance in US adults. Neurotoxicology 2009;30:231–9.
139. Bryant J, Meng Q, Davis JA, et al. A multi-level model of blood lead as a function of air lead. Sci Total Environ 2013;416-462:207–13.
140. Ahluwalia N, Dwyer J, Terry A, et al. Update on NHANES dietary data: focus on collection, release, analytical considerations, and uses to inform public policy. Adv Nutr 2016;7:121–34.
141. National Center for Environmental Health, Division of Laboratory Sciences, CDC, 2nd National Report on Biochemical Indicators of Diet and Nutrition in

the U.S. Population, 2012. Available at: https://www.cdc.gov/nutritionreport/pdf/Nutrition_Book_complete508_final.pdf. Accessed October 26, 2017.

142. Center for Disease Control and Prevention. National Report on Human Exposure to Environmental Chemicals. 2017. Available at: https://www.cdc.gov/exposurereport/index.html. Accessed November 14, 2017.
143. Koru-Sengul T, Clark JD, Ocasio MA, et al. Utilization of the National Health and Nutrition Examination (NHANES) survey for symptoms, tests, and diagnosis of chronic respiratory diseases and assessment of second hand smoke exposure. Epidemiology (Sunnyvale) 2011;1(2). https://doi.org/10.4172/2161-1165.1000104.
144. Whittaker-Brown SA, Liu B, Taioli E. The Relationship between Tobacco Smoke Exposure and Airflow obstruction in US Children-Analysis of the National Health and Nutrition Examination Survey (2007-2012). Chest 2017 [pii:S0012-3692(17) 32893-3]. Epub ahead of print.
145. Kurd KS, Gelfand JM. The prevalence of previously diagnosed and undiagnosed psoriasis in US adults: results from NHANES 2003-2004. J Am Acad Dermatol 2009;60:218–24.
146. National Health and Nutrition Examination Survey. New proposal guidelines. Available at: https://www.cdc.gov/nchs/nhanes/proposal_guidelines.htm. Accessed November 14, 2017.
147. National Health and Nutrition Examination Survey. 3A. Second Exam Files for Dietary Recall, Examination, Laboratory, Additional Laboratory Analytes (July 1999). Available at: https://wwwn.cdc.gov/nchs/nhanes3/datafiles.aspx#core. Accessed November 14, 2017.
148. National Health and Nutrition Examination Survey. Lead-Dust. Available at: https://wwwn.cdc.gov/Nchs/Nhanes/1999-2000/LAB20.htm. Accessed November 14, 2017.
149. National Health and Nutrition Examination Survey. Volatile Organic Compounds-Water and Related Questionnaire Items. Available at: https://wwwn.cdc.gov/Nchs/Nhanes/2007-2008/VOC_E.htm. Accessed November 14, 2017.
150. National Health and Nutrition Examination Survey. Allergens- Household Dust Available at: https://wwwn.cdc.gov/Nchs/Nhanes/2005-2006/ALDUST_D.htm. Accessed November 14, 2017.
151. Jackson SL, Cogswell ME, Zhao L, et al. Association between urinary sodium and potassium excretion and blood pressure among adults in the United States: National Health and Nutrition Examination Survey, 2014. Circulation 2017. https://doi.org/10.1161/CirculationAHA.117.029193.
152. National Health and Nutrition Examination Survey. Physical activity and cardiovascular fitness tutorial. Available at: https://www.cdc.gov/nchs/tutorials/PhysicalActivity/index.htm. Accessed November 14, 2017.
153. US National Center for Health Statistics. National Health and Nutrition Examination Survey. Historical summary of component content over time: NHANES I (1971-75) through NHANES 2005-06. Available at: https://www.cdc.gov/nchs/data/nhanes/Historical_NHANES_component_matrix.pdf. Accessed October 26, 2017.
154. National Health and Nutrition Examination Survey 1999–2016 Survey Content Brochure. Available at: https://wwwn.cdc.gov/nchs/data/nhanes/survey_contents.pdf. Accessed November 1, 2017.
155. George MD, McGill NK, Baker JF. Creatine kinase in the U.S. population, impact of demographics, comorbidities, and body composition on the normal range. Medicine 2016;95(33):e4344.

156. Hollowell JG, Staehling NW, Flanders WD, et al. Serum TSH, T4, and thyroid antibodies in the United States population (1988 to 1994): National Health and Nutrition Examination Survey (NHANES III). J Clin Endocrinol Metab 2002;87: 489–99.
157. Satoh M, Chan EKL, Ho LA, et al. Prevalence and sociodemographic correlates of antinuclear antibodies in the United States. Arthritis Rheum 2012;64:2319–27.
158. Rubio-Tapia A, Ludvigsson JF, Brantner TL, et al. The prevalence of celiac disease in the United States. Am J Gastroenterol 2012;107:1538–44.
159. Barinas-Mitchell EB, Pietropaolo S, Zhang YJ, et al. Islet cell autoimmunity in a triethnic adult population of the third National Health and Nutrition Examination Survey. Diabetes 2004;53:1293–302.
160. McQuillan GM, McLean JE, Chiappa M, et al. National Health and Nutrition Examination Survey Biospecimen program: NHANES III (1988–1994) and NHANES 1999–2014. Vital Health Stat 2 2015;(170):1–14.
161. National Center for Health Statistics. NHANES genetic data. Hyattsville, MD. 2011. Available from: http://www.cdc.gov/nchs/nhanes/genetics/genetic.htm. Accessed November 12, 2017.
162. National Health and Nutrition Examination Survey. 1988-2014 data documentation: prescription medications-drug information (RXQ_DRUG). Available at: https://wwwn.cdc.gov/Nchs/Nhanes/1999-2000/RXQ_DRUG.htm. Accessed November 15, 2017.
163. Gu Q, Dillon CF, Burt VL. Prescription drug use continues to increase: U.S. prescription drug data for 2007-2008. NCHS Data Brief 2010;42:1–8.
164. Overman RA, Yeh UY, Deal CL. Prevalence of oral glucocorticoid usage in the United States: a general population perspective. Arthritis Care Res (Hoboken) 2013;65:294–8.
165. Choi HK, Seeger JD. Glucocorticoid use and serum lipid levels in US adults: the third National Health and Nutrition Examination Survey. Arthritis Rheum 2005;53: 528–35.
166. Dillon CF, Paulose-Ram R, Hirsch R, et al. Skeletal muscle relaxant use in the united states: data from the third National Health and Nutrition Examination Survey (NHANES III). Spine 2004;29:892–6.
167. Buettner C, Davis RB, Leveille SG, et al. Prevalence of musculoskeletal pain and statin use. J Gen Intern Med 2008;23:1182–6.
168. Buettner C, Rippberger MJ, Smith JK, et al. Statin use and musculoskeletal pain among adults with and without arthritis. Am J Med 2012;125:176–82.
169. Ervin RB, Wright JD, Kennedy-Stephenson J. Use of dietary supplements in the United States, 1988–94. Vital Health Stat 11 1999;244:1–20.
170. Kantor ED, Rehm CD, Mengmeng M, et al. Trends in dietary supplement use among US adults from 1999-2012. JAMA 2016;316:1464–74.
171. Gu Q, Dillon CF, Eberhardt MS, et al. Preventive aspirin and other antiplatelet medication use among U.S. Adults aged ≥40 years: data from the National Health and Nutrition Examination Survey, 2011-2012. Public Health Rep 2015; 130:643–54.
172. Farina EK, Austin GK, Lieberman HR. Concomitant dietary supplement and prescription medication use is prevalent among us adults with doctor-informed medical conditions. J Acad Nutr Diet 2014;114:1784–90.
173. Wilson PB. Dietary supplementation is more prevalent among adults with arthritis in the United States population. Complement Ther Med 2016;29:152–7.
174. Paulose R, Hirsch R, Dillon C, et al. Prescription and non-prescription analgesic use among the U.S. adult population: results from the Third National

Health & Nutrition Examination Survey (NHANES III). Pharmacoepidemiol Drug Saf 2003;12:315–26.
175. Paulose-Ram R, Hirsch R, Dillon C, et al. Frequent monthly use of selected non-prescription and prescription non-narcotic analgesics among U.S. adults. Pharmacoepidemiol Drug Saf 2005;14:257–66.
176. Agodoa LY, Francis ME, Eggers PW. Association of analgesic use with prevalence of albuminuria and reduced GFR in US adults. Am J Kidney Dis 2008; 51:573–83.
177. Plantinga L, Grubbs V, Sarkar U, et al. Nonsteroidal anti-inflammatory drug use among persons with chronic kidney disease in the United States. Ann Fam Med 2011;9:423–30.
178. National Health and Nutrition Examination Survey. NHANES III, 1A. Interview and Exam Components (July 1997). Household adult file. Available at: https://wwwn.cdc.gov/nchs/nhanes3/datafiles.aspx#core. Accessed November 15, 2017.
179. National Health and Nutrition Examination Survey. Physical activity (PAQ). Available at: https://wwwn.cdc.gov/Nchs/Nhanes/1999-2000/PAQ.htm. Accessed November 15, 2017.
180. Wang CY, Haskell WL, Farrell SW, et al. Cardiorespiratory fitness levels among US adults 20-49 years of age: findings from the 1999-2004 National Health and Nutrition Examination Survey. Am J Epidemiol 2010;171:426–35.
181. National Health and Nutrition Examination Survey. NHANES physical activity and cardiovascular fitness tutorial. Available at: https://www.cdc.gov/nchs/tutorials/PhysicalActivity/index.htmhttps://wwwn.cdc.gov/nchs/nhanes/search/nnyfs12.aspx. Accessed November 15, 2017.
182. Smuck M, Tomkins-Lane C, Ith MA. Physical performance analysis: a new approach to assessing free-living physical activity in musculoskeletal pain and mobility-limited populations. PLoS One 2017;12(2):e0172804.
183. National Center for Health Statistics. Plan and operation of a health examination survey of U.S. Youths 12-17 years of age. Vital Health Stat 1 1969;8:1–86.
184. National Health and Nutrition Examination Survey. NNYFS 2012. Available at: https://wwwn.cdc.gov/nchs/nhanes/search/nnyfs12.aspx. Accessed November 15, 2017.
185. National Health and Nutrition Examination Survey. Physical Functioning (PFQ). Available at: https://wwwn.cdc.gov/Nchs/Nhanes/1999-2000/PFQ.htm. Accessed November 15, 2017.
186. National Health and Nutrition Examination Survey. Social Support (SSQ.) Available at: https://wwwn.cdc.gov/Nchs/Nhanes/1999-2000/SSQ.htm. Accessed November 15, 2017.
187. Fleisch MA, Illescas AH, Hohl BC, et al. Relationships between social isolation, neighborhood poverty, and cancer mortality in a population-based study of US adults. PLoS One 2017;12(3):e0173370.
188. Watt RG, Heilmann A, Sabbah W, et al. Social relationships and health related behaviors among older US adults. BMC Public Health 2014;14:533.
189. National Health and Nutrition Examination Survey. NHANES III, 1A. Interview and exam components (July 1997). Examination file. Available at: https://wwwn.cdc.gov/nchs/nhanes3/datafiles.aspx#core. Accessed November 15, 2017.
190. Ostchega Y, Dillon CF, Lindle R, et al. Isokinetic leg muscle strength in older Americans and its relationship to a standardized walk test: data from the national health and nutrition examination survey 1999-2000. J Am Geriatr Soc 2004;52:977–82.

191. Kalyani RR, Tra Y, Yeh HC, et al. Quadriceps strength, quadriceps power, and gait speed in older U.S. adults with diabetes mellitus: results from the National Health and Nutrition Examination Survey, 1999-2002. J Am Geriatr Soc 2013;61: 769–75.
192. Loenneke JP, Loprinzi PD. Statin use may reduce lower extremity peak force via reduced engagement in muscle-strengthening activities. Clin Physiol Funct Imaging 2018;38(1):151–4.
193. Ostchega Y, Porter KS, Hughes J, et al. Resting pulse rate reference data for children, adolescents, and adults: United States, 1999-2008. Natl Health Stat Rep 2011;41:1–16.
194. Drizd T, Dannenberg AL, Engel A. Blood pressure levels in persons 18–74 years of age in 1976-80, and trends in blood pressure from 1960 to 1980 in the United States. Vital Health Stat 11 1986;(234):1–76.
195. Hoffman HJ, Dobie RA, Ko CW, et al. Americans hear as well or better today compared with 40 years ago: hearing threshold levels in the unscreened adult population of the United States, 1959–1962 and 1999–2004. Ear Hearing 2010;31:725–34.
196. Kuczmarski RJ, Ogden CL, Guo SS, et al. 2000 CDC growth charts for the United States: methods and development. Vital Health Stat 11 2002;(246): 1–201.
197. Fryar CD, Gu Q, Ogden CL. Anthropometric reference data for children and adults: United States, 2007–2010. National Center for Health Statistics. Vital Health Stat 11 2012;252:1–48.
198. Hankinson JL, Odencrantz JR, Fedan KB. Spirometric reference values from a sample of the general U.S. population. Am J Respir Crit Care Med 1999;159: 179–87.
199. Looker AC, Wahner HW, Dunn WL, et al. Updated data on proximal femur bone mineral levels of US adults. Osteoporos Int 1998;8:468–89.
200. Kanis JA, McCloskey EV, Johansson H, et al. A reference standard for the description of osteoporosis. Bone 2008;42:467–75.
201. Long LR, Antani S, Lee DJ, et al. Biomedical information from a National Collection of Spine X-Rays: film to content-based retrieval. Proc of SPIE Medical Imaging: PACS and Integrated Medical Information Syst 2003;5033:70–84. Available at: https://lhncbc.nlm.nih.gov/files/archive/pub2003010.pdf. Accessed November 1, 2017.
202. Hsu W, Sameer Antani S, Long RL, et al. SPIRS: a web-based image retrieval system for large biomedical databases. Int J Med Inform 2009;8(Suppl 1): S13–24.
203. Gururajana A, Kamalakannana S, Sari-Sarrafa H, et al. On the creation of a segmentation library for digitized cervical and lumbar spine radiographs. Comput Med Imaging Graph 2011;35:251–65.
204. Qian X, Tagare HD, Fulbright RK, et al. Optimal embedding for shape indexing in medical image databases. Med Image Anal 2010;14:243–54.
205. Ostchega Y, Harris TB, Hirsch R, et al. Reliability and prevalence of physical performance examination assessing mobility from the National Health and Nutrition Examination Survey III. J Am Geriatr Soc 2000;48:1132–5.
206. Cook CE, Richardson JK, Pietrobon R. Dimensionality, internal consistency, and item analysis of the national health and nutrition examination surveys activities of daily living instrument among patients with report of low back pain. J Manipulative Physiol Ther 2006;29:183–9.

207. Cook CE, Richardson JK, Pietrobon R, et al. Validation of the NHANES ADL scale in a sample of patients with report of cervical pain: factor analysis, item response theory analysis, and line item validity. Disabil Rehabil 2006;28:929–35.
208. US National Health and Nutrition Examination Survey. Questionnaires, Datasets, and Related Documentation. Available at: https://www.cdc.gov/nchs/nhanes/nhanes_questionnaires.htm. Accessed November 1, 2017.
209. US National Health and Nutrition Examination Survey. NHANES Web Tutorials. Available at: https://www.cdc.gov/nchs/tutorials/Nhanes/index.htm. Accessed November 1, 2017.
210. US National Center for Health Statistics. Current Publications. Available at: https://www.cdc.gov/nchs/products/index.htm. Accessed November 14, 2017.
211. Curtin LR, Mohadjer LK, Dohrmann SM, et al. National health and nutrition examination survey: sample design, 2007–2010. Vital Health Stat 2 2013;160:1–23.
212. Lohr SL. Sampling: design and analysis. Boston: Duxbury Press; 1999. p. 266–8.
213. National Center for Health Statistics. Surveys and data collection systems. Available at: https://www.cdc.gov/nchs/surveys.htm. Accessed November 14, 2017.
214. US National Health and Nutrition Examination Survey. Survey Methods and Analytic Guidelines. Available at: https://wwwn.cdc.gov/Nchs/Nhanes/AnalyticGuidelines.aspx. Accessed November 14, 2017.
215. Curtin LR, Kruszon-Moran D, Carroll M, et al. (2006), Estimation and analytic issues for rare events in NHANES, proceedings of the survey research methods section. ASA; 2006. p. 2893–903. Available at: https://www.researchgate.net/profile/Margaret_Carroll2/publication/253720335_Estimation_and_Analytic_Issues_for_Rare_Events_in_NHANES/links/0c960529f2813e6bb5000000.pdf?disableCoverPage=true&inViewer=true&origin=publication_detail&pdfJsDownload=true. Accessed November 1, 2017.
216. Burt CW, Hing E. Making patient-level estimates from medical encounter records using a multiplicity estimator. Statist Med 2007;26:1762–74.
217. Sacks JJ, Helmick CG, Luo YH. Prevalence of and annual ambulatory health care visits for pediatric arthritis and other rheumatologic conditions in the United States in 2001–2004. Arthritis Rheum 2007;57:1439–45.
218. US Centers for Disease Control and Prevention. NHANES analytic guidelines, the third national health and nutrition examination survey, NHANES III (1988–94). Hyattsville (MD): National Center for Health Statistics; 1996 [cited 2011]. Available at: http://www.cdc.gov/nchs/data/nhanes/nhanes3/nh3gui.pdf. Accessed October 26, 2017.
219. Parker JD, Talih M, Malec DJ, et al. National Center for health statistics data presentation standards for proportions. Vital Health Stat 2 2017;175:1–22.
220. US National Health and Nutrition Examination Survey. Continuous NHANES web tutorial: variance estimation. Available at: http://www.cdc.gov/nchs/tutorials/nhanes/SurveyDesign/VarianceEstimation/intro.htm. Accessed November 1, 2017.
221. Helmick CG, Lawrence RC, Pollard RA, et al. Arthritis and other rheumatic conditions: who is affected now, who will be affected later? National Arthritis Data Workgroup. Arthritis Care Res 1995;8:203–11.
222. Murphy LB, Cisternas MG, Greenlund KJ, et al. Defining arthritis for public health surveillance: methods and estimates in four US population health surveys. Arthritis Care Res (Hoboken) 2017;69:356–67.

223. Centers for Disease Control and Prevention (CDC). Monitoring progress in arthritis management-United States and 25 states, 2003. MMWR Morb Mortal Wkly Rep 2005;54:484–8.
224. Centers for Disease Control and Prevention (CDC). Adults who have never seen a health-care provider for chronic joint symptoms-United States, 2001. MMWR Morb Mortal Wkly Rep 2003;52:416–9.
225. Balamuth E, Shapiro S. Health interview responses compared with medical records. Vital Health Stat 2 1965;7:1–81.
226. Madow WG. Interview data on chronic conditions compared with information derived from medical records. Vital Health Stat 2 1967;(23):1–84.
227. Madow WG. Net differences in interview data on chronic conditions and information derived from medical records. Vital Health Stat 2 1973;57:1–58.
228. Edwards WS, Winn DM, Kurlantzick V, et al. National Center for Health Statistics. Evaluation of National Health Interview Survey diagnostic reporting. Vital Health Stat 2 1994;120:1–116.
229. Schenker N, Raghunathanb TE, Bondarenkoc I. Improving on analyses of self-reported data in a large-scale health survey by using information from an examination-based survey. Statist Med 2010;29:533–45.
230. Stommel M, Schoenborn CA. Accuracy and usefulness of BMI measures based on self- reported weight and height: findings from the NHANES & NHIS 2001-2006. BMC Public Health 2009;9:421.
231. Lazo M, Hernaez R, Eberhardt MS, et al. Prevalence of nonalcoholic fatty liver disease in the United States: the Third National Health and Nutrition Examination Survey, 1988-1994. Am J Epidemiol 2013;178:38–45.
232. Hernaez R, McLean J, Lazo M, et al. Association between variants in or near PNPLA3, GCKR, and PPP1R3B with ultrasound-defined steatosis based on data from the third National Health and Nutrition Examination Survey. Clin Gastroenterol Hepatol 2013;11:1183–90.e2.
233. Simard JF, Mittleman MA. Prevalent rheumatoid arthritis and diabetes among NHANES III participants aged 60 and older. J Rheumatol 2007;34:469–73.
234. Demmer RT, Molitor JA, Jacobs DR Jr, et al. Periodontal disease, tooth loss and incident rheumatoid arthritis: results from the First National Health and Nutrition Examination Survey and its epidemiological follow-up study. J Clin Periodontol 2011;38:998–1006.
235. Sparks JA, Karlson EW. The Roles of Cigarette Smoking and the Lung in the Transitions between Phases of Preclinical Rheumatoid Arthritis. Curr Rheumatol Rep 2016;18(3):15.
236. del Puente A, Knowler WC, Pettitt DJ, et al. The incidence of rheumatoid arthritis is predicted by rheumatoid factor titer in a longitudinal population study. Arthritis Rheum 1988;31:1239–44.
237. Nielsen SF, Bojesen SE, Schnohr P, et al. Elevated rheumatoid factor and long term risk of rheumatoid arthritis: a prospective cohort study. BMJ 2012;345:e5244.
238. Landgren O, Graubard BI, Kumar S, et al. Prevalence of myeloma precursor state monoclonal gammopathy of undetermined significance in 12372 individuals 10-49 years old: a population-based study from the National Health and Nutrition Examination Survey. Blood Cancer J 2017;7:e618.
239. Hannan MT, Felson DT, Pincus T. Analysis of the discordance between radiographic changes and knee pain in osteoarthritis of the knee. J Rheumatol 2000;27(6):1513–7.

240. Bedson J, Croft PR. The discordance between clinical and radiographic knee osteoarthritis: a systematic search and summary of the literature. BMC Musculoskelet Disord 2008;9:116.
241. Lo GH, McAlindon TE, Hawker GA, et al. Symptom assessment in knee osteoarthritis needs to account for physical activity level. Arthritis Rheumatol 2015; 67:2897–904.
242. Verbrugge LM, Rennert C, Madans JH. The great efficacy of personal and equipment assistance in reducing disability. Am J Public Health 1997;87: 384–92.
243. Turczyn KM, Drury TF. An inventory of pain data available from the national center for health statistics. Vital Health Stat 1 1992;26:1–75.
244. Hochberg MC, Borenstein DG, Arnett FC. The absence of back pain in classical ankylosing spondylitis. Johns Hopkins Med J 1978;143:181–3.
245. Gladman DD. Psoriatic arthritis. Rheum Dis Clin North Am 1998;24:829–44.
246. Bandinelli F, Manetti M, Ibba-Manneschi L. Occult spondyloarthritis in inflammatory bowel disease. Clin Rheumatol 2016;35:281–9.
247. Queiro R, Maiz O, Intxausti J, et al. Subclinical sacroiliitis in inflammatory bowel disease: a clinical and follow up study. Clin Rheumatol 2000;19:445–9.
248. Jennings F, Lambert E, Fredericson M. Rheumatic diseases presenting as sports-related injuries. Sports Med 2008;38:917–30.
249. Kobak S, Sever F, Ince O, et al. The prevalence of sacroiliitis and spondyloarthritis in patients with sarcoidosis. Int J Rheumatol 2014;2014:289454.
250. Colmenero JD, Ruiz-Mesa JD, Sanjuan-Jimenez R, et al. Establishing the diagnosis of tuberculous vertebral osteomyelitis. Eur Spine J 2013;22(Suppl 4): 579–86.
251. Ishizaka N, Sohmiya K, Miyamura M, et al. Infected aortic aneurysm and inflammatory aortic aneurysm-in search of an optimal differential diagnosis. J Cardiol 2012;59:123–31.
252. Antonelli MJ, Magrey M. Sacroiliitis mimics: a case report and review of the literature. BMC Musculoskelet Disord 2017;18:170.
253. Pehlivan Y, Kisacik B, Sayiner ZA, et al. Inflammatory back pain in patients treated with isotretinoin. J Rheumatol 2011;38:2690.
254. Schliep KC, Mumford SL, Peterson CM, et al. Pain typology and incident endometriosis. Hum Reprod 2015;30:2427–38.
255. Holton KF, Denard PJ, Yoo JU, et al. Diffuse idiopathic skeletal hyperostosis (DISH) and its relation to back pain among older men: the MrOS study. Semin Arthritis Rheum 2011;41:131–8.
256. Kuperus JS, de Gendt EEA, Oner FC, et al. Classification criteria for diffuse idiopathic skeletal hyperostosis: a lack of consensus. Rheumatology (Oxford) 2017; 56:1123–34.
257. Hassoon A, Bydon M, Kerezoudis P, et al. Chronic low-back pain in adults with diabetes: NHANES 2009-2010. J Diabetes Complications 2017;31:38–42.
258. Raastad J, Reiman M, Coeytaux R, et al. The association between lumbar spine radiographic features and low back pain: a systematic review and meta-analysis. Semin Arthritis Rheum 2015;44:571–85.
259. Bacon RM, Kugeler KJ, Mead P. Surveillance for Lyme disease–United States, 1992-2006. MMWR Surveill Summ 2008;57:1–9.

Qualitative Methods to Advance Care, Diagnosis, and Therapy in Rheumatic Diseases

Lesley Ann Saketkoo, MD, MPH[a,b,c,*],
John D. Pauling, BMedSci, BMBS, PhD, FRCP[d,e]

KEYWORDS

- Qualitative • Focus group • Interview • Patient perspective • Phenomenology
- Coding • Ethnography • Conceptual framework

KEY POINTS

- Qualitative research is an indispensable form of research vital information that impacts the biopsychosocial burden of chronic illness and in improved health care operations.
- Qualitative research is often used as a foundation or to complement more traditional quantitative research methods to augment knowledge of rheumatic diseases.
- Qualitative research, although inherently subjective, is a robust process that can be evaluated and held to a high standard of quality.

Not everything that can be counted counts, and not everything that counts can be counted.

—William Bruce Cameron, Professor of Sociology, 1963

INTRODUCTION

The last 2 centuries of medical research advancements were driven by the systematic collection of measurable assessments relying on quantifiable constructs and

---

Disclosure Statement: Neither author has any conflicts of interest to disclose relevant to the contents of this article.

[a] Division of Pulmonary Medicine and Critical Care, Tulane University School of Medicine, Lung Center, 1430 Tulane Avenue, New Orleans, LA 70112, USA; [b] New Orleans Scleroderma and Sarcoidosis Patient Care and Research Center, New Orleans, LA 70112, USA; [c] University Medical Center, Comprehensive Pulmonary Hypertension Center, New Orleans, LA 70112, USA; [d] Royal National Hospital for Rheumatic Diseases, Royal United Hospitals, Upper Borough Walls, Bath BA1 1RL, UK; [e] Department of Pharmacy and Pharmacology, University of Bath, Bath BA11RL, UK
* Corresponding author. Division of Pulmonary Medicine and Critical Care, Tulane University School of Medicine, 1430 Tulane Avenue, New Orleans, LA 70130.
E-mail address: lsaketk@tulane.edu

Rheum Dis Clin N Am 44 (2018) 267–284
https://doi.org/10.1016/j.rdc.2018.01.004
rheumatic.theclinics.com

producing measurable variables within populations. Quantitative research has far progressed medical science, but tells us little about the opinions and experiences of living with disease that could provide actionable insight but are less amenable to quantification. Qualitative research, in contrast, provides valuable insight into patient experiences, attitudes, behavior, meaning, and thoughts, and broadens our understanding of human disease. Thus, in recent years, qualitative research has carved a bona fide position as valuable science in health care operations and understanding of disease (**Fig. 1**).[1,2] This position has been hard won for a science that inherently relies on subjectivity in both data collection and analysis, and, although it endeavors to be free of bias, will always be guided by investigator perception and sensitivity. Although recently less so, qualitative research still faces challenges in obtaining research funding and a difficulty publishing in high-impact journals persisting to some extent.[3]

This article reviews the underpinnings, usefulness, and validity of qualitative methods; punctuated with examples of how they have been applied in rheumatic disease research. To optimally define qualitative methodology, it is contrasted in this article with its counterpart, quantitative methodology, to which all readers have an acquaintanceship, hopefully making it easier to assimilate the less familiar ideas of qualitative research, revealing how these seemingly diverse schools are, in fact, interdependent, with high-quality research often using both approaches. This review is addressed to a broad spectrum of readers, ranging from those wishing to better appraise the burgeoning number of published qualitative studies to researchers considering the role qualitative methods might play in answering their own research questions. We hope to inspire serious interest—and perhaps dedicated careers—in applying these methods to deciphering a deeper understanding of the biopsychosocial burden of rheumatic disease and how qualitative research methods might support the development of incremental management strategies[4] to improve health-related quality of life, and perhaps even survival.[5]

WHAT IS QUALITATIVE RESEARCH?

Qualitative research explores the meaning attached to health-related experiences, cultures, views, opinions, and practices by individuals within their personal social

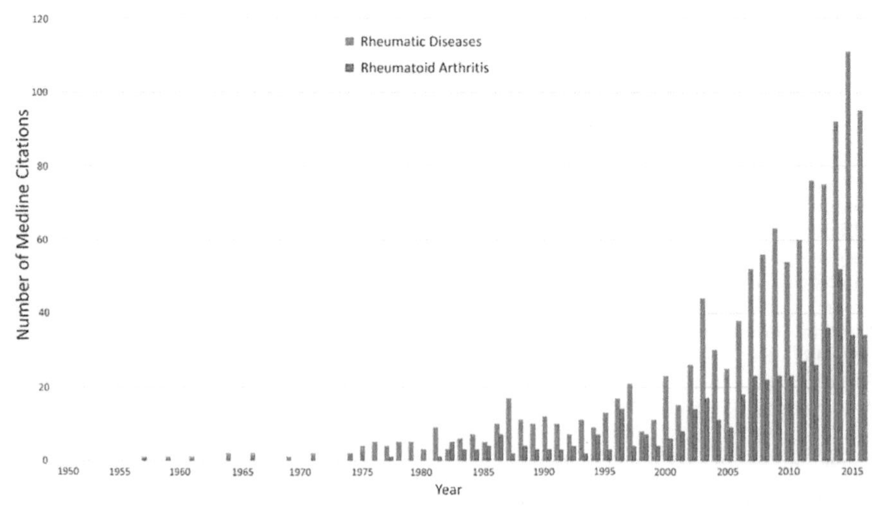

Fig. 1. Number of Medline citations identified for a search of qualitative research and rheumatic disease from 1950 to 2015.

and cultural context.[6] Although data are represented by words that reflect recorded speech and behavior (in contrast with the numerical quantity, distribution, magnitude, and frequency of quantitative research methods), qualitative methods are marked by careful, deliberate strategies of robust and systematic data collection, organization, and interpretation of these nonnumerical data. Where quantitative research predominantly examines the relationships between independent, dependent, and extraneous variables represented by numerical values, the corresponding qualitative analytical units are themes and concepts that arise through discussion, observation or document review. In contrast with quantitative research methods, the interactive nature of qualitative research enables investigators to actively participate in the quest for enhanced understanding (not necessarily definitive answers) and unexpected scientific lines of inquiry can emerge within the process of data acquisition[1] (**Table 1**).

Investigation typically takes the form of open-ended survey answers, field note observations, and/or anonymized transcripts obtained in focus group, or semistructured individual patient interviews[1] to form the descriptive raw data of the research from which the interpretation is derived.[7] Qualitative methods can be applied to any study of human interactions, patient experiences, communication, diagnostic evaluation, disease activity definitions, and health measurement scale development relevant to disease management[1] focusing directly on the health condition itself, or any other aspect of care, including technical or operational facets. Pharmaceutical companies routinely apply qualitative research methods to health care providers and patients for marketing purposes, and recently have been more involved in funding the development of patient-reported outcome measures for use in clinical trials within diseases of interest to them.

However, the main use of qualitative methods in health care is to evaluate and understand the perspectives of patients and health care providers as a means to heighten knowledge of disease processes, diagnostic evaluation, and management to improve health outcomes and health-related quality of life. In the rheumatic diseases these include physician and patient treatment decision making in rheumatoid arthritis (RA) and osteoarthritis,[8–10] prescribing practices for musculoskeletal pain,[11] family and relationships in RA,[12] parenting and arthritis,[13,14] experiences of juvenile idiopathic arthritis,[15] patient–health care provider interactions,[16–23] perceived health benefits of treatment/intervention,[24–26] adherence to the intervention,[26–29] as well as developing research priorities.[30] Increasingly, qualitative research has become more focused on specific disease manifestations that might only affect a minority of patients within a disease entity, for example, body image dissatisfaction in patients with cutaneous lupus,[31] or potentially common but hitherto neglected experiences of diseases, such as fatigue in osteoarthritis.[32] However, qualitative investigations are not limited to patient experiences and might include any person related to any part of the disease process or health care experience, depending on the question to be answered (**Box 1**). Subjects might, therefore, include family, friends, caregivers, clinicians, community health care providers, laboratory scientists, specialist nurses, rehabilitation specialists, trainees, and administrative staff. Qualitative research is an inquisitive process, capturing motivation/adherence, emotions, needs, perceptions, experience, or opinions in words, but otherwise follows a similar degree of robust and systematic data collection, organization, and interpretation.

WHEN TO CHOOSE QUALITATIVE METHODS

Quantitative methods have formed the mainstay of biomedical research and are generally applied when there is sufficient information to form a hypothesis that can

Table 1
Similarities and differences between qualitative and quantitative research methods

Concept	Quantitative	Qualitative
Goals	Generate comparisons and correlations of attributes	Investigate human perspectives
Level of investigation	Broad, impersonal	Deep, personal
Level of data detail	Concise, numerical summation	Richly, detailed description
Focus	Relationship of numerical values	Personal experience
Driver	To prove/predict a hypothesis	Discovery/exploration
Research question	Hypothesis statement often proving a single predicted outcome to measure descriptive, causal, or associative/relational occurrences or states resulted in units of magnitude, quantity or frequency	Exploratory question seeking new understanding of human experience in dynamic, yet unquantifiable and in specifically described situations and settings
Sample size	Large; focused on precise trends across large groups	Small; focused on collected case content
Sample recruitment	Random, representative, generalizable	Purposeful, not necessarily representative nor generalizable
Setting of data collection	Experimental; may occur in 'the field' with descriptive studies	Usually from where the participants are, that is, 'the field,' natural environment
Instruments	May be surveys with closed-ended questions May use equipment such as beakers, pipettes, serum testing etc	The interviewer or observer are the instruments with open-ended queries
Method types	Descriptive Correlative Causal Comparative Inferential	Historical analysis using archival data Phenomenology Ethnography/participant observation (direct or indirect) Action research
Data units/coding	Numerical whether nominal, ordinal, interval, or ratio data	Words/concepts
Analytical approach	Deductive: based on existing theories or established views	Inductive; allows data to emerge and guide the researcher and often takes researcher back to data collection phase to clarify/further explore a concept
Analysis	Statistical modeling to confirm accuracy and reproducibility	Interpretive and Identification of concepts and creation of themes
Design	Highly structured, experimental and quasiexperimental; design is fully committed before implementation	'Emergent,' that is, responsive to data collection and subject to change depending on initial findings

(continued on next page)

Table 1
(continued)

Concept	Quantitative	Qualitative
Design perspective	Objective, outcome oriented	Subjective, process oriented
Data sources	Variable, objective medical data, quantifiable subjective data reduced to data points	Interviews, observation, audio/visual clips or documents
Data collection platform	Spreadsheets or other formulaic templates	Recording transcriptions generating volumes of narrative
Data	Scalable Easy to understand/interpret Easy to generate comparisons	Not scalable Difficult to analyze and interpret Collect more than 1 type to get holistic, comprehensive understanding to answer 1 question
Success indicator	Predetermine/predict an outcome	Saturation of newly discovered concepts
Conclusion	Strongly formulated with generalizability	Tentative
Presentation of data	Often follows a formulaic statistical report that is central with some narrative describing background, arguments regarding relevance of results and conclusions drawn	Narrative, interpretative, often contains direct participant quotes or behavior descriptions, also with brief background and conclusion
Resource consumption	Variable, depending on source of data	Time/labor intensive
Data collection	Minimal, calculations often set as formulas run on computers	Time/labor intensive
Data analysis	Commonly formulaic, able to require minimal effort	Requires several people to evaluate the same data
Data reporting		Requires high level narrative and literary skills

Box 1
Applications and goals of qualitative research methods

Procurement of data sufficient to generate hypotheses for future quantitative investigation

Conceptual framework to characterize/facilitate understanding of a disease, issue, or area of concern/phenomena

Emergence of recurrent themes for actionable attention

Protocols, policy, educational materials

Classification system/taxonomy

Survey instruments to measure relevance, importance, intensity of qualitative concepts, for example, patient-reported outcome measures be tested using quantifiable comparative, associative, hierarchical, or interval-type assessments. Qualitative strategies might be used when there are insufficient data to form a stable hypothesis or quantitative assessment, and the attainment of more information might help to formulate one. Alternately, quantitative results might be available, but there is a need to understand the personal human relevance/motivation that drives the results. Both qualitative and quantitative research methods provide important tools that complement each other toward larger goals, with many research projects adopting a mixed methods approach for comprehensiveness.

The preferred methodology for any given project is determined by the goals of the overall research question (discussed elsewhere in this article). Increasingly, the dovetailing of qualitative with more traditional quantitative research methods in a complementary fashion has been proven to support broader research goals. An integrated mixed methods approach has become the mainstay of PROM development throughout medical and rheumatic disease research.[2,33] An example of innovative blending of qualitative and quantitative methods, is the McMaster Toronto Arthritis (MACTAR) patient preference questionnaire.[34] The MACTAR captures both qualitative and quantitative data on patient priorities of physical function by enabling patients to set and quantify their own health-related priorities. The MACTAR identified a number of domains relating to functional impairment in patients with systemic sclerosis (SSc) that are not captured in the Health Assessment Questionnaire-Disability Index, highlighting the importance of patient participation in outcome measure design, content development, and adoption.[35]

The incorporation of qualitative methods is particularly relevant to PROM development, where capturing the patient experience is paramount to the success of the instrument, leading to regulatory bodies such as the US Food and Drug Administration establishing that engaging the target patient population in PROM development should be used to support labeling claims and marketing authorization.[36,37] The importance of the patient voice has led to patient research partners coining the phrase, "Nothing about us, without us!"[38]

One of several examples of qualitative patient data influencing outcomes is the derivation of a minimal set of outcome measure for clinical trials in connective tissue disease-related interstitial lung disease.[39] The project sought qualitative perspectives from both experts and patients with their relationships to the emerged concepts that were examined and cross-examined subsequently with quantitative strategies to gauge their degree of importance. The qualitative input from patients altered the direction of the entire study and the final product; further, it drew physician experts' attention to the symptom of cough as central to the interstitial lung disease experience, inspiring further independent quantitative investigations on potential causes, therapeutic implications, and potential methods for capturing the severity and impact of cough in connective tissue disease-related interstitial lung disease.[39,40] The integration of quantitative and qualitative research studies can be challenging and less readily amenable to traditional metaanalytical approaches of aggregating data from multiple studies.[3,41,42] Nonetheless, applying mixed method approaches expands the boundaries of research enabling a more complete assessment of most aspects of human disease.[41] Examples of effective integration of applied methods are presented in **Box 2**.

APPROACHES TO QUALITATIVE RESEARCH METHODS

Qualitative research methods include a variety of techniques for systematically collecting, organizing, and interpreting human experiences captured through open

Box 2
Examples of mixed methods production motifs

1. Patient-reported outcome measures development
   Qualitative *focus group* data collection/analysis with isolation of concepts >> Quantitative testing of concepts for relevance/important in larger group >> Qualitative *focus group/ interview field testing* of best language >> Qualitative *action research* with patients to develop a set of questions >> Quantitative testing of questions using factor analysis, test–retest, etc
2. *Phenomenologic* experience of living with a rheumatic health condition:
   Qualitative *focus group* experience of living with *x* condition with analysis yielding *y* as prevalent interfering symptom >> Quantitative assessment of *y* as a reliable marker of disease activity in *x* in randomized, controlled clinical trial
3. *Phenomenologic* experience with *historical analysis* of published blogs of people living with a specific manifestation of an autoimmune health condition:
   Qualitative *focus groups* with analysis yielding unexpected pervasive self-management technique >> (a) *action research* working with patients to develop anticipatory guidance strategies for safety *and* (b) quantitative testing of self-management technique for efficacy
4. *Ethnography* combined with focus groups to learn barriers to health care access in a rural area:
   Qualitative *focus groups* with analysis of perceived power differences between health care providers and patients as a barrier >> recorded *observation of behavior* of patients and providers within health system identifying specific areas of concern >> qualitative *action research* with patient and providers to develop strategies that create equanimity in communication >> quantitative assessment of effectiveness of new strategies versus prior behavior

discussion and observation.[1] Phenomenology, the study of human experience, is the overarching concept of qualitative research and drives almost all methods of performing qualitative research in health care, typically using interviews and focus groups, and can unearth unexpected experiences considered important by patients, otherwise overlooked by clinicians. For example, focus groups in RA revealed that a recurrent and pervasive theme that arose in the focus group data was the symptom of fatigue. The strong emergence of this caused subsequent research to quantify the magnitude of intensity, frequency, and correlation of fatigue in RA resulting in the quantitative discovery of fatigue as a reliable indicator of RA disease activity.[43]

Ethnography is systematic study based on observation of people and has been more often used for cultural or social research cultures. It can take the form of direct observation by a nonparticipatory party or indirect by the researcher actually taking part in the natural setting in which the behavior is observed. There have been few ethnographic studies, but it is an application becoming more common, especially in combination with interview methods. One of the few studies in RA used ethnography to understand the barriers to arthritis care in a Mayan community.[44] This study observed both people with arthritis and health care providers of varying levels, revealing that the availability and attainability of access was further complicated by patient acceptability of the diminishing levels of quality of life that seemed to be related to indigenous versus nonindigenous power imbalances. The study concluded that accessibility strategies that are culturally sensitive and developed with Mayans are needed to increase Mayans accessing care.[18] Another ethnographic study investigated self-injection practices, yielding important insight to suboptimal injection practices identifying improvement areas for patient performance and health care team behavior.[44,45]

Action research may involve observation and/or interview techniques and sets out to develop a product (policy, educational materials, etc) by engaging the expertise of the participants to solve a problem. This approach has been applied successfully to developing a handbook by patients for patients with RA[46] and to developing goal roadmaps for the operational enhancement of scleroderma centers.[47]

Historical analysis is another application that examines often historical and usually published narrative data, such as newspapers and journals, for data relevant to answering a question in qualitative research. The expansion of digital blogs and forums could lead to an expansion of the use of this tool in chronic illnesses. The patient experience of disease can also be captured in nontextual form as exemplified by examination of the later works of Klee, Renoir, Hugué, and Gaudi, who each expressed their experiences of living with debilitating health and fear of mortality at the hands of autoimmune diseases.[48–50]

Regardless of the chosen strategy, qualitative methods are at best implemented or supervised by those who might have received dedicated academic training such as medical anthropologists, psychologists, and social workers, or someone recognized as being experienced in this field, the inclusion of which is often a quality indicator of the research. Because this multidisciplinary nature is an important quality indicator of the research, health care providers and lay people, such as patients, can be trained to implement the components of qualitative research such as information gathering and analytical methods. However, qualitative research demands the same level of respect and rigor as other scientific endeavors in medical research; in fact, it is arguably a more challenging task to crystalize the "true" voice when expressing both the common and disparate experiences of a group of subjects, whatever the context.

The Research Question

The careful construction of the research question is crucial to good yield of data and efficiency in both qualitative and quantitative research. A good question defines the goal of the data collection and frames the existing research gap while at the same time delineating the confines of the research scope (**Boxes 3–5**). An excellent question guides research design and choice of methodology, and supports project planning and assessing resources. Further, it serves to rein in the focus when the qualitative exploration reveals so many interesting and tempting distractors. Finally, a good research question facilitates the delivery of the published findings by framing the reportable content (publication) of the analysis and results.

The subject of the research question deserves considerable thought; focusing on the most essential stakeholders to answer the question or questions at hand. For

Box 3
Examples of general topics for qualitative research in health care

Understanding barriers/facilitators to accessing or learning something (eg, online patient portals, quality health care, obtaining appropriate therapy, improving physical function etc)

Motivation for behaviors (eg, patient medication adherence, provider prescribing practices, providing health education and counseling, etc)

Social, home, employment, or health care team dynamics (stress-related situations, communication, etc)

Beliefs, perceptions or priorities (eg, patient beliefs surrounding methotrexate use or vaccines, health care provider beliefs surrounding pain in osteoarthritis, patient priorities in health care provision, etc.)

Box 4
The anatomy of the qualitative research question

Inductive and incites exploration

Framed as a question (what, why, how) or an aim (infinitive verb, eg, 'to explain,' 'to identify,' etc)

Clear focus on singular and distinct phenomenon

Neutral language that is open

Stated subject of interest

Target patient population well-defined

Setting well-defined

certain research questions, the perspectives of very different stakeholders may be required to accurately and comprehensively address the issue. Further, sometimes a 360° perspective of all potential stakeholders is useful. This strategy is frequently used when developing disease specific Core Sets for the International Classification of Functioning, Health and Disability and developed on the converging insights of patients, family members, physicians, rehabilitation therapists, social workers, and psychologists, such as a mixed methods approach in ankylosing spondylitis to develop a quantifiable health index.[51]

Focus Groups and Interviews

Interviews and focus groups are the main, most commonly used methods of data collection in health care related phenomenological research. They provide rich detail of personal perspective in narrative data form; however, each method has different qualities and dynamics that generally yield different depths and expanses of insight. A combination of approaches, applied in an iterative fashion can support researchers seeking rich and varied data to answer a specific research question. For instance, a series of interviews might initially collect insights that can be further explored in a focus group, or the focus group might generate themes that require more in-depth probing in an interview format. The choice of strategy depends on the sensitivity of the subject, among other factors. Interviews and focus groups require a skill, sensitivity, and sensibility to conduct and typically comprise unstructured or semistructured interview

Box 5
Examples of qualitative research questions

To understand system-level and interpersonal factors of prolonged prednisone use and delay of disease-modifying antirheumatic drug optimization in young African American women with systemic lupus erythematosus.

To identify barriers to early diagnosis of systemic lupus erythematosus of Hispanic population in Milwaukee.

To characterize the daily life experience of systemic sclerosis patients living with calcinosis.

What are the most disabling aspects to patients diagnosed with rheumatoid arthritis in the first 3 years?

What are the expectations of scleroderma patients, patient families and scleroderma specialists in a scleroderma center of excellence?

techniques adhering to a planned topic or question guide (discussed elsewhere in this article). Important environmental considerations, especially for people with rheumatic diseases, must include ease of access to a venue and comfort with attention to room temperature, seating, availability of water, and proximity to lavatories, as well as knowing when participants are getting tired.

Focus groups induce narrative data through discussion of an issue or topic that is common to a group of people with shared experiences.[52,53] Focus groups facilitate discussion and debate among participants, clarifying convergent and divergent views expressed.[54] The group strategy helps to characterize common and divergent cultural and social experiences in health care, while simultaneously providing reassurance to group members by dispelling the sense that "nobody knows how I feel" in relation to the subject of interest. The group dynamics and interactions of a focus group can create a relaxed setting and also widen the range of response compared with individual interviews, because each member, in addition to sharing their own perspective, hears others' perspectives processing them against their own perspective. This comparison with other perspectives arising in the group ignites a deepening of participants' self-exploration and sharing.[53]

Group discussion also sparks recollection of details for participants that might have been forgotten or overlooked by the participant in an interview setting. Focus groups also provide an opportunity to capture language and phrasing that target populations adopt to describe experiences. The vocabulary and descriptive phrases can prove particularly valuable if goals include developing patient-reported outcome measures, patient education materials, or manuals for health care providers and others.[40,55] The size and composition of the group will influence the narrative. A group that is too large may impair the depth of expression or completion of communication, and some participants may not have a chance to speak at all. Other important considerations when assembling groups are factors that might interfere with comfortable and free expression, for example, hierarchical differences when examining barriers in the operational flow of clinic, or gender when examining sexual health. In these situations, separate focus groups should accommodate each member type (so-called strata).

Audio-recording with subsequent verbatim transcription of study data enables independent verification of the study findings.[3] The researcher or assistant should also take field notes to observe and document tone, emotionality, and physical behaviors that emphasize, clarify, seemingly contradict, or add to a participant's voiced perspective.

Purposive sampling techniques to ensure broad participation from within the target patient population can be applied to maximize the transferability (external validity) of the study interpretation and the specific patient populations to which they pertain.[3] In contrast with quantitative research methods, diversity within the study population can be a strength, because the findings are not necessarily meant to be transferable across large population groups.[3] A complete description of the study population (and the extent to which a priori purposive sampling framework was achieved), site and context provides clarity and context on the sample population to which the interpretations purport.[3]

Whether focus groups or individual interviews are adopted, an a priori purposive sampling framework can help to ensure a representative sample of patients with respect to clinical phenotype and demographics, while also ensuring adequate diversity of the cohort in terms of ethnic, geographic, and cultural participation. Qualitative research methods do not adhere to traditional sample size calculations and generally involve smaller sample sizes than their quantitative counterparts. There is not a minimum number of interview subjects or focus groups for any given subject. Instead, the choice of qualitative research method and subject sample size is dictated by the research question and goal of achieving thematic saturation.[56] Large sample sizes are not always appropriate and can complicate analysis with a single case study design sometimes proving an adequate and effective method for tackling a specific research question.[7]

Qualitative researchers need to be alert to many of the same biases that befall quantitative research, such as sampling, analysis, and selective presentation of data.[42] The unique role of the investigator in data acquisition (eg, interviewing style and topic guide) and their own personal characteristics (eg, age, gender, social status, personality, and health [disabled or able]) can influence the participant experience and the quality of data collection.[42,57] It is acknowledged that investigator's personal experiences, values, perceptions, and preconceived concepts influence the data acquisition process in the semistructured interviews in a focus group setting. Although the effects of this bias are not easily eliminated, investigators should use reflexive reporting to openly describe investigator's preconceptions and how these assumptions were challenged or supported during the course of data collection and analysis.[3,55]

Topic and Question Guide Development and Application

The topic guide is a carefully constructed flow of the interview questions, which is the backbone of active data collection, and ideally should be published with the results of study. Interview questions are open-ended queries that should be clear, simple, and easy to understand when posed out loud. If questions are more complex, consider choreographing pauses in the midst of the question to allow for comprehension and reflection before completing the question. After writing a question, ask it aloud to other research team members to afford opportunities to modify awkward-sounding questions. Poorly constructed questions can cause the group to falter in momentum. The order of questions can be important, and is based on cultivating comfort and then fostering an openness of communication that might occur naturally when encountering new people in nonresearch daily life. Brief opening questions that are straightforward and easy for interviewee or group members to answer helps to establish rapport between interviewer/moderator and the interviewee/group, allowing time for participants to feel comfortable with speaking are good to begin sessions. Subsequent transitioning questions continue to warm the participant to speaking as well as sharing one's own and responding to others' perspectives, both of which serve to ease the discussion into the sharper focus on the central/key questions necessary to procure material that address the overall research question. A smaller number of key questions that target the data collection is likely to procure a higher quality and more comprehensive yield than many key questions. In our research, we often use the technique of beginning certain key questions by asking the participant to "think back." For example, "think back to the time, when you first new something was not right with your health (leaving a pause here), what were the changes to your health you noticed?" The application of this and similar techniques helps to guide the participant's mind, placing them in the midst of the situation/experience of interest and sensitizing the participant to reexperience and thus to more readily recall and share important details.

Back up and probe questions are exactly what their names imply, and are used to keep a discussion progressing when group members might be shy or uncertain what to say, or to follow up on a particular remark more deeply. With regard to probing remarks further, we avoid direct questions that might sound harsh; instead we might say, "That's interesting, can you comment further on your remark?" The tone of the moderator can make all the difference in the same words, either creating defensiveness or sounding inviting. Our goal is to maintain a tone that is soft, friendly, and interested. Eye contact with each participant is important and should be gentle, reflecting the qualities of the prior sentence.

QUALITATIVE DATA ANALYSIS

Irrespective of the qualitative research method, the raw "data" are typically in narrative form and include transcripts, reflective notes, and field notes together to form the descriptive raw "data" of the research, but cannot provide an interpretation[4,7] without rigorous analytical application.

The assembling of the analytical team is vital to the success and perceived quality of the study. A multidisciplinary team with varying fields of expertise is exemplary, affording the opportunity to see the narrative from diverse perspectives. In the ideal situation, the team is led by someone with significant experience in conducting, supervising, and, if possible, comfort in teaching qualitative methods. Regardless of the scientific discipline, with practice, the sensitivity and capability of the researcher deepens; the data are only as reliable as the care, accuracy, and as much objectivity as the situation allows, as implemented by the researcher.

The most common approach to qualitative data analysis is grounded theory, which is the purest of inductive approaches whereby the data are approached without preconceived codes by the researcher; thus, the researcher analyzes with naïve eyes, allowing the data to speak and to be the driver of the emerging framework.[58] The theories produced by the research are "grounded" only in the data collected, with no input from prior studies. Here, codes are developed as part of the ongoing analytical process and they are modified and refined with new discoveries in the data. There is constant reengagement with already coded sections, a dynamic that is part of most qualitative analyses called constant comparative analysis. Although various approaches to systematic analysis of qualitative data exist, each involves the process of decontextualization (compiling repositories of shared experiences using individual components lifted from the data) and recontextualization (ensuring these defined experiences collate with the context from which they were originally identified to avoid issues around data fragmentation related decontextualization).[7]

Virtually all qualitative analytical methods are derived from grounded theory. Other methods range from the start list method, whereby the analysts develop a list of preconceived codes based on past studies to which new codes are added during the analysis.[59] Such approaches can help expedite the process when preexisting data are available. At the far end is the more deductive spectrum, with a definitive code list applied.[1,2,7,60] This method can be seen in the strict application of International Classification of Functioning, Health and Disability coding to a focus group transcript. Such studies gauge frequency of occurrence and, therefore, sit on the borderline between being qualitative and quantitative in nature. Analytical approaches are dictated by what is already known, what the question is, and the overall goal of the research.

The analysis and interpretation of qualitative data is subjective and complex in nature, and a difficult, time-intensive task. It is an iterative process returning to the same script repeatedly as an individual analyst and as a team of analysts, with several independent analysts performing identical tasks on the same manuscript or manuscripts—repeatedly—and the team discussing and comparing coding of their individual efforts until the final analysis is settled (**Fig. 2**).

The process of data analysis runs continuously in parallel with data acquisition; investigators are often present and active participants in the process of capturing experiences.[7] Analysis of the textual data needs to be systematic and thorough, and is

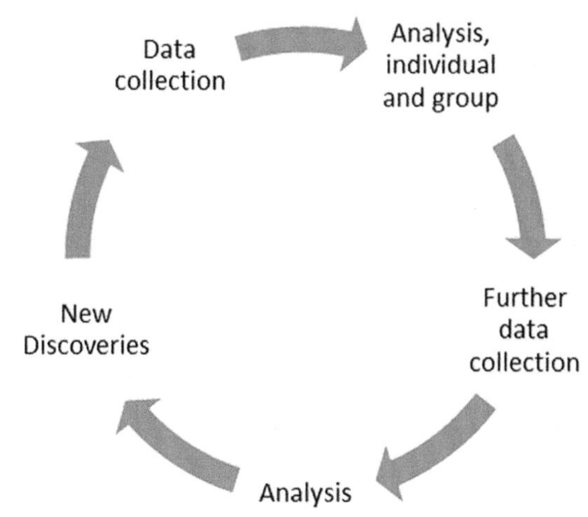
Data
collection
Analysis,
individual
and group
Further
data
collection
Analysis
New
Discoveries

Fig. 2. Schematic of dynamics between data collection and analysis: a continually iterative in both intraanalysis and interanalysis that integrates new data and continually refine existing data.

therefore labor intensive and time consuming.[7] In striking contraindication to best quantitative practices, it is only through analysis that the halt of data collection is signaled. No new information arising in the analyses signals that saturation has been reached and data collection can be discontinued.

The process begins with each analyst conducting an overview of a virgin transcript or recording, developing a receptiveness to the narrative as the first step in analysis, called familiarization, allows concepts and themes to emerge.[2] This step is achieved by reading the narrative in its entirety without yet attempting to code. After appreciating the scope, depth, and evolution of ideas, the manuscript is marked line by line for discrete "thought units," which are chunks of text that reflect a single concept. Thought units may become filed under "codes." Codes are labels consisting of a single word or discrete phrase that embody the essence of an important element of the narrative. Coding is an integral component in categorizing data and building a framework in a way that explains the diversity of experiences expressed in the data.[2,7] The identification of contrary experiences ("deviant" or negative opinions) enables investigators to interrogate their data with greater scrutiny, challenging and qualifying hypotheses, and refining interpretations.[7] Iterative testing on new or expanded samples can be used to confirm propositions derived from earlier analyses.[7]

Codes relevant to the research question are assembled into "code structures." Code structures make categorical sense of emerging themes and are often displayed in outline form. Remembering that qualitative research is in all spheres an iterative process, the code structure will continually change and be modified until a final conceptual framework emerges after all the narratives have been coded. The framework is often used to provide both understanding of a phenomenology as well as future directions in research and care.

Alternatively, there is also a place for quantification in some strictly qualitative studies. Johnson and colleagues[61] sought to understand physician expert perceptions of disease subtyping in SSc using semistructured interviews to collect qualitative insight and, after applying qualitative analytical methods, were able to calculate the frequency of discrete codes correlated with individual participants. This combined analytical technique was also used to understand the experiences of patients living with SSc-related calcinosis[62]; the calculation of quantifiable frequency data facilitated understanding that is useful both in supporting normative assumptions as well as providing direction for actionable deliverables in care. In this case, learning that many patients routinely extract calcinosis by either self-instrumentation or warm water soaking and extrusion provoked the not yet tested, but safe enough, anticipatory guidance regarding topical antibiotic use.

Several computer software programs are available to assist with the organization, retrieval, and reorganization of data.[7] However, the rigor of the analysis and the development of the framework depends the researcher only. If the software program interferes with the essential intimacy the researcher must have with the narrative, then it is best to revert to non–software-assisted analysis until those skills and sensibilities are more deeply set. The beauty of such software is to afford a researcher already intimate with the data more avenues of exploration that confer a deeper intimacy of relational associations.[7]

QUALITATIVE RESEARCH AS AN EMERGING, ACCEPTED, AND ESSENTIAL METHOD IN HEALTH SCIENCES

The quality indicators of quantitative methods are not the quality indicators of qualitative method and require a unique set of indicators to ensure qualitative rigor.[1,3,63] Qualitative studies, expectedly, are not completely reproducible in another group of participants; given the smaller, nonrandomized, purposeful sample sizes and more personal nature of the data, the data inherently lack unadulterated generalizability. In qualitative research, bias is virtually inescapable because the analysis relies on the sensibilities of the analyst, although working hard to be objective; it is through empathy that coding is signaled. A very messy—very human—but scientifically sound business!

It is crucial that qualitative research methods consider many of the same quality standards governing quantitative research, such as the validity (credibility), objectivity (confirmability), and generalizability (transferability) of the research findings.[3] Attention should also be drawn to the inevitable influence of bias on the relevance and validity of the study findings.[3] The researcher's personal and professional preconceptions cannot be entirely negated, but a complete and transparent account of the role and effect of the researcher at each step of the research process ensures bias can be accounted for in the interpretation of the study findings.[3]

Articles should include the relevance of the question and rationale of the approach, for example, why qualitative and why the particular applications and sampling strategy selected as well as the principal of saturation. Inclusion of the actual interview guide as well as information on the analysis (eg, number of coders, multidisciplinary team, the code structure, and management of divergent cases) is essential information when reporting the research.[64,65] Thus, to ensure rigor, protocols and guidelines have been presented. The most accepted of these is the COREQ. The COREQ is a 32-item checklist that is used for prepublication in some journals to ensure that qualitative research has been conducted with utmost rigor.[66] The COREQ consists of 3 domains with several questions under each: (a) the study team, (b) the study design, and (c) the analysis and findings.[66] The first study exploring the Raynaud experience in SSc demonstrating that current SSc patient-reported outcome measures do not capture the complex burden on morbidity[67] is a clear example of data summarization formatted for ease of quality evaluation. It is important to recognize that some of the items are arguably controversial for example, member checking; however, an overall guidance for quality assurance is necessary, providing an opportunity for the team to explain their process.

SUMMARY

The acceptance of qualitative research has been a long road fraught with criticism, but the scientific community has begun to appreciate the value of the unquantifiable. In many regards, the comparatively recent emergence of qualitative research methods in health science research reflects a return to pre-20th century medicine. Then, as now, clinicians appreciated the huge wealth of information that can be derived from observing and listening to patients recounting personal experiences of illness and qualitative research methods provide an important reminder of the complementary art and science of medicine. Over the course of this century, qualitative research has provided patients, carers, and health care workers with a greater voice, ensuring their personal experiences contribute to knowledge development, clinical assessments, and the shaping of future health care services.[42]

REFERENCES

1. Malterud K. The art and science of clinical knowledge: evidence beyond measures and numbers. Lancet 2001;358(9279):397–400.
2. Bradley EH, Curry LA, Devers KJ. Qualitative data analysis for health services research: developing taxonomy, themes, and theory. Health Serv Res 2007; 42(4):1758–72.
3. Malterud K. Qualitative research: standards, challenges, and guidelines. Lancet 2001;358(9280):483–8.
4. Gawande A. The heroism of incremental care. The New Yorker: Annals of Medicine 2017.
5. Saketkoo LA. Wildflowers abundant in the garden of systemic sclerosis research, while hopeful exotics will one day bloom. Rheumatology (Oxford) 2017. [Epub ahead of print].
6. Ong BN, Richardson JC. The contribution of qualitative approaches to musculoskeletal research. Rheumatology (Oxford) 2006;45(4):369–70.
7. Pope C, Ziebland S, Mays N. Qualitative research in health care. Analysing qualitative data. BMJ 2000;320(7227):114–6.
8. Suter LG, Fraenkel L, Holmboe ES. What factors account for referral delays for patients with suspected rheumatoid arthritis? Arthritis Rheum 2006;55(2):300–5.
9. Ballantyne PJ, Gignac MAM, Hawker GA. A patient-centered perspective on surgery avoidance for hip or knee arthritis: lessons for the future. Arthritis Rheum 2007;57(1):27–34.
10. Kroll TL, Richardson M, Sharf BF, et al. "Keep on truckin'" or "it's got you in this little vacuum": race-based perceptions in decision-making for total knee arthroplasty. J Rheumatol 2007;34(5):1069–75.
11. Klein D, MacDonald A, Drummond N, et al. A qualitative study to identify factors influencing COXIB prescribed by family physicians for musculoskeletal disorders. Fam Pract 2006;23(6):659–65.
12. Mann C, Dieppe P. Different patterns of illness-related interaction in couples coping with rheumatoid arthritis. Arthritis Rheum 2006;55(2):279–86.
13. Barlow JH, Cullen LA, Foster NE, et al. Does arthritis influence perceived ability to fulfill a parenting role? Perceptions of mothers, fathers and grandparents. Patient Educ Couns 1999;37(2):141–51.

14. Backman CL, Smith LD, Smith S, et al. Experiences of mothers living with inflammatory arthritis. Arthritis Rheum 2007;57(3):381–8.
15. Degotardi PJ, Revenson TA, Ilowite NT. Family-level coping in juvenile rheumatoid arthritis: assessing the utility of a quantitative family interview. Arthritis Care Res 1999;12(5):314–24.
16. Sanders C, Donovan JL, Dieppe PA. Unmet need for joint replacement: a qualitative investigation of barriers to treatment among individuals with severe pain and disability of the hip and knee. Rheumatology (Oxford) 2004;43(3):353–7.
17. Rhodes LA, McPhillips-Tangum CA, Markham C, et al. The power of the visible: the meaning of diagnostic tests in chronic back pain. Soc Sci Med 1999;48(9): 1189–203.
18. Donovan JL, Blake DR. Qualitative study of interpretation of reassurance among patients attending rheumatology clinics: "just a touch of arthritis, doctor?". BMJ 2000;320(7234):541–4.
19. Haugli L, Strand E, Finset A. How do patients with rheumatic disease experience their relationship with their doctors? A qualitative study of experiences of stress and support in the doctor-patient relationship. Patient Educ Couns 2004;52(2): 169–74.
20. Ward V, Hill J, Hale C, et al. Patient priorities of care in rheumatology outpatient clinics: a qualitative study. Musculoskeletal Care 2007;5(4):216–28.
21. Hay MC, Cadigan RJ, Khanna D, et al. Prepared patients: internet information seeking by new rheumatology patients. Arthritis Rheum 2008;59(4):575–82.
22. Arthur V, Clifford C. Rheumatology: the expectations and preferences of patients for their follow-up monitoring care: a qualitative study to determine the dimensions of patient satisfaction. J Clin Nurs 2004;13(2):234–42.
23. Hale ED, Treharne GJ, Lyons AC, et al. "Joining the dots" for patients with systemic lupus erythematosus: personal perspectives of health care from a qualitative study. Ann Rheum Dis 2006;65(5):585–9.
24. Marshall NJ, Wilson G, Lapworth K, et al. Patients' perceptions of treatment with anti-TNF therapy for rheumatoid arthritis: a qualitative study. Rheumatology (Oxford) 2004;43(8):1034–8.
25. Woolhead GM, Donovan JL, Dieppe PA. Outcomes of total knee replacement: a qualitative study. Rheumatology (Oxford) 2005;44(8):1032–7.
26. Thorstensson CA, Roos EM, Petersson IF, et al. How do middle-aged patients conceive exercise as a form of treatment for knee osteoarthritis? Disabil Rehabil 2006;28(1):51–9.
27. Campbell R, Evans M, Tucker M, et al. Why don't patients do their exercises? Understanding non-compliance with physiotherapy in patients with osteoarthritis of the knee. J Epidemiol Community Health 2001;55(2):132–8.
28. Veenhof C, van Hasselt TJ, Koke AJA, et al. Active involvement and long-term goals influence long-term adherence to behavioural graded activity in patients with osteoarthritis: a qualitative study. Aust J Physiother 2006;52(4):273–8.
29. Sale JE, Gignac M, Hawker G. How "bad" does the pain have to be? A qualitative study examining adherence to pain medication in older adults with osteoarthritis. Arthritis Rheum 2006;55(2):272–8.
30. Tallon D, Chard J, Dieppe P. Exploring the priorities of patients with osteoarthritis of the knee. Arthritis Care Res 2000;13(5):312–9.
31. Hale ED, Treharne GJ, Norton Y, et al. 'Concealing the evidence': the importance of appearance concerns for patients with systemic lupus erythematosus. Lupus 2006;15(8):532–40.

32. Power JD, Badley EM, French MR, et al. Fatigue in osteoarthritis: a qualitative study. BMC Musculoskelet Disord 2008;9:63.
33. Adamson J, Gooberman-Hill R, Woolhead G, et al. 'Questerviews': using questionnaires in qualitative interviews as a method of integrating qualitative and quantitative health services research. J Health Serv Res Policy 2004;9(3):139–45.
34. Tugwell P, Bombardier C, Buchanan WW, et al. The MACTAR Patient Preference Disability Questionnaire—an individualized functional priority approach for assessing improvement in physical disability in clinical trials in rheumatoid arthritis. J Rheumatol 1987;14(3):446–51.
35. Mouthon L, Rannou F, Berezne A, et al. Patient preference disability questionnaire in systemic sclerosis: a cross-sectional survey. Arthritis Rheum 2008;59(7):968–73.
36. US Department of Health and Human Services (DHHS), US Food and Drug Administration (FDA). Guidance for industry: patient-reported outcome measures: use in medical product development to support labeling claims. 2009. Available at: http://www.fda.gov/downloads/Drugs/GuidanceComplianceRegulatoryInformation/Guidances/UCM193282.pdf. Accessed June 01, 2016.
37. Bottomley A, Jones D, Claassens L. Patient-reported outcomes: assessment and current perspectives of the guidelines of the Food and Drug Administration and the reflection paper of the European Medicines Agency. Eur J Cancer 2009;45(3):347–53.
38. Chu LF, Utengen A, Kadry B, et al. "Nothing about us without us": patient partnership in medical conferences. BMJ 2016;354:i3883.
39. Saketkoo LA, Mittoo S, Huscher D, et al. Connective tissue disease related interstitial lung diseases and idiopathic pulmonary fibrosis: provisional core sets of domains and instruments for use in clinical trials. Thorax 2014;69(5):428–36.
40. Saketkoo LA, Mittoo S, Frankel S, et al. Reconciling healthcare professional and patient perspectives in the development of disease activity and response criteria in connective tissue disease-related interstitial lung diseases. J Rheumatol 2014;41(4):792–8.
41. Morgan DL. Practical strategies for combining qualitative and quantitative methods: applications to health research. Qual Health Res 1998;8(3):362–76.
42. Lempp H, Kingsley G. Qualitative assessments. Best Pract Res Clin Rheumatol 2007;21(5):857–69.
43. Minnock P, Kirwan J, Bresnihan B. Fatigue is a reliable, sensitive and unique outcome measure in rheumatoid arthritis. Rheumatology 2009;48(12):1533–6.
44. Loyola-Sanchez A, Richardson J, Wilkins S, et al. Barriers to accessing the culturally sensitive healthcare that could decrease the disabling effects of arthritis in a rural Mayan community: a qualitative inquiry. Clin Rheumatol 2016;35(5):1287–98.
45. Schiff M, Saunderson S, Mountian I, et al. Chronic disease and self-injection: ethnographic investigations into the patient experience during treatment. Rheumatol Ther 2017;4(2):445–63.
46. Prothero L, Georgopoulou S, de Souza S, et al. Patient involvement in the development of a handbook for moderate rheumatoid arthritis. Health Expect 2017;20(2):288–97.
47. Jaeger VK, Aubin A, Baldwin N, et al. Optimizing scleroderma centers of excellence: perspectives from patients and scleroderma (SSc) experts. Arthritis Rheum 2014;66:S1180–1.
48. Hinojosa-Azaola A, Alcocer-Varela J. Art and rheumatology: the artist and the rheumatologist's perspective. Rheumatology (Oxford) 2014;53(10):1725–31.

49. Pou MA, Diaz-Torne C, Azevedo VF. Manolo Hugue: from sculpture to painting due to arthritis. Rheumatol Clin 2011;7(2):135–6 [in Spanish].
50. Suter H. Paul Klee's illness (systemic sclerosis) and artistic transfiguration. Front Neurol Neurosci 2010;27:11–28.
51. Kiltz U, van der Heijde D, Boonen A, et al. Development of a health index in patients with ankylosing spondylitis (ASAS HI): final result of a global initiative based on the ICF guided by ASAS. Ann Rheum Dis 2015;74(5):830–5.
52. O'Sullivan R. Focus groups as qualitative research, 2nd edition. Sociology 1998; 32(2):418–9.
53. Morgan D. Focus groups as qualitative research. 2nd edition. Thousand Oaks (CA): Sage Publications; 1997. Available at: http://methods.sagepub.com/book/focus-groups-as-qualitative-research. Accessed December 19, 2017.
54. Krueger R, Casey M. Focus groups: a practical guide for applied research. 3rd edition. Thousand Oaks (CA): Sage; 2000.
55. Hale ED, Treharne GJ, Kitas GD. Qualitative methodologies I: asking research questions with reflexive insight. Musculoskeletal Care 2007;5(3):139–47.
56. Guest G, Bunce A, Johnson L. How many interviews are enough? An experiment with data saturation and variability. Field Method 2006;18:59–82.
57. Benestad B, Vinje O, Veierod MB, et al. Quantitative and qualitative assessments of pain in children with juvenile chronic arthritis based on the Norwegian version of the pediatric pain questionnaire. Scand J Rheumatol 1996;25(5):293–9.
58. Glaser BG, Strauss AL. The discovery of grounded theory: strategies for qualitative research. London, UK: Weidenfeld and Nicolson; 1968.
59. Miles MB, Huberman AM. Qualitative data analysis: an expanded sourcebook. Thousand Oaks (CA): Sage; 1994.
60. Stamm TA, Mattsson M, Mihai C, et al. Concepts of functioning and health important to people with systemic sclerosis: a qualitative study in four European countries. Ann Rheum Dis 2011;70(6):1074–9.
61. Johnson SR, Fransen J, Khanna D, et al. There is a need for new systemic sclerosis subset criteria. a content analytic approach. Ann Rheum Dis 2015;74:1141.
62. Christensen AM, Khalique S, Cenac S, et al. Systemic sclerosis (Ssc) related calcinosis: patients provide what specialists want to learn development of a calcinosis patient reported outcome measure (PROM). Ann Rheum Dis 2015;74:600.
63. Mays N, Pope C. Qualitative research in health care. Assessing quality in qualitative research. BMJ 2000;320(7226):50–2.
64. Giacomini MK, Cook DJ. Users' guides to the medical literature: XXIII. Qualitative research in health care B. What are the results and how do they help me care for my patients? Evidence-Based Medicine Working Group. JAMA 2000;284(4): 478–82.
65. Giacomini MK, Cook DJ. Users' guides to the medical literature: XXIII. Qualitative research in health care A. Are the results of the study valid? Evidence-Based Medicine Working Group. JAMA 2000;284(3):357–62.
66. Tong A, Sainsbury P, Craig J. Consolidated Criteria for Reporting Qualitative Research (COREQ): a 32-item checklist for interviews and focus groups. Int J Qual Health Care 2007;19(6):349–57.
67. Pauling JD, Domsic RT, Saketkoo LA, et al. A multi-national qualitative research study exploring the patient experience of Raynaud's phenomenon in systemic sclerosis. Arthritis Care Res, in press.

Similarity Network Fusion

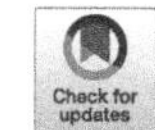

A Novel Application to Making Clinical Diagnoses

Andréanne N. Zizzo, MD, MSc, FRCPC[a,*], Lauren Erdman, MSc[b], Brian M. Feldman, MD, MSc, FRCPC[c], Anna Goldenberg, PhD[b]

KEYWORDS

• Similarity network fusion • Analysis • Classification • Immune-mediated disease

KEY POINTS

- Similarity Network Fusion (SNF) is a useful analytical tool to group patients together and understand patient characteristics.
- SNF uses different data types and is therefore helpful in classifying patients when diagnoses may be difficult to determine or understand.
- SNF represents a novel computational analytical method that may assist with understanding similarities and differences between patients and extends beyond classification criteria and working diagnoses.

INTRODUCTION

Systemic autoimmune processes are challenging conditions to diagnosis accurately, monitor, and treat. Many of these conditions present within the pediatric age range and can contribute to significant morbidity if not diagnosed promptly and managed appropriately. Systemic lupus erythematosus (SLE) represents one such condition that affects 3.3 to 8.8 cases per 100,000 children.[1] It is a noncurative disease with many systemic features that are burdensome to the child and those involved in his or her care. It is diagnosed using a set of clinical and serologic classification features

Disclosure Statement: The authors have no commercial or financial affiliation to disclose pertaining to the content of this article.

[a] Department of Pediatrics, Division of Gastroenterology and Hepatology, Western University, Children's Hospital, London Health Sciences Centre, 800 Commissioners Road East, B1-162, London, Ontario N6A 5W9, Canada; [b] Genetics and Genome Biology, Department of Computer Science, The Hospital for Sick Children, Peter Gilgan Centre for Research and Learning (PGCRL), University of Toronto, 686 Bay Street, Toronto, Ontario M5G 0A4, Canada; [c] Department of Pediatrics, Division of Rheumatology, University of Toronto, The Hospital for Sick Children, 555 University Avenue, Toronto, Ontario M5G 1X8, Canada

* Corresponding author.

E-mail address: andreanne.zizzo@lhsc.on.ca

Rheum Dis Clin N Am 44 (2018) 285–293

https://doi.org/10.1016/j.rdc.2018.01.005

rheumatic.theclinics.com

that were officially developed in 1971 but continue to evolve and to be revised.[2,3] The waxing and waning pattern of this chronic disease poses a challenge to those involved with monitoring its course, since the disease also progresses and symptoms evolve over time.

Similarly, many autoimmune conditions are diagnosed based on an established constellation of clinical and serologic features. The broad spectrum of presenting symptoms within which to identify diagnostic features can pose a challenge in knowing how to best manage and classify patient diseases. For example, autoimmune hepatitis (AIH) can present with a combination of fatigue, abdominal pain, weight loss, anorexia, fever, and jaundice.[4] These symptoms are also found in patients with rheumatologic disorders such as systemic lupus erythematosus (SLE). In this instance, the nonspecific features make a clinical diagnosis difficult to achieve.

Immune-mediated diseases can also progress to involve additional organs that would not classically be attributed to the working diagnosis. Because autoimmune conditions tend to predispose patients to developing other autoimmune conditions, clinicians may find themselves wondering whether new organ involvement represents a severe form of the primary disease or the first presentation of an additional autoimmune disorder. A better understanding of what the evolving process of such conditions should be and what should be considered a separate disease entity is necessary. This would enable more accurate prognostication and explanation to patients and families around the management of their chronic disease. As an example, the etiology of liver involvement in patients with SLE represents one of these unanswered challenges.

Initially coined lupoid hepatitis, autoimmune hepatitis (AIH) represents one such condition.[5] Numerous conflicting studies have tried to describe the extent of liver disease that could be attributed to SLE before its features would be better defined as a primary liver disease. The conclusion from Runyon and colleagues[6] is that liver disease can be significant in SLE and that a separate entity termed lupoid hepatitis should not be considered. Gibson and colleagues[7] had the opposite feeling and concluded that liver disease was mainly subclinical in SLE and that anything more pronounced would correspond to a separate disease entity. A prospective study by Miller and colleagues[8] supported both MacKay's initial paper and the conclusion drawn by Gibson and colleagues, finding that only mild liver disease could be attributed to the spectrum of SLE. The medical advances of the next 2 decades only contributed additional confusion to the description of what should be considered lupoid hepatitis and what should be labeled SLE-associated hepatitis (or lupus hepatitis). Little distinguishes the 2 clinical presentations to this day.

The difficulty in defining these 2 diseases as distinct entities is that there are more unifying than dividing features. The clinical presentations, the liver biopsy findings and the autoantibody profile appear to be interchangeable between diseases.[9–16] The same conflicting findings have been evident within the pediatric literature.[14,17–19] Another challenge may be attributed to the fact that these diseases are diagnosed according to classifications of features determined by consensus expert opinion.[3,20–22]

There is the potential for an inherent flaw in defining these diseases based on expert opinion-driven clinical criteria. Clinically, patients with autoimmune diseases that manifest with multiorgan involvement may receive a diagnosis based on the specialist to whom they are initially referred. The patient who presents with elevated liver enzymes and systemic features may be referred to a hepatologist and be given a diagnosis of autoimmune hepatitis (AIH). The same patient could be given the diagnosis of SLE with liver involvement if first referred to a rheumatologist. Both clinicians are challenged with the task of applying complex predefined classification to best explain the patient's presenting features. Without a clear understanding of the liver disease, clinicians are left with an incomplete picture with which to make important decisions that could affect management.

In order to best address this type of clinical challenge, it is first important to identify an alternate way of making sense of these patients' complex constellation of features outside of current classification criteria. This exercise sets up a paradigm shift of removing a patient's working diagnosis and finding an analytical method that would provide insight into how to more accurately classify patients with immune-mediated processes. As mentioned, the spectrum of liver involvement in rheumatic diseases may be 1 such challenge that remains unanswered. Another may relate to whether certain features at presentation in a patient with a working diagnosis SLE could determine overall disease progression. Regardless of the clinical scenario posing the dilemma, thinking about patient features more broadly than the current scope of classification criteria proposes a more neutral perspective from which to find a solution on how to better understand these patients.

The analytical challenge with this type of clinical question lies in the need to find a statistical method that first allows for the integration of multiple different data types. For instance, patients would need to be characterized and grouped based on clinical features, biochemical data, imaging features, serologic antibody titers, and liver biopsy information where available. Second, the application of an analysis to the retrospective nature of these studies also requires that the statistical method used would be able to incorporate the maximal amount of data variables available even when not all patients may have the same information collected.

SUMMARY AND DISCUSSION OF METHODOLOGICAL TECHNIQUE

A computational method known as Similarity Network Fusion (SNF) is a novel machine-learning method that has demonstrated its capacity for data integration when different data measurement types are being used simultaneously. It can be used to better understand diseases.[23] Most clustering techniques are more adept at integrating similar forms of data, either all categorical variables or all continuous. In this type of clinical dilemma, data are dichotomous, with multiple categories, and continuous in nature. Therefore, the ideal approach is to use a technique that enables integration of different data sources into 1 network analysis.

SNF has been shown to successfully integrate patient networks together based on multiple data types, while maintaining strong connections between patients based on their individual data types. It subsequently allows for clustering of the integrated network. SNF also has a built-in method for imputation, which means that one can use any data available from each patient rather than only the data from patients with no missing observations.

Application of this analytical tool is performed using the SNFtool package.

In SNF analysis, patients are grouped together based on the similarities shared in their collected data in the form of a patient network. The construction of this network is achieved in a 2-step process. First, each data type is used separately to build a network of patients based on variables belonging to that data type. For example, a similarity network may be constructed using biochemical data alone, another using clinical symptoms alone, another using autoimmune features alone. These networks can be visually depicted through a heatmap made up of multiple cells. Each cell along the X and Y axis of the heatmap corresponds to an individual patient interaction for the particular data type analyzed and the higher the similarity between the 2 patients, the darker the color depicted (**Fig. 1**). The individual heatmaps or similarity matrices are

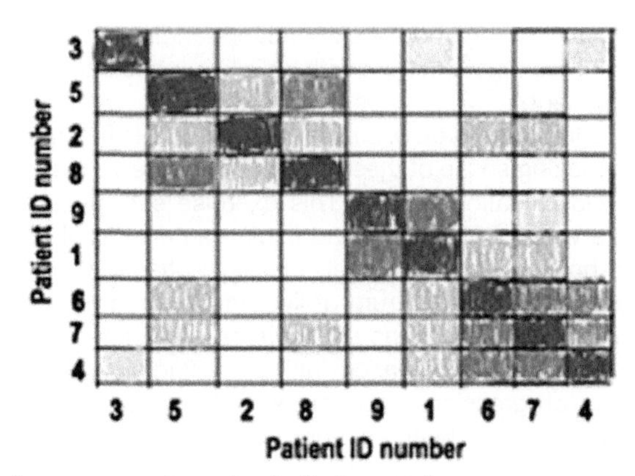

Fig. 1. Diagramatic representation of a similarity matrix.

generated using agglomerative hierarchical or spectral clustering to show the grouped patient-patient similarity for each data type.

Agglomerative hierarchical clustering looks at each observation as its own initial cluster and subsequently builds pairs of clusters that are merged as one. The analysis continues to compare these newly merged pairs of clusters with the subsequent observation until each observation has been assessed and organized relative to each other based on how similar or dissimilar it is to the rest of the observations. The number of groups is then chosen based on some criterion (eg, silhouette statistical, Dunn index), and groups are formed with more similar patients grouped closer together and the more dissimilar patients further apart. Patients are aligned along the X and Y axes in such a way that the diagonal corresponds to each patient being compared (ie, perfectly similar and therefore depicting the darkest color in **Fig. 1**).

Different to the agglomerative hierarchical clustering is spectral clustering. Spectral clustering uses K-means clustering of the first p principal components from the similarity matrix to identify K patient clusters. This technique is applied for the second step of the SNF analysis described next.

In the second step, each of the similarity matrices is integrated into a single network to identify how patients group together based on all of their provided data. The integration of the similarity matrices is an iterative process that adds information on the similarities between patients provided by each data type. This iterative process sequentially adds the information provided from each data source in order to ensure that the added value of each additional data source builds upon the previous one. This allows for the final similarity network to capture the contribution of different data sources to patient clustering and assist in identifying how the data drive similarities among patients. In the integrated heatmap (ie, that iteratively added each data type), the groups are visually depicted using spectral clustering that draws the groups of patients to the diagonal of the heatmap. Like the individual heatmaps based on each type of data, the integrated heatmap is also made up of multiple cells, where each cell on the X and Y axis corresponds to the interaction between a pair of patients. The stronger the similarity between patients, the closer they are grouped together and the darker the color shown (eg, **Fig. 2**).

A strength of this technique as compared with other clustering techniques is that each data point provided by a particular patient contributes to the network analysis. As such, this analysis does not solely rely on only variables collected on all patients to be included in the analysis. For example, even if some patients do not have

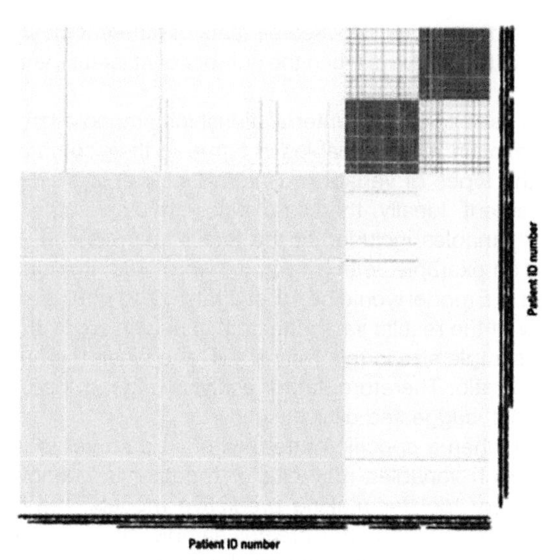

Fig. 2. Diagramatic representation of the integrated heatmap.

recorded data on variable "A" but others do, the information provided on the patients who do have variable "A" measured can still be included in the final network. Each data point collected on each patient contributes to the final network. In doing so, this method provides a more comprehensive view of how to aggregate all of the data provided by a particular patient and draw similarities and differences among the patients within the network. Furthermore, this technique has also been validated as an effective tool when used for small sample sizes.[23]

A brief review of how other cluster analysis techniques could be used to address the type of clinical dilemma (eg, latent class analysis, K-means clustering, factor analysis, principal component analysis [PCA] and classification and regression tree [CART]), may assist is further supportive the value of SNF as a novel clinical method.

Latent class analysis works most effectively when categorical or dichotomous variables are primarily used. This method is indicated when trying to classify people into unmeasured groups based on chosen variables. For example, using this technique could help to categorize people into different types of travelers, or latent classes, based on their choice of destinations within the past 5 years. Latent class analysis is also used when the goal of the analysis is to identify subtypes within a group or diagnostic subcategories. In order to be used, latent class analysis relies on the assumption that those within the same class share the same homogeneous set of observed responses and cannot be distinguished based on these. It also relies on a large number of cases in order to be used effectively. Although this analytical technique has some abilities to answer the type of clinical dilemma presented, it appears to work most effectively when data can be divided dichotomously (eg, yes or no). Because most retrospective data of patient groups are defined by more than dichotomous variables (ie, continuous variables) and do not share the same homogeneous set of observations, latent class analysis may not be an effective technique to objectively cluster patients based on the available data.

K-means clustering is used to partition a number of observations n into a number of clusters k when you can determine how many clusters to use a priori.[24] This technique is helpful to minimize differences between patients grouped within the same cluster while maximizing the differences between patients of different clusters. The limitation of using this analytical technique is when the number of clusters cannot be determined a priori.

Factor analysis is used to analyze interrelationships among a large number of variables and aims to explain these variables in terms of their common underlying factors.[25,26] Usually, the types of variables used in factor analysis are assumed to be numeric in measurement. Ideally, the sample size should also be greater than 100, and the number of variables included in the factor analysis should not exceed the rule of the 10:1. As an example, with a sample size of 100, the maximum number of variables *n* included in a model would be 10, so that 100:10 = 10. Using factor analysis may limit the quality of the results when the data variables are both numeric and categorical, when the sample size is relatively small, and when the number of variables exceeds the desired ratio. Therefore, factor analysis may not be the ideal statistical analysis in the authors' suggested clinical scenario.

PCA can be used when a specific pattern within a data set is unknown and also when the way in which variables may cluster together is unknown. Although it is used as an exploratory tool for making predictive models, the limitation in using PCA is that populations studied with greater sample sizes (in the thousands) will have better success at finding trends within the same data pool.[25] It also requires that each data point used in the analysis be measured for each study participant and otherwise removed from the analysis. Because retrospective study data in rheumatic diseases likely represent a smaller sample size, the aim should be to use a technique that can maintain as many patients as possible in the study population in order to allow data integration that would avoid losing important data in generating the clusters.

CART analysis is equipped to use different types of variables. This cluster analysis technique is indicated when there is little a priori knowledge of how variables interact. Decision trees are generated based on the contribution of each subsequent data variable added.[27,28] How each data variable leads to the next associated variable is usually determined based on an outcome of interest (eg, in order to predict a particular outcome). In the type of clinical scenario described, one is blinded to the outcome of interest, the final diagnosis, in order to assess how patients objectively cluster together. This form of analysis is called unsupervised. In this way, CART analysis would not be a helpful technique to address the clinical challenge presented.

Despite its many strengths and capabilities, SNF analysis is limited by the quality of the data used to determine patient groups. As such, the insight gained from the final network results is only as helpful as the quality of the information provided in the analysis. A measure of the quality of this information is provided by a tool used by the SNF analysis called calculation of mutual information (calNMI). This measure provides insight into why the final heatmap appears the way it does and how much each data type contributes to the final groups.

For example, when looking at patients with immune-mediated liver diseases, it may be hypothesized that the autoantibody profile will provide a lot of information about how patient groups are formed. Other types of data included in the analysis may be clinical features, imaging features, and demographic data. The sequential addition of information from each individual heatmap generated for the final SNF analysis can be quantified as a calNMI value. Therefore, if the calNMI value was much higher for data provided for patient groups that combined clinical features, demographic data, and antibody profile as compared with the calNMI value calculated from the data provided from the combined information of clinical features and demographic data alone, then the hypothesis would be confirmed. The contribution of information from antibody profile would largely contribute to how patients group together. If the subsequent addition of imaging features did not yield a large additional difference in calNMI value, then it would imply that imaging data did not have a great contribution to how the patients in the study sample differed one from the other.

SNF presents many strengths when looking at potential clinical applications. First, it is able to assist with better understanding patient disease by objectively analyzing collected data and identifying similar groups of patients without the influence of expert opinion or preconceived notions pertaining to how patients should group together. Second, SNF has also been shown to generate clusters that are predictive of patient outcomes and identify which characteristics drive the newly defined patient groups and thus, a given clinical outcome.[23] This can further assist with establishing predictive models addressing severity of disease and predicting overall outcomes. Therefore, using SNF analysis becomes helpful as a tool in perfecting clinical understanding of patients, the behavior of their diseases, and its potential outcomes in terms of response to treatment, complications, and survival.

The ability of SNF analysis to use each of the data points contributed by each patient within the study sample represents an important strength when one considers the limitations of missing data with retrospective studies. The literature on controlling for missing values uses a minimum of 80% of the data available as the preferred cutoff before potential imputing strategies would lead to too much error within conclusions drawn.[29–31] In the introductory paper on SNF,[23] a cutoff of 20% missing data was also used to have a patient included in the analysis. SNF analysis added considerable strength to a retrospective data set by allowing each data variable with 20% or less of the data to be kept in the analytical pool. What this meant practically was that regardless of which patient contributed a data point to a certain variable, as long as 20% or less of the data on a particular variable was complete, then the information could be included in the analysis. As a result, this analytical tool becomes useful when seeking that patients contribute as much information as possible to an analytical question without using methods of data imputation.

Despite its many strengths as an analytical tool and potential for future clinical classification of diseases, there is some anticipated resistance in seeing SNF becoming a more largely accepted clinical tool. One clear potential challenge lies in the difficulty in providing the usual nomenclature and paradigm of statistical significance measures. Although standard *P*-value calculation for univariate analysis can be achieved for the different variables contributing to the patient group assignment, it becomes challenging to provide the same expected statistical significance calculation for an overall patient network. One method used to overcome this represents the calNMI value explained earlier. Another method involves applying a boot-strapping technique to validate the findings of the network analysis. Further methods may also consider using regression tree analysis to test the predictive ability of the model with further similar patients encountered. Regardless of the method used, SNF does require a paradigm shift in how one thinks about patients and also how one approaches making data analysis meaningful.

In conclusion, computer-driven methodological analyses like SNF become insightful as one broadens the understanding of how patient diseases may differ from current understanding and classification. This novel approach to network analysis is hypothesis-generating and strives to remove any potential (mis)conception of disease that may be deeply rooted in current clinical frameworks. As physicians become more familiar with the strength of this form of computational analysis, they will have found yet another sophisticated tool to addresses some of the limitations of other cluster analytical techniques and provide a deeper knowledge into how to understand patient diseases and predict outcomes. Ultimately, it may allow one to determine nuances in clinical presentations that up to this point may not have yielded as much insight into the patient's overall disease trajectory.

REFERENCES

1. Kamphuis S, Silverman ED. Prevalence and burden of pediatric-onset systemic lupus erythematosus. Nat Rev Rheumatol 2010;6(9):538–46.
2. Heinlen LD, McClain MT, Merrill J, et al. Clinical criteria for systemic lupus erythematosus precede diagnosis, and associated autoantibodies are present before clinical symptoms. Arthritis Rheum 2007;56(7):2344–51.
3. Hochberg MC. Updating the American College of Rheumatology revised criteria for the classification of systemic lupus erythematosus. Arthritis Rheum 1997; 40(9):1725.
4. Czaja AJ. Current concepts in autoimmune hepatitis. Ann Hepatol 2005;4(1): 6–24. Available at: http://ovidsp.ovid.com/ovidweb.cgi?T=JS&PAGE=reference&D=emed7&NEWS=N&AN=15798657.
5. Mackay IR, Taft LI, Cowling DC. Lupoid hepatitis. Lancet 1956;271:1323–6.
6. Runyon BA, LaBrecque DR, Anuras S. The spectrum of liver disease in systemic lupus erythematosus. Report of 33 histologically-proved cases and review of the literature. Am J Med 1980;69(2):187–94. Available at: http://www.ncbi.nlm.nih.gov/pubmed/7405944. Accessed September 25, 2013.
7. Gibson T, Myers AR. Subclinical liver disease in systemic lupus erythematosus. J Rheumatol 1981;8(5):752–9. Available at: http://www.ncbi.nlm.nih.gov/pubmed/7310775. Accessed January 24, 2014.
8. Miller MH, Urowitz MB, Gladman DD, et al. The liver in systemic lupus erythematosus. Q J Med 1984;211:401–9.
9. Forman MB, Levy H, Gear AJ, et al. Hepatic involvement in systemic lupus erythematosus. A case report. S Afr Med J 1981;59:726–8.
10. Mackay IR. Auto-immune (lupoid) hepatitis: an entity in the spectrum of chronic active liver disease. J Gastroenterol Hepatol 1990;5(3):352–9. Available at: http://www.ncbi.nlm.nih.gov/pubmed/2103416.
11. Hall S, Czaja AJ, Kaufman DK, et al. How lupoid is lupoid hepatitis? J Rheumatol 1986;13(1):95–8. Available at: http://www.ncbi.nlm.nih.gov/pubmed/3701746. Accessed November 29, 2013.
12. Arnett FC, Reichlin M. Lupus hepatitis: an under-recognized disease feature associated with autoantibodies to ribosomal P. Am J Med 1995;99(5):465–72. Available at: http://www.ncbi.nlm.nih.gov/pubmed/7485202. Accessed September 30, 2013.
13. Leggett BA. The liver in systemic lupus erythematosus. J Gastroenterol Hepatol 1993;8:84–8.
14. Mariniello G, Russo G, Carlomagno R, et al. Liver involvement in juvenile systemic lupus erythematosus (SLE). Pediatr Rheumatol 2011;9(suppl 1):254.
15. Piga M, Vacca A, Porru G, et al. Liver involvement in systemic lupus erythematosus: incidence, clinical course and outcome of lupus hepatitis. Clin Exp Rheumatol 2010;28:504–10.
16. Atsumi T, Sagawa A, Jodo S, et al. Severe hepatic involvement without inflammatory changes in systemic lupus erythematosus: report of two cases and review of the literature. Lupus 1995;4:225–8.
17. El-Shabrawi MH, Farrag MI. Hepatic manifestations in juvenile systemic lupus erythematosus. Recent Pat Inflamm Allergy Drug Discov 2014;8(1):36–40.

18. Deen MEJ, Porta G, Fiorot FJ, et al. Autoimmune hepatitis and juvenile systemic lupus erythematosus. Lupus 2009;18(8):747–51.
19. Usta Y, Gurakan F, Akcoren Z, et al. An overlap syndrome involving autoimmune hepatitis and systemic lupus erythematosus in childhood. World J Gastroenterol 2007;13(19):2764–7.
20. Alvarez F, Berg PA, Bianchi FB, et al. International Autoimmune Hepatitis Group report: review of criteria for diagnosis of autoimmune hepatitis. J Hepatol 1999; 31(5):929–38. Available at: http://www.ncbi.nlm.nih.gov/pubmed/10580593.
21. Ebbeson RL, Schreiber RA. Diagnosing autoimmune hepatitis in children: is the International Autoimmune Hepatitis Group scoring system useful? Clin Gastroenterol Hepatol 2004;2(10):935–40. Available at: http://www.ncbi.nlm.nih.gov/pubmed/15476158.
22. Petri M. Review of classification criteria for systemic lupus erythematosus. Rheum Dis Clin North Am 2005;31(2):245–54, vi.
23. Wang B, Mezlini AM, Demir F, et al. Similarity network fusion for aggregating data types on a genomic scale. Nat Methods 2014;11(3):333–7.
24. Moore A. K-means and hierarchical clustering. 2016. Available at: https://www.autonlab.org/tutorials/kmeans.html. Accessed March 3, 2015.
25. Norman GR, Streiner DL. Principal components and factor analysis: fooling around with factors. In: Norman GR, Streiner DL, editors. Biotatistics: the bare essentials. 3rd edition. Hamilton, Ontario: B.C. Decker, Inc; 2008. p. 194–209.
26. O'Brien K. Factor analysis: an overview in the field of measurement. Physiother Can 2007;59:142–55.
27. Loh W-Y. Classification and regression tree methods. In: Ruggeri F, Kennett RS, Faltin FW, editors. Encyclopedia of statistics in quality and reliability. Madison (WI): Wiley; 2008. p. 315–23. Available at: https://www.researchgate.net/profile/Wei-Yin_Loh/publication/227993005_Classification_and_Regression_Tree_Methods/links/004635241a5885c605000000.pdf.
28. Lewis RJ. An introduction to classification and regression tree (CART) analysis. 2000. Available at: http://citeseerx.ist.psu.edu/viewdoc/download?doi=10.1.1.95.4103&rep=rep1&type=pdf. Accessed June 1, 2015.
29. Cheema JR. Some general guidelines for choosing missing data handling methods in educational research regular articles. J Mod Appl Stat Methods 2014;13(2):53–75.
30. Dong Y, Peng CJ. Principled missing data methods for researchers. Springerplus 2013;2(1):222.
31. Sterne JAC, Carlin JB, Royston P, et al. Multiple imputation for missing data in epidemiological and clinical research: potential and pitfalls. Br Med J 2009; 338:b2393.

Randomized Trials, Meta-Analyses, and Systematic Reviews: Using Examples from Rheumatology

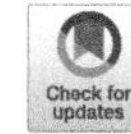

Janet E. Pope, MD, MPH, FRCPC[a,*], Glen S. Hazlewood, MD, PhD[b,c]

KEYWORDS

- Randomized controlled trial • Meta-analysis • Network meta-analysis
- Systematic review • Quality • Inclusion criteria • Blinding • Rheumatic diseases

KEY POINTS

- Randomized controlled trials should follow established methodology and be registered.
- Sample size calculations are based on primary outcomes and possibly some key secondary outcomes.
- Meta-analyses provide summary estimates of a treatment effect (benefits or side effects) across all trials.
- Network meta-analyses allow for comparisons between different treatments, even if they have not been directly compared in a randomized trial.

INTRODUCTION

This article introduces contemporary ideas and standards for clinical research in rheumatology for randomized trials, systematic reviews, and meta-analyses. Various definitions, trial designs, and illustrations are provided within rheumatic diseases research.

CONFOUNDING

When treatments are used in clinical practice, there are many factors that influence our decision to use a particular treatment. In rheumatoid arthritis (RA), for example, the

---

Disclosure: J.E. Pope has no potential conflict of interest but consults for many pharmaceutical companies. G.S. Hazlewood has no potential conflict of interest to declare. G.S. Hazlewood is supported by a CIHR New Investigator Salary Award and The Arthritis Society Young Investigator Salary Award.
[a] Rheumatology, University of Western Ontario, St. Joseph's Health Care, D2, 268 Grosvenor Street, London, Ontario N6A 4V2, Canada; [b] Department of Medicine, University of Calgary, 1820 Richmond Road SW, Calgary, Alberta T2T 5C7, Canada; [c] Department of Community Health Sciences, University of Calgary, 1820 Richmond Road SW, Calgary, Alberta T2T 5C7, Canada
* Corresponding author.
E-mail address: Janet.pope@sjhc.london.on.ca

Rheum Dis Clin N Am 44 (2018) 295–305
https://doi.org/10.1016/j.rdc.2018.01.006 rheumatic.theclinics.com
0889-857X/18/

selection of a treatment is dependent on patient factors, such as disease activity, as well as patient and physician preference.[1,2] If these variables are also associated with the outcomes of interest, and are not on the causal pathway, then they are referred to as confounders. For example, patients with higher disease activity may be more likely to receive intensive treatment. Simply comparing the treatment outcomes of the "intensive" versus "nonintensive" groups will be biased, as the patient groups are inherently different.

Dealing with confounding is perhaps the biggest challenge of clinical research on interventions. Observational studies address this by measuring and adjusting for potential confounders; however, investigators may be unaware of confounders or they may be difficult to measure. The strength of randomized controlled trials (RCTs) is that by randomly assigning patients to groups, they ensure that the patient groups are similar across potential confounders, both measured and unmeasured. For this reason, RCTs have been considered the gold standard for evaluating the effects of interventions. RCTs are thought to be higher levels of evidence than nonrandomized/observational studies (**Box 1**).[3]

RANDOMIZED CONTROLLED TRIALS

Randomization

There are necessary procedures required for the conduct of high-quality RCTs. First, there is randomization, which helps to reduce confounding, by allowing for chance allocation of patients (subjects) to one treatment or another. The randomization procedure should not allow for anyone participating in the trial to manipulate the treatment allocation. Although sealed envelopes can be used, there is a potential for tampering, and central randomization is now the norm. With central randomization, a computer-generated number is given through a central site, often using a call after a patient has consented and passed the screening of inclusion and exclusion criteria.

Box 1
Levels of evidence (from low to high)

Expert Opinion

Case series

Case-control study

Cohort study

Randomized controlled trial (RCT)
- Critically appraised articles
- Evidence synthesis (critically appraised topic)

Systematic Reviews
- Systematic review of case series, registries, cohorts
- Meta-analysis of RCTs
- Network meta-analysis of RCTs

Indented items are more recent additions to studies on levels of evidence. This is only a guide, as some RCTs may be of poor quality and small and some systematic reviews may not include many studies. A RCT may have stronger evidence than a systematic review of case series.

Data from Walden University Library. Evidence-Based Practice Research: Levels of Evidence Pyramid. Evidence Levels of evidence pyramid. Secondary Levels of evidence pyramid. Available at: http://academicguides.waldenu.edu/healthevidence/evidencepyramid. Accessed February 6,2018.

Randomization does not need to be a 50/50 chance of treatment or placebo, but can be varied. For instance, in early-phase trials, there may be several doses of a drug being tested, and randomization may be every 4 subjects: 3 people on active treatment (1 person for each dose) and 1 person on placebo, yielding a 3-to-1 chance of active to placebo.

With completely random assignment of patients, there is a risk that one group will, through chance, have too many or too few patients. This will not bias the results, but may lead to a study that is underpowered, particularly when trials have few patients per arm. For this reason, randomization is often done in blocks. If randomization is done 1:1 and conducted in blocks of 6, then every block of 6 patients will have 3 patients assigned to each group. If the first 3 patients are randomly assigned to the first group, then the next 3 will be automatically assigned to the second. This approach can potentially lead to study investigators predicting allocation assignment, which would bias the randomization process. As such, the blocks are typically varied and randomly chosen (eg, variable block sizes of 4 and 6 patients).

Stratification

For large trials with several sites, randomization may need to be stratified by site or country to have approximately equal numbers enrolled in the strata if there could be differences in treatment. For instance, systemic lupus erythematosus trials will have country differences, as more patients receive background corticosteroids in Europe compared with North America and conversely North America uses more background immunosuppression.[4] There also may be stratification on an important variable, such as rheumatoid factor (RF) positivity. This could be the case in rituximab trials in RA, in which the response to treatment is better if the RF is positive.[5,6]

Bias

Randomization reduces bias due to confounding, but there are several other potential sources of bias in an RCT, even when randomization is done well. A selection bias exists if the population under study is not chosen at random from the target population. For example, if only adherent patients are randomized, the estimation of the treatment effect may be biased. This may be due to the adherence itself, or because adherence is often related to other factors that can impact treatment outcomes. Nonadherent patients also may lack a reimbursement plan and cannot afford other treatments. Other types of bias include the following: reporting bias (not reporting negative outcomes), publication bias (negative trials are less likely to be published and take longer to publish), or survivor bias (patients doing poorly drop out, which may be different between groups, such as with more patients in the placebo arm having treatment failure or more in the active having serious adverse events). There can be analytical or statistical bias if the patients who drop out are not accounted for. This is especially important in long trials (such as a 2-year study with D-penicillamine vs placebo in systemic sclerosis)[7] or a study with a mandatory escape if patients are not achieving a certain improvement before the primary end point, as was the case in an RCT of certolizumab pegol in RA.[8]

Blinding

Blinding is also known as masking. Blinding is important, as knowledge of the treatment assignment may bias the findings.[9] This may occur through influencing the delivery of the intervention, follow-up, or outcome assessment. For example, if a physician knows a patient with RA is in the control arm, the physician may be more likely to consider a joint tender or swollen, and more likely to use adjunctive treatments allowed by the trial (eg, nonsteroidal anti-inflammatory drugs, corticosteroids) or withdraw the patient from the trial.

The bias introduced by a lack of blinding can impact any outcome, as it may influence the delivery of the intervention. However, the anticipated impact of unblinding also depends on the outcome being assessed.[10] Patient-reported or physician-reported outcomes will be most susceptible to bias. Objective outcomes, such as radiographic damage, will be less susceptible to bias, particularly if the outcome assessors are blinded. It is important that clinical trials report exactly who is and is not blinded, as this is important in assessing the validity of the findings.[11]

There are instances in which blinding is not feasible or unethical. Some studies are single blinded, where only the subject (or investigator) is unaware of treatment allocation. In a trial of surgery versus no surgery for knee osteoarthritis, the patient knew treatment allocation but the assessor was blinded.[12] In a trial of autologous stem cell transplantation in active systemic sclerosis, this treatment was compared with cyclophosphamide.[13,14] Blinding also may be difficult if active treatment has a fast effect, such as dropping c-reactive protein quickly, such as with several biologics or if there is a common side effect on active treatment. Often a pharmacist at each site is unblinded to prepare a drug if it is an intravenous infusion and there may be another person involved in the trial who sees the laboratory reports for safety but also to maintain investigator blinding of the inflammatory markers.

In an unblinded trial, it is important to consider the potential impact of this in the interpretation of the findings. A placebo effect can be quite striking. In 2 RCTs of vertebroplasty for acute osteoporotic compression fractures, investigators went to great lengths to ensure adequate blinding of patients.[15,16] This included the use of sham procedures, including ensuring patients in the control could smell the same noxious cement agent. The findings were dramatic. Although prior observational studies had suggested a large effect from vertebroplasty,[17] the RCTs essentially showed no difference between vertebroplasty and the sham procedure.

In some cases, a trial may be unblinded, but the expected direction of the bias would tend to support the conclusion of the trial. For example, a recent unblinded trial compared tapering treatment to usual care in patients with RA who were in sustained remission.[18] The investigators postulated that the lack of blinding would be expected to result in a greater detection of treatment flares in the intervention arm. Given the results showed treatment tapering was noninferior to usual care for major flares, the investigators postulated that, if the trial were blinded, tapering would still be expected to be noninferior; the direction of the bias is expected to favor the control arm.[18]

Choice of Comparator

The choice of comparator in an RCT requires careful consideration and can vary substantially. With new treatments, a placebo comparator is used to ensure the drug has an effect over no treatment. A placebo has no active ingredients. It is supposed to look, feel, smell, and taste identical to the active comparator. Some trials have difficulty with a placebo as the active drug, such as a biologic is a protein and slightly more viscous than the placebo. Alternatively, the control treatment can be an active treatment, or an add-on to standard of care. RA trials frequently compare with a placebo, such as in methotrexate (MTX)-inadequate responders in which a placebo is added to background MTX. Examples of the different types of comparators can be seen in clinical trials of a recently approved therapy for RA. Trials of tofacitinib have compared 2 doses of the drug with placebo in MTX-inadequate responders[19]; tofacitinib monotherapy versus MTX in MTX-naive patients[20]; tofacitinib added to various disease-modifying drugs[21]; tofacitinib used in biologic-inadequate responders[22];

tofacitinib used as monotherapy[23]; tofacitinib added to MTX; or tofacitinib monotherapy against an active comparator (adalimumab) added to MTX or in a noninferiority design.[24]

Study Design

Most RCTs are parallel where each participant is in one group. Other designs are less common, such as crossover trials, in which a treatment is allocated and after a certain time the subject is switched to the other treatment in random order, with or without a washout. This design has been frequently used in Raynaud trials.[25] There are other types of trials, such as cluster design, where, for example, a geographic area is randomized. A factorial design can be used when 2 interventions are studied (eg, randomizing patients to rituximab [2 doses] or placebo, and then randomizing also to concomitant oral, intravenous corticosteroids or both).[6] This can allow for comparisons in more treatment groups and to determine the added effect of another intervention.

Most trials are designed to demonstrate that an intervention is superior to the control group (superiority). The control in these cases is usually a placebo or standard of care and the intervention is active treatment or an add-on to standard of care. When 2 active treatments are studied, such as tofacitinib versus adalimumab or baricitinib versus adalimumab, the design is often noninferiority.[26] Noninferiority assumes that one (new) treatment is no worse than the other (established) treatment. Interestingly, in the study protocol of the baricitinib versus adalimumab trial, if noninferiority occurred, there was a hierarchy of analyses to also determine subsequently if superiority of one active drug could be determined compared with the other.[26] Equivalence studies are rare and test that the interventions are indistinguishable from one another. The latter could be done if one intervention was equivalent but less costly.

Inclusion and Exclusion Criteria

Most protocols have several inclusion and exclusion criteria. Inclusion criteria are typically based on active disease, the proper diagnosis, and an age range, whereas exclusion criteria are typically based on safety considerations and inclusion of only a specific population. These criteria can affect the generalizability of the study. Most trials have unnecessary exclusions that also affect the feasibility of enrolling patients.[27] Occasionally there is an upper limit for randomizing a certain group of patients. In patients with RA, those experienced on tumor necrosis factor (TNF) inhibitors are more difficult to treat (have attenuated responses) compare with those who are TNF inhibitor naïve. This has occurred in some RA trials, whereby the percentage of TNF inhibitors exposed was limited to a small proportion, such as 20% to 30% of the total sample size.[28,29]

Analyses

The statistical analyses should be written in advance, with the primary and secondary outcomes and analysis plan outlined. With a randomized trial, the primary analysis is typically straightforward, as confounding has been addressed by randomization. However, adjustment for covariates that may be distributed unevenly due to chance is often done, and may increase the power of the clinical trial. The analysis plan also should state how missing data will be handled. Sometimes all dropouts are considered failures even if they are responding but stop a medication because of a side effect.

For trials designed to demonstrate a difference between trial arms (ie, a superiority trial), it is standard practice to use an intention-to-treat analysis. In an intention-to-treat analysis, all patients are analyzed according to the arm in which they were randomized, regardless of which intervention they actually receive. This is a more conservative approach, and minimizes the chance of a Type I error, concluding there is a difference when there actually is not. It also ensures greater generalizability of the findings, as all patients are included. There are modified intent-to-treat analyses in which only patients who receive at least 1 dose of a study drug are analyzed.

In comparison, an on-treatment analysis is typically used for noninferiority trials.[30] This again is a more conservative approach, as the intention is to conclude that the 2 treatment approaches are sufficiently similar. Consider a situation in which no (or very few) patients actually adhered to the intervention. In this setting, the outcomes of the 2 groups would be the same (or very similar), outside of chance variability. With an intention-to-treat analysis, one may erroneously conclude that the treatment approaches are similar.

Sample Size Calculation

When designing a trial, it is important to enroll enough patients so that the results will either prove or disprove the hypothesis was a sufficient degree of certainty. This is determined usually at a 95% probability (P = .05). The sample size calculation will depend on the estimated outcomes in the active treatment and control groups, the randomization approach (eg, 1:1 vs 2:1), and the hypothesis being evaluated. The sample size is then inflated by, for example, 20% if there are suspected to be 20% dropouts during the study. There are online calculators for sample size calculations.

Consent

For most trials, a patient is explained what the study involves and signs a consent after reading a letter of information. This occurs before any trial procedure is conducted. In these trials, there should not be any treatment administered without consent. Often trials report that full written consent was obtained, but it is more accurate to state that the trial was explained, questions were answered, and the patient provided written consent, as it is difficult to ascertain if full consent was obtained due to the complicated letters of information in trials that are now routinely more than 15 pages long.[31] There are rarely studies whereby consent may be waived. Examples include emergency situations in which patients are unable to consent and receive 2 different standards of care (which is not the case in rheumatology trials), or with certain cluster randomized trials in which all the patients in a region receive a type of care compared with another region in which the care would be considered routine or standard.

Trial Quality

The quality of clinical trials can be assessed using a number of approaches. The Cochrane Risk of Bias tool is commonly used.[10] With this approach, reviewers rate the risk of bias of a randomized trial as "high," "unclear," or "low," across several different domains (eg, random sequence generation, allocation concealment). An overall judgment regarding the risk of bias also can be made. Other scales for rating the risk of bias also exist. With the Jadad scale, trials are scored out of 5 based on randomization (up to 2 points), blinding (up to 2 points), and how dropouts are analyzed (1 point).[32]

Registration of Trials

Most RCTs will not be published if they have not been registered before the conduct of the trial. This is a way to check that the reporting of trials follows the analysis plan. A common site to register a trial is ClinicalTrials.gov.

Ethical Considerations

A clinical trial is a special circumstance, and there may be ethical considerations. Trials should be large enough to demonstrate a true effect if there is one, but not so large that more patients are exposed to unnecessary harms or to ineffective treatment (the latter in the placebo arm). Overpowering of trials is common in RA treatment trials.[33] This may be done partially to determine if secondary outcomes are different between the treatment groups (such as American College of Rheumatology 70% (ACR70) response criteria), or to do subset analyses (eg, TNF inhibitor failures vs TNF inhibitor–naïve patients in RA trials or MTX users vs nonusers in psoriatic arthritis trials).[33]

Phases of Trials

New therapeutic agents typically progress through multiple stages of clinical trials. Phase I trials are dose ranging and often conducted on healthy volunteers looking for major safety signals. Phase II is conducted on patients and tries to determine efficacy and studies safety and side effects. Phase III is large and tries to determine precise effect on efficacy at a specific dose or doses and safety. These are larger trials and the drug is assumed to have a positive treatment effect. Phase IV studies are after a drug is approved (post marketing) and may study longer-term benefit, other side effects, and possibly study other populations (eg, with more comorbidities, other background medications).

SYSTEMATIC REVIEWS AND META-ANALYSES OF RANDOMIZED CONTROLLED TRIALS

The goal with a systematic review is to answer a specific research question by summarizing all relevant literature. For questions related to effects of interventions, systematic reviews are often limited to RCTs. After identifying all relevant existing literature, the included studies are then critically appraised for their quality and relevance to the clinical question. If the studies are of sufficient quality and similarity in their methods, then the results of the studies can be pooled in a meta-analysis to determine a summary estimate of the treatment effect for any outcome.

When the trials are pooled in a meta-analysis, the main assumption is that any effect modifiers are balanced across the trials. An effect modifier is any variable that affects the relative effects of 2 treatments. This is important to distinguish from prognostic variables that impact the absolute probability of an outcome, but do so equally to both treatment arms. For example, patients with higher disease severity will typically have worse outcomes. Disease severity will be an effect modifier only if the difference in outcomes between 2 treatments (treatment effect) varies with disease severity. If effect modifiers are not balanced across the trials, there is said to be heterogeneity. For instance, MTX-naïve patients should be more treatment responsive than those who have failed MTX or a previous biologic. These groups are typically analyzed separately in meta-analyses.[34–36]

Evaluating the trials for potential heterogeneity is a critical step when deciding whether to pool trials and requires knowledge of the disease and condition, as well as application of common sense. Trials should be sufficiently similar in their design, such that potential effect modifiers are similar across trials and a pooled estimate could be sensibly applied to the target population. Statistical measures, such as I^2, can be used to compare the variability of results between trials to gauge how likely any observed variation was due to chance.[37] Although these tests are useful, it is essential not to rely on them exclusively for deciding whether to pool trials.[10] To illustrate this, consider an extreme example. Suppose American College of Rheumatology 50% (ACR50) response criteria were similar between a trial of a TNF inhibitor in patients with RA and another trial in patients with psoriatic arthritis. If these studies were pooled, the statistical heterogeneity would be low. However, it is clearly not appropriate to pool the results, as the summary estimate would not be meaningful.

NETWORK META-ANALYSIS

A major challenge with a traditional meta-analysis is that the trials often do not address the clinical questions in which we are interested. Trials often compare treatments to placebo, whereas we are interested in the comparative benefits and harms between active treatments. Even if trials with an active comparator have been performed, they are typically fewer in number than the placebo-controlled trials and, like any trial, may have important biases. Thus, relying solely on these active-controlled trials also may not provide the best estimates of the underlying true treatment effects.

Network meta-analyses provide a mechanism for considering the entire body of available evidence to make comparisons between all treatments of interest.[38] They consider both direct evidence (head-to-head trials) and indirect evidence to provide comparisons between any 2 treatments. Indirect evidence exists when 2 treatments have not been directly compared with each other, but have both been compared with the same treatment (eg, placebo). Longer chains of indirect evidence are also possible if there is more than 1 treatment linking the treatments (eg, trials of A-B, B-C, and C-D providing indirect evidence between treatments A and D). A network meta-analysis considers the entire body of evidence to provide comparisons between all treatments. As such, their use has been growing in popularity.

ASSUMPTIONS AND POTENTIAL BIASES WITH NETWORK META-ANALYSIS

The main theory underlying a network meta-analysis is a logical argument. If we know the true treatment effect for treatment A compared with treatment B, and treatment B compared with treatment C, then we know the true treatment effect of treatment A compared with treatment C. Error introduced in the *measurement* of the true treatment effects, either systematic or random, may bias the results, but this is a limitation of any study or meta-analysis. Minimizing the potential biases of a network meta-analysis requires an understanding of the assumptions required.[39]

The main assumption made when pooling trials in a traditional meta-analysis is that any effect modifiers are balanced across the trials. The additional assumption with a network meta-analysis is that the effect modifiers are balanced across different comparisons.[40] There are 2 possibilities in which this is true. First, effect modifiers may be balanced across all studies, regardless of the comparison made. In this case, the heterogeneity of any traditional meta-analysis would be low, and a network meta-analysis will yield unbiased estimates. In the second case, the effect modifiers are somewhat unbalanced in the direct comparisons, but the imbalance is similar across different comparisons. In this case, there is heterogeneity within each direct comparison, but because it is similar across comparisons, the estimates in a network meta-analysis will not be subject to any additional biases other than those required in pooling the direct evidence. If the studies in the direct comparisons were judged to be appropriate to pool, then it would be equally appropriate to perform a network meta-analysis.[40] An example of a network meta-analysis after treatment with MTX in RA was recently published to determine the relative ranking of several post-MTX treatment possibilities that have been studied in RA.[36,41]

The final case is one in which the effect modifiers are unbalanced across the direct evidence for different comparisons.[40] For example, if disease activity was an effect modifier and trials of treatment A and B were performed in patients with low disease activity, and trials of treatments B and C were performed in patients with high disease activity, then pooling the comparisons would yield biased estimates for a comparison of treatment A and C. In this case, there is said to be inconsistency or intransitivity in the evidence, as the indirect evidence would differ from a direct head-to-head trial of treatments A and C.

SUMMARY/DISCUSSION

This article demonstrates new ideas in the conduct of RCTs, meta-analyses, and larger systematic reviews, such as network meta-analyses. The design of these higher-order studies has changed and continues to evolve as comparative statistical tests and standards vary. Illustrations with respect to rheumatology provide examples of types of RCTs and systematic reviews.

REFERENCES

1. Harris JA, Bykerk VP, Hitchon CA, et al. Determining best practices in early rheumatoid arthritis by comparing differences in treatment at sites in the Canadian Early Arthritis Cohort. J Rheumatol 2013;40:1823–30.
2. Hazlewood GS, Thorne JC, Pope JE, et al. The comparative effectiveness of oral versus subcutaneous methotrexate for the treatment of early rheumatoid arthritis. Ann Rheum Dis 2016;75(6):1003–8.
3. Levels of evidence pyramid. Secondary levels of evidence pyramid. Available at: http://academicguides.waldenu.edu/healthevidence/evidencepyramid. Accessed February 6, 2018.
4. Furie R, Petri M, Zamani O, et al. A phase III, randomized, placebo-controlled study of belimumab, a monoclonal antibody that inhibits B lymphocyte stimulator, in patients with systemic lupus erythematosus. Arthritis Rheum 2011;63:3918–30.
5. Cohen SB, Emery P, Greenwald MW, et al. Rituximab for rheumatoid arthritis refractory to anti-tumor necrosis factor therapy: results of a multicenter, randomized, double-blind, placebo-controlled, phase III trial evaluating primary efficacy and safety at twenty-four weeks. Arthritis Rheum 2006;54:2793–806.
6. Emery P, Fleischmann R, Filipowicz-Sosnowska A, et al. The efficacy and safety of rituximab in patients with active rheumatoid arthritis despite methotrexate treatment: results of a phase IIB randomized, double-blind, placebo-controlled, dose-ranging trial. Arthritis Rheum 2006;54:1390–400.
7. Clements PJ, Furst DE, Wong WK, et al. High-dose versus low-dose D-penicillamine in early diffuse systemic sclerosis: analysis of a two-year, double-blind, randomized, controlled clinical trial. Arthritis Rheum 1999;42:1194–203.
8. Keystone E, Heijde D, Mason D Jr, et al. Certolizumab pegol plus methotrexate is significantly more effective than placebo plus methotrexate in active rheumatoid arthritis: findings of a fifty-two-week, phase III, multicenter, randomized, double-blind, placebo-controlled, parallel-group study. Arthritis Rheum 2008;58:3319–29.
9. Karanicolas PJ, Farrokhyar F, Bhandari M. Practical tips for surgical research: blinding: who, what, when, why, how? Can J Surg 2010;53:345–8.
10. Higgins JP, Altman DG, Gotzsche PC, et al. The Cochrane collaboration's tool for assessing risk of bias in randomised trials. BMJ 2011;343:d5928.
11. Moher D, Hopewell S, Schulz KF, et al. CONSORT 2010 explanation and elaboration: updated guidelines for reporting parallel group randomised trials. BMJ 2010;340:c869.
12. Kirkley A, Birmingham TB, Litchfield RB, et al. A randomized trial of arthroscopic surgery for osteoarthritis of the knee. N Engl J Med 2008;359:1097–107.

13. Hung EW, Mayes MD, Sharif R, et al. Gastric antral vascular ectasia and its clinical correlates in patients with early diffuse systemic sclerosis in the SCOT trial. J Rheumatol 2013;40:455–60.
14. van Laar JM, Farge D, Sont JK, et al. Autologous hematopoietic stem cell transplantation vs intravenous pulse cyclophosphamide in diffuse cutaneous systemic sclerosis: a randomized clinical trial. JAMA 2014;311:2490–8.
15. Buchbinder R, Osborne RH, Ebeling PR, et al. A randomized trial of vertebroplasty for painful osteoporotic vertebral fractures. N Engl J Med 2009;361: 557–68.
16. Kallmes DF, Comstock BA, Heagerty PJ, et al. A randomized trial of vertebroplasty for osteoporotic spinal fractures. N Engl J Med 2009;361:569–79.
17. Ploeg WT, Veldhuizen AG, The B, et al. Percutaneous vertebroplasty as a treatment for osteoporotic vertebral compression fractures: a systematic review. Eur Spine J 2006;15:1749–58.
18. van Herwaarden N, van der Maas A, Minten MJ, et al. Disease activity guided dose reduction and withdrawal of adalimumab or etanercept compared with usual care in rheumatoid arthritis: open label, randomised controlled, non-inferiority trial. BMJ 2015;350:h1389.
19. Kremer JM, Cohen S, Wilkinson BE, et al. A phase IIb dose-ranging study of the oral JAK inhibitor tofacitinib (CP-690,550) versus placebo in combination with background methotrexate in patients with active rheumatoid arthritis and an inadequate response to methotrexate alone. Arthritis Rheum 2012;64:970–81.
20. Fleischmann RM, Huizinga TW, Kavanaugh AF, et al. Efficacy of tofacitinib monotherapy in methotrexate-naive patients with early or established rheumatoid arthritis. RMD Open 2016;2:e000262.
21. Kremer J, Li ZG, Hall S, et al. Tofacitinib in combination with nonbiologic disease-modifying antirheumatic drugs in patients with active rheumatoid arthritis: a randomized trial. Ann Intern Med 2013;159:253–61.
22. Charles-Schoeman C, Burmester G, Nash P, et al. Efficacy and safety of tofacitinib following inadequate response to conventional synthetic or biological disease-modifying antirheumatic drugs. Ann Rheum Dis 2016;75:1293–301.
23. Fleischmann R, Cutolo M, Genovese MC, et al. Phase IIb dose-ranging study of the oral JAK inhibitor tofacitinib (CP-690,550) or adalimumab monotherapy versus placebo in patients with active rheumatoid arthritis with an inadequate response to disease-modifying antirheumatic drugs. Arthritis Rheum 2012;64: 617–29.
24. Fleischmann R, Mysler E, Hall S, et al. Efficacy and safety of tofacitinib monotherapy, tofacitinib with methotrexate, and adalimumab with methotrexate in patients with rheumatoid arthritis (ORAL Strategy): a phase 3b/4, double-blind, head-to-head, randomised controlled trial. Lancet 2017;390:457–68.
25. Thompson AE, Pope JE. Calcium channel blockers for primary Raynaud's phenomenon: a meta-analysis. Rheumatology (Oxford) 2005;44:145–50.
26. Taylor PC, Keystone EC, van der Heijde D, et al. Baricitinib versus placebo or adalimumab in rheumatoid arthritis. N Engl J Med 2017;376:652–62.
27. Yuen SY, Pope JE. Learning from past mistakes: assessing trial quality, power and eligibility in non-renal systemic lupus erythematosus randomized controlled trials. Rheumatology (Oxford) 2008;47:1367–72.
28. Pope JE, Haraoui B, Rampakakis E, et al. Treating to a target in established active rheumatoid arthritis patients receiving a tumor necrosis factor inhibitor: results from a real-world cluster-randomized adalimumab trial. Arthritis Care Res (Hoboken) 2013;65:1401–9.

29. Weinblatt ME, Fleischmann R, Huizinga TW, et al. Efficacy and safety of certolizumab pegol in a broad population of patients with active rheumatoid arthritis: results from the REALISTIC phase IIIb study. Rheumatology (Oxford) 2012;51: 2204–14.
30. Matilde Sanchez M, Chen X. Choosing the analysis population in non-inferiority studies: per protocol or intent-to-treat. Stat Med 2006;25:1169–81.
31. Pope JE, Tingey DP, Arnold JM, et al. Are subjects satisfied with the informed consent process? A survey of research participants. J Rheumatol 2003;30: 815–24.
32. Jadad AR, Moore RA, Carroll D, et al. Assessing the quality of reports of randomized clinical trials: is blinding necessary? Control Clin Trials 1996;17:1–12.
33. Celik S, Yazici Y, Yazici H. Are sample sizes of randomized clinical trials in rheumatoid arthritis too large? Eur J Clin Invest 2014;44:1034–44.
34. Singh JA, Hossain A, Tanjong Ghogomu E, et al. Biologics or tofacitinib for people with rheumatoid arthritis unsuccessfully treated with biologics: a systematic review and network meta-analysis. Cochrane Database Syst Rev 2017;(3):CD012591.
35. Singh JA, Hossain A, Mudano AS, et al. Biologics or tofacitinib for people with rheumatoid arthritis naive to methotrexate: a systematic review and network meta-analysis. Cochrane Database Syst Rev 2017;(5):CD012657.
36. Hazlewood GS, Barnabe C, Tomlinson G, et al. Methotrexate monotherapy and methotrexate combination therapy with traditional and biologic disease modifying anti-rheumatic drugs for rheumatoid arthritis: a network meta-analysis. Cochrane Database Syst Rev 2016;(8):CD010227.
37. Higgins JP, Thompson SG. Quantifying heterogeneity in a meta-analysis. Stat Med 2002;21:1539–58.
38. Jansen JP, Fleurence R, Devine B, et al. Interpreting indirect treatment comparisons and network meta-analysis for health-care decision making: report of the ISPOR task force on indirect treatment comparisons good research practices: part 1. Value Health 2011;14:417–28.
39. Ades A. ISPOR states its position on network meta-analysis. Value Health 2011; 14:414–6.
40. Jansen JP, Naci H. Is network meta-analysis as valid as standard pairwise meta-analysis? It all depends on the distribution of effect modifiers. BMC Med 2013;11:159.
41. Hazlewood GS, Barnabe C, Tomlinson G, et al. Methotrexate monotherapy and methotrexate combination therapy with traditional and biologic disease modifying antirheumatic drugs for rheumatoid arthritis: abridged Cochrane systematic review and network meta-analysis. BMJ 2016;353:i1777.

"Big Data" in Rheumatology

Intelligent Data Modeling Improves the Quality of Imaging Data

Robert B.M. Landewé, MD[a,b,*], Désirée van der Heijde, MD[c]

KEYWORDS

- Imaging • Statistical analysis • Reliability • Variability
- Generalized estimating equations • Generalized linear mixed model

KEY POINTS

- Signal-to-noise ratio is a valuable concept in imaging to describe warranted effects (change, signal) in relation to unwarranted erratic effects (noise). For most imaging techniques, signal-to-noise ratio is poor.
- In cohort studies and trials, precautions are taken in the process of obtaining and scoring images to avoid spurious (biased) results. These precautions include protocolled image acquisition, use of multiple readers, and concealed (random) time order.
- Imaging studies in trials and long-term extension studies thereof and in observational studies often include different read sessions. These read sessions may include different time points, so that the same time points of each patient are scored multiple times by different readers and in several read sessions.
- Multilevel longitudinal data analysis making use of all individual data of all read sessions may account for correlated data at different levels, assures optimal data usage, and may lead to increased precision and statistical power.

INTRODUCTION

Imaging is an integral part of studying the course and outcome of inflammatory diseases in rheumatology. The topic is broad. Imaging may help to get an impression about the activity of the disease at a certain point: assessment of disease activity.

Disclosure Statement: The authors do not have any commercial or financial conflict of interest to disclose in relation to the work described here, nor have they received funding for the work described in this article.
[a] Amsterdam Rheumatology and Clinical Immunology Center, Amsterdam, the Netherlands; [b] Zuyderland Medical Center Heerlen, Heerlen, the Netherlands; [c] Leiden University Medical Center, Leiden, the Netherlands
* Corresponding author. Department of Rheumatology and Clinical immunology, Amsterdam Rheumatology and Immunology Center, Academic Medical Center, PO Box 2260, Amsterdam 1100DD, the Netherlands.
E-mail address: landewe@rlandewe.nl

Rheum Dis Clin N Am 44 (2018) 307–315
https://doi.org/10.1016/j.rdc.2018.01.007
rheumatic.theclinics.com
0889-857X/18/

But imaging data may also visualize and quantify the consequences of chronic inflammation over time: assessment of structural changes. In terms of outcome measurement, disease activity (and imaging data reflecting it) is volatile and reversible and therefore considered a process measure, whereas structural change is permanent and (largely) irreversible and therefore considered an outcome measure.

Imaging may be used in studies for many reasons: in randomized, controlled trials (RCTs) to investigate some aspects of tested drugs, in observational studies to investigate predictive associations and disease outcomes, or in studies investigating the pathophysiology of a disease.

It is good to realize that the term imaging entails the technique itself and a (quantifying) score reflecting the result. Both technical factors (equipment and technicians, processing of images) and factors related to scoring (methodologic factors) determine the quality of the imaging product (usually a score).

These scores are sensitive to many disturbing factors. In clinical practice, the merits of the technique are often overstated ("the new technique is highly sensitive"), and the limitations regarding reliability are downplayed. In clinical studies, there is more appreciation for methodologic fallacies and for analytical requirements. This article describes integrated analysis of imaging data as an example to better deal with imaging data against a background of well-known and inherent methodologic fallacies of imaging.

CONCEPT OF SIGNAL-TO-NOISE RATIO

Signal-to-noise ratio is a scientific concept used in electronic engineering that compares the level of a desired signal to the level of background noise. Used metaphorically, it may refer to the ratio of useful information over false or irrelevant data, for instance, in the interpretation of imaging results (or other clinical assessments). It is obvious that imaging data, such as data on radiographic progression in patients with rheumatoid arthritis, combine useful data (the signal) and irrelevant data (the noise). Imaging data classically have a rather poor signal-to-noise ratio for several reasons. Here are described 3 sources of imaging variability using an example of radiographic progression in rheumatoid arthritis (RA).

The measure of radiographic changes, scored on consecutive radiographs of hands and feet obtained from patients with RA, is currently considered the regulatory standard for proving if a new drug has the ability to slow or stop the occurrence or progression of structural changes.[1] Abnormalities (erosions, joint space narrowing) are subtle and equivocal (judgmental), and changes over time are even subtler. This situation requires optimal imaging quality and consistent quality over time for proper comparison and interpretation. Subtle changes in positioning, exposure, windowing, and others (noise) may jeopardize a proper interpretation, and changes that are caused by technical flaws can easily be interpreted as true changes (signal). This type of noise can hardly be distinguished from true signal. In the context of a randomized clinical trial, it is to be expected that technical noise is a random process that works similarly in both treatment arms and that the true treatment effect (the nominator of the signal-to-noise ratio) is not affected. But random variation (noise) will still affect the denominator of the signal-to-noise ratio, and thus the statistical power to detect a difference between treatment arms. It is obvious that in uncontrolled observational studies, the effects of noise are not erased, and expectations of readers about the most probable (or wished) change may influence the interpretation of an imaging result (expectation bias). Examples in the rheumatologic literature (with commercial connotations) are paramount but not always recognized.

In addition to technical noise, there is random variation invoked by the reader who judges the images and provides a score.[2] The random variation is best visualized by test-retest experiments in which the same reader scores the same images twice without notice. Such experiments consistently prove that 80% to 90% of the variability in scoring observed between cases constitutes true variation between patients but 10% to 20% of it is owing to random (intrareader) error. Intrareader variability affects the denominator and deflates the signal-to-noise ratio.

A third source of variability is interreader variability.[2] Two readers who provide a change score on a pair (2 time points) of radiographs in the same patient hardly, if ever, arrive at exactly the same result. Readers may be conservative (they only score change if they are very certain) or sensitive (they score change already at a far lower threshold of certainty), and even if similar personalities are paired, results may differ substantially.

Technical variability, intrareader variability, and interreader variability are different sources of variability. They are hard to distinguish but together constitute a significant level of noise compared with an often subtle true signal. This situation complicates the statistical detection of a treatment effect in an RCT. In fact, this means that the interpretation of an imaging result (either in a single patient in clinical practice or in a group of patients in an RCT) should always include a proper consideration of the signal-to-noise ratio. In practice, this belief is sharply at odds with the common clinical belief that an imaging result is the product of technical innovation and should therefore gain more credit than any type of clinical data. The uncontested expansion of ultrasound scan in clinical rheumatology testifies to such a belief.

METHODOLOGIC PRECAUTIONS TO CONSTRAIN THE EFFECTS OF NOISE

Statisticians working for regulatory bodies (more than clinical researchers) are well aware of the inherent shortcomings of imaging data. They have implemented a set of measures aiming at a better elimination of the effects of noise in the interpretation of drug effects. Below are measures that aim at avoiding the spurious effects of noise in clinical trial settings.

1. Images should be obtained under protocolled conditions. These protocols prescribe standard procedures to be used all over the world to avoid too much technical noise. This is one of the reasons that radiographic progression—although being a rather old-fashioned technique compared with MRI, ultrasound scan, and positron emission tomography—is still the regulatory standard for measuring radiographic progression in RCTs.
2. Images should be scored by at least 2 readers. This procedure (and derivations thereof) can be considered an elaboration of the central limit theorem stating that the average of scores of multiple readers gives a more truthful representation of true change than the score of 1 incidental reader.[3] It likely gives a better approximation of the truth and provides better insight into interreader variability that can be assessed by reliability statistics (intra–class correlation coefficients, κ statistics, and smallest detectable change).[2]
3. Images should be scored double blindly. *Double blind* means that readers not only are blind to the treatment allocated to a patient in an RCT when they score the images, but also that they are not aware of the time order of the images that they see on their screens. Although this latter requirement effectively avoids expectations (eg, wishful thinking) influencing the change score, it may be at the cost of the strength of the signal. We know that reading

with known time order results in the detection of more change while not increasing bias.[4]

Many have asked why only imaging is subjected to these rigorous precautions, as clinical assessments may suffer similar limitations if not worse.[5] This finding is true, and there are many explanations (eg, feasibility), but for the purpose of this article, it suffices to state that these precautions importantly add to the credibility of imaging results of clinical trials.

CURRENT IMAGING PRACTICE IN STUDIES

Sponsors developing new treatments in a particular chronic disease and clinical researchers following up with a prospective cohort of patients usually do not want to wait 5 to 10 years before they can analyze their results. They rather split these analyses up into different parts, usually with a different main aim. A sponsor, for instance, is interested in a timely approval of their new drug and wants imaging data to be available at the shortest time interval that is still acceptable for regulatory authorities. In our example of radiographic progression in RA, that interval is usually after a follow-up of at least 6 months. For this purpose, images are read in so-called read sessions (or campaigns), in which 2 time points (random time order unknown to the reader) are compared in 1 session. An analysis of this time interval may serve then to approve a particular new drug if it proves superior over placebo or an active comparator drug.

But trials and cohort-studies usually do not stop after the first interval. and additional study questions may arise and provoke subsequent read sessions (eg, maintenance of effect).

A subsequent read session is always considered a standalone, which means that every subsequent read session will not only include the latest (new) time point, but also a re-read of one or more previous time points. This is also not an unusual practice in observational cohorts of patients. Because of constraints in time and resources, 1 or more time points are frequently excluded in later read sessions. Of note, such a procedure may occur several times in a trial or a cohort study, providing a multitude of data exploring different time points per reading session, as seen in **Table 1**. All scores have been obtained under the same conditions, namely, concealed time order and concealed treatment allocation. Also, because of limitations in the availability of readers over a significant period, readers may differ across (usually not within) read sessions. This means that often in 1 study database, data of different read sessions spanning different timeframes, sometimes including different readers, are available (see **Table 1**; **Table2**).

Table 1
Example of a study with 200 patients starting at baseline and followed up for 36 months and the planning of 4 read sessions, each including different time points

	Time Point				
Read Session	**Baseline**	**6 mo**	**12 mo**	**24 mo**	**36 mo**
First (R1, R2)	X	X	—	—	—
Second (R1, R2)	X	—	X	—	—
Third (R1, R2)	X	X	—	X	—
Fourth (R2, R4, R5)	X	—	X	—	X
Patients in study	200	200	150	100	75

Abbreviation: R, reader.

Table 2
Comparison of the number of scores to be analyzed between a conventional completers-only analysis and a 3-level integrated analysis approach using the patient numbers and the read sessions from Table 1

	Time Point				
Type of Analysis	**Baseline**	**6 mo**	**12 mo**	**24 mo**	**36 mo**
Completers-only analysis with constructed scores	200 scores	X	150 scores	X	75 scores
Three-level integrated analysis using all data	4800 scores	800 scores	900 scores	200 scores	225 scores

Constructed scores: aggregated score per time point based on a decision rule (eg, mean readers' score).

ANALYTICAL DILEMMAS

Investigators have to make a decision about which read sessions to choose for a particular study question. Because the availability of the last time point usually determines the choice for a particular read session, data of previous sessions will usually be ignored (intentional data loss), and the choice of the read sessions is based on the argument that a particular time point score is only present in the last read sessions. While such a choice is completely rational from a logistic standpoint, it implies a preference and introduces a well-known bias that from the principle of methodologic rigor would preferably be avoided: bias by study completion.

A second dilemma that leads to intentional data loss is the use of decision algorithms. Often, investigators rely on consensus among readers. For instance, in case of discrete decisions (positive vs negative) the final verdict is based on an "at least 2 out of 3" decision rule. Such a consensus decision may add to the truthfulness of an individual patient's score, but also ignores the score of the deviating third reader, thus ignoring one source of reader variability. Theoretically, it will depend on the type of study and the research question whether the advantage of a better estimate of the signal will outweigh the disadvantage of ignoring part of the noise. By any means, appreciating full data will be fairer, because it is less influenced by guided decisions.

We have built the argument that imaging data are not free of bias and uncertainty. And we have argued that—appreciating the different sources of bias that may play a role in obtaining imaging scores—it may be preferable to use as much data as possible in obtaining the best estimate for an imaging result (or a derivative of that such as a change score). In the absence of a proper gold standard, the best estimate of the truth will always be the aggregated mean score, appreciating the conditions under which these scores have been obtained.

The final argument to mention is the argument of statistical power. Imaging change scores are often subtle compared with clinical change scores, jeopardizing statistical power to detect small effects. Statistical power is among others dependent on sample size, and using as much data as available will add to it (this is an important argument used by big-data protagonists) even though we are dealing with repeated assessments in the same patients.

AGGREGATING DATA

The simplest way of aggregating data is to combine all available data of all different read sessions and calculate grand mean scores irrespective of data correlation. Such a procedure, although statistically powerful, is fallible for several statistical principles regarding correlated data and may yield spurious results. Different read sessions of different time periods should be considered independent studies within the same study. There are many reasons for this. Readers may score patients differently when they are confronted with 4 instead of 2 time points. Different readers may score the same patient differently. Readers may score differently 5 years earlier than today, for example. In addition, 1 session may include 2 time points (eg, baseline and month 6), whereas a second session may include one other time point (eg, baseline and month 12, but not month 6).

Still, when aggregating the data, the dataset should statistically be considered as a dataset of correlated data (statistical dependence), and precautions should be taken to adjust for correlated data to avoid spurious results.

Different levels of correlation can be distinguished:

1. The first level of correlation is the level of the patient. This means that a patient's score on month 6 can be largely predicted by knowing the same patient's score at baseline (and vice versa). In conventional analyses, this type of correlation is usually adjusted for by simply applying change scores over time (subtract the score at baseline from the score at 6 months to obtain the 6-month change score). In longitudinal statistical models with time as a covariate (see later discussion) change over time is analyzed by obtaining the parameter estimate (regression coefficient) for the covariate time while adjusting for within-patient correlation.
2. The second level of correlation is at the level of the reader. Different readers scoring the same set of images may still arrive at different scores. Although part of this variability can be considered random, the same reader will repeatedly apply the same rule with her own interpretation and will consistently do that in different patients and in different read sessions. A good example is a sensitive reader, who interprets equivocal changes as real changes and scores them accordingly, versus the conservative reader, who only scores changes if they are "crystal clear." *Sensitive* and *conservative* are terms that reflect readers' attitudes, like personality traits, and can be recognized across different studies. In conventional analysis, the spurious effects of between-reader variation are usually eliminated by taking the mean readers' scores in computations. In longitudinal models, these mean scores can and usually will be used for modeling the data, but one may choose to model the individual reader's scores separately and approach the problem as a 2-level model.
3. The third level of correlation is the level of read session. Obviously, there is a high level of statistical dependence across read sessions because they include the same patients and part of the same time points. Still, as argued above, it is different to score 4 sets of images from one patient compared with only 2 sets, and these differences are indeed reflected in (subtly) different scores. In addition, read sessions may be performed several years apart, and the same reader may have increased experience or may have slightly changed her attitude toward scoring changes. The argument becomes entirely clear if over time different readers have been used. Many imaging studies have been analyzed using longitudinal models appreciating the first 2 levels of correlation. But until recently, we have not seen models in which the effects of variability at the third level have been taken into consideration. However, the practice of the investigator making a convenient choice of analyzing only the read session that includes the time points of main interest (often the latest time point) is still most common. It can be argued that this practice leads to unwarranted loss of information, whereas the presence of sophisticated models allows the handling of all available data at once.

MULTILEVEL SOLUTIONS

Longitudinal data analysis implies the proper handling of correlated data to avoid spurious estimates of the effect size (eg, mean change) and variability (eg, 95% confidence interval [CI]). Essentially, 2 types of models are available for analyzing longitudinal data with a multilevel template such as described in this report. These models are generic models, widely available in popular statistical software that is used in industry and academia and can be used to analyze all kinds of longitudinal data. The application propagated here is absolutely not new, as it stems from work in social sciences, econometrics, and education (in which multilevel approaches are paramount). In longitudinal clinical studies, however, multilevel databases are sparsely applied, probably because of interpretational problems. Clinical studies, such as RCTs, focus on fixed effects (eg, the effects of a treatment on an outcome), whereas multilevel studies rather describe (or at least adjust for) random effects (here: effects in a subgroup of patients, effects per read sessions, effects per reader).

The 2 types of modeling that exist are:

1. Generalized estimating equations (GEEs) modeling allows for the correlation between observations without using a particular likelihood for the model that explains the origin of the correlations (correlation structure, or variance-covariance matrix).[6] In fact, GEEs allow the analyst to specify one overall working correlation structure that should suffice across all levels of correlation (eg, 3 levels of correlation). It is therefore rather simple but potentially more sensitive to wrong choices. GEE is said to be most suitable when the investigator is interested in the average response of the population (here: the mean group change over time) rather than in the regression parameters that enable the prediction of effect in a particular subgroup of the population. At first glance, GEE seems less suitable for imaging data with a structure outlined in this report (3 levels of correlation).
2. Generalized linear mixed models (GLMMs) are well known in rheumatology because they allow the proper handling of correlated data, which are so inherent to follow-up studies in patients.[7] These models are also known as *multilevel models* or *mixed models* and are sometimes impurely referred to as *random-effects models*. GLMMs include random effects in the predictor-function, which may help getting insight into the origin of correlations and predict estimates in individual patients or subgroups of patients with a particular baseline characteristic (prediction analysis). GLMMs are computationally far more complex than GEEs, and, unlike GEEs, require the specification of several correlation structures.

EXAMPLES OF 3-LEVEL INTEGRATED ANALYSIS

We have applied integrated 3-level longitudinal data analysis, spanning different read sessions, using different readers, in 2 studies with multiple read sessions in 2 cohorts.

The first cohort was a database with clinical trial data of 2 clinical drug trials (adalimumab), and open-label extensions thereof, spanning 7 read sessions (10 years) of 1 study and 6 read sessions (10 years) of the second study.[8] Both studies analyzed radiographic progression in patients with RA. Both started as drug-registration trials and were extended to 10 years of follow-up. The data were integrated using a 3-level GLMM. The results of the integrated 3-level approach were compared with the results of the conventional 10-year completer's analysis. In general, main effects were not different regardless of the method of analysis. GLMM using all read sessions, however, allowed us to draw reasonably robust conclusions on subgroups of prognostic interest despite rather low numbers of patients per subgroup.

The second (inception) cohort-study delivered data from a nationwide French study (DESIR) including patients with chronic back pain suggestive of axial spondyloarthritis. The main question underlying this prospective cohort study was whether inflammation of the sacroiliac joints measured by MRI would eventually lead to radiographic changes measured on pelvic radiographs, and this question has been solved appropriately using conventional analysis.[9] But the study also included 3 subsequent read sessions with multiple readers for MRI and different readers for pelvic radiographs. All read sessions included baseline, but the other time points were covered by different read sessions. Changes over time in MRI and radiographic sacroiliitis were analyzed by GEEs (linear and dichotomous scores) as well as GLMMs (linear scores), and included a comparison between the integrated analysis, a conventional completers analysis with individual readers scores, and a completers analysis with combined readers scores based on decision algorithms. The main findings in this study were that effect sizes (parameter estimates) depended somewhat on the method chosen, as were estimates of variability (here: 95% CIs). But the signal-to-noise ratio was not affected importantly.[10] The biggest advantage of the integrated analysis compared with the completers-only analysis (with or without decision algorithms) was that available data were used far more completely and in an entirely assumption-free manner, without losing precision. An additional benefit observed in this analysis was that associations with rare findings (ie, only occurring in a few patients) obtained more robust (narrower 95% CIs) estimates using the integrated analysis than one of the completers analyses, suggesting that for rare events as many observations as possible are required.

THE PLACE OF INTEGRATED ANALYSIS IN THE INTERPRETATION OF IMAGING DATA

Should integrated longitudinal data analysis become the standard for analyzing imaging data in rheumatology? This is not an easy question because it involves issues of precision and issues of feasibility, which may easily conflict. From a standpoint of scientific rigor, integrated analysis should be preferred mainly for theoretic reasons. We plea for the use of all available data, because any decision or choice regarding the usability of particular data sets implies a potential bias, and convenient data are more likely to be chosen than inconvenient data. An assumption-free analysis that includes all data that have once been obtained conveys greater credibility than a dataset that has been selected based on investigators' preferences.

However, the clinical audience will not easily understand integrated analyses. It will be relatively easy to convince statistical experts of the merits of integrated analyses, but clinical consumers will more likely rely on analyses that they understand rather than on data that reach them in statistically manipulated manners. The phrase that statisticians may "torture the data till they confess" stems from clinicians that are statistically illiterate and therefore mistrust statistical methodology.

This argument extends to reviewers of articles in the review process of scientific papers submitted to our scientific journals. Very few reviewers are able to scrutinize articles built by statisticians, and many of these articles will be mistrusted and rejected.

We are believers of the dictum that data should be presented comprehensibly to clinical readership. Still we think that integrated analysis should have a place in the objective interpretation of imaging data from RCTs, long-term extensions thereof, and clinical cohort studies. Therefore, we do not plea for refraining from conventional analysis of imaging data, but rather recommend to use conventional analysis and integrated analysis side by side, to make optimal use of all available data without facing the risk that results are too biased by choices based on expectations, beliefs, and wishful thinking.

SUMMARY

Analysis of imaging data in rheumatology is a challenge. Reliability of scores is an issue for several reasons. Signal-to-noise ratio of most imaging techniques is rather unfavorable (too little signal in relation to too much noise). Optimal use of all available data may help to increase credibility of imaging data, but knowledge of complicated statistical methodology and the help of skilled statisticians is required. Clinicians should appreciate the merits of sophisticated data modeling and liaise with statisticians to increase the quality of imaging results, as proper imaging studies in rheumatology imply more than a supersensitive imaging technique alone.

REFERENCES

1. van der Heijde D, Landewé R. Are conventional radiographs still of value? Curr Opin Rheumatol 2016;28:310–5.
2. Landewé RB, van der Heijde DM. Principles of assessment from a clinical perspective. Best Pract Res Clin Rheumatol 2003;17(3):365–79.
3. Fries JF, Bloch DA, Sharp JT, et al. Assessment of radiologic progression in rheumatoid arthritis. A randomized, controlled trial. Arthritis Rheum 1986;29:1–9.
4. van Tuyl LH, van der Heijde D, Knol DL, et al. Chornological reading of radiographs in rheumatoid arthritis increases efficiency and does not lead to bias. Ann Rheum Dis 2014;73:391–5.
5. Lassere MN, van der Heijde D, Johnson KR, et al. Reliability of measures of disease activity and disease damage in rheumatoid arthritis: implications for samllest detectable difference, minimum clinically important difference, and anlysis of treatment effects in randomized controlled trials. J Rheumatol 2001;28:892–3.
6. Hanley JA, Negassa A, Edwardes MD, et al. Statistical analysis of correlated data using generalized estimating equations: an orientation. Am J Epidemiol 2003; 157(4):364–75.
7. Fitzmaurice GM, Laird NM, Ware J. Applied longitudinal analysis. 2nd edition. John Wiley & Sons; 2011. ISBN 0-471-21487-6.
8. Landewe R, Ostergaard M, Keystone EC, et al. Analysis of integrated radiographic data from two long-term, open-label extension studies of adalimumab for the treatment of rheumatoid arthritis. Arthritis Care Res (Hoboken) 2015;67: 180–6.
9. Dougados M, Sepriano A, Molto A, et al. Sacroiliac radiographic progression in recent onset axial spondyloarthritis: the 5-year data of the DESIR cohort. Ann Rheum Dis 2017;76:1823–8.
10. Sepriano A, Ramiro S, van der Heijde D, et al. Integrated longitudinal analysis increases precision and reduces bias: a comparative 5-year analysis in the DESIR cohort. Arthritis Rheumatol 2017 [abstract no: 2806].

Strategies for Dealing with Missing Accelerometer Data

Samantha Stephens, PhD[a,*], Joseph Beyene, PhD[b], Mark S. Tremblay, PhD[c], Guy Faulkner, PhD[d], Eleanor Pullnayegum, PhD[e], Brian M. Feldman, MD, MSc, FRCPC[f]

KEYWORDS

• Imputation • Missing • Data • Physical activity • Measurement

KEY POINTS

- Missing data poses a threat to the validity, reliability, and generalizability of data from physical activity trials.
- Consideration for the type and amount of missing data is necessary to select appropriate imputation methods.
- Multiple imputation should be used to replace missing physical activity data because it has been shown to give the most unbiased estimates.

INTRODUCTION

Participation in recommended levels of physical activity has been associated with important clinical outcomes in youth and adults with rheumatologic conditions, such as improved physical function, joint pain, disability, and overall quality of life.[1–4] Yet, youth and adults with rheumatologic conditions are highly inactive.[1–3,5] It is necessary to understand the optimal dose of physical activity to understand and measure its effect on health in youth and adults with rheumatologic conditions. Accelerometry, an

---

Disclosures: The authors have no conflicts of interest or disclosures to declare in relation to this article.

[a] Neurosciences and Mental Health, Pediatric M.S., Neuroinflammatory Disorders Program, Center for Brain and Mental Health, Peter Gilgan Centre for Research and Learning, The Hospital for Sick Children, 686 Bay Street, Room 8.9830, Toronto, Ontario M5G 0A4, Canada; [b] Department of Clinical Epidemiology and Biostatistics, 208 Michael G. DeGroote Centre for Learning, McMaster University, 1280 Main Street W., Hamilton, Ontario L8S 4K1, Canada; [c] Children's Hospital of Eastern Ontario Research Institute, University of Ottawa, Ottawa, Ontario, Canada; [d] Canadian Institutes of Health Research, Public Health Agency of Canada, Applied Public Health, University of British Columbia, D. H. Copp Building, Room 4606 2146 Health Sciences Mall, Vancouver, BC V6T1Z3, Canada; [e] Child Health Evaluative Sciences, The Hospital for Sick Children, Public Health Sciences, The University of Toronto, Toronto, Ontario, Canada; [f] Child Health Evaluative Sciences, The Hospital for Sick Children, Department of Pediatrics, Institute of Health Policy Management and Evaluation, The Dalla Lana School of Public Health, The University of Toronto, Toronto, Ontario, Canada
* Corresponding Author.
E-mail address: Samantha.stephens@sickkids.ca

Rheum Dis Clin N Am 44 (2018) 317–326
https://doi.org/10.1016/j.rdc.2018.01.012
0889-857X/18/

objective and unobtrusive method for determining physical activity patterns, has proven a valid outcome measurement tool that overcomes many of the methodologic limitations of subjective methods (eg, self-reports), such as recall bias.[6,7] Despite quality control methods a particular challenge to physical activity measurement with accelerometers is missing data.

Missing data is a universal measurement problem that threatens the integrity of study results by calling into question the interpretation, reliability, and generalizability of the findings. Regardless of the outcome measurement tool used, missing data can introduce bias and challenge the interpretation of study findings. Accelerometer missing data poses a unique problem, however, because many times partial data exist for the participant involved in the study. For example, data may be missing for a position of the day (eg, a participant took off the monitor for a brief period) or entire days of data may be missing (eg, 2 out of 7 days).

To properly address missing data it is important to differentiate between the mechanisms of missingness that one may encounter, because imputation strategies to deal with missingness are dependent on the mechanism. According to Little and Rubin[8] there are three mechanisms of missing data: (1) missing completely at random (MCAR), (2) missing at random (MAR), and (3) not missing at random (NMAR). Data considered MAR suggest that the pattern of missingness is systematically related to some unobserved characteristic of the missing variable.[8] To classify missing data as MCAR, it must be established that the missingness is completely unrelated to the variables that are being studied.[8] Thus, the proportion of the total sample with missing data cannot be differentiated from the sample with complete data. Finally, NMAR is designated when the missingness is neither MAR nor MCAR, or the reason for the missing observations is related to the unobserved outcome.

In this article we describe the problem of missing data in the context of conducting research involving the measurement of physical activity via accelerometry as an outcome. We describe the different statistical approaches that have been used, and describe the benefits and detriments of each of the statistical approaches with consideration given to the missingness mechanism.

PHYSICAL ACTIVITY OUTCOME MEASUREMENT AND DATA PROCESSING

New technologies have been developed to more accurately measure physical activity at the individual and population level in an objective manner. The accelerometer, one such technology, has gained popularity as an objective outcome measure of physical activity that allows the user to derive time stamped and sequenced data on body movements in real time while the subject is in their own environment. Many studies use accelerometers to capture and describe physical activity behaviors, from quantifying time spent in varying intensities of physical activity to describing patterns of physical activity, such as weekdays versus weekends in varying populations. Accelerometry has proven to be a valid and reliable measure of physical activity measurement in healthy children and adults.[7,9–11] Quality control and data reduction procedures have been developed to enhance robustness and validity of data captured from the accelerometer.[12] For example, decision rules, algorithms, and methods to identify nonwear periods and spurious data have been established and some have been incorporated into software packages.[13,14]

Strategies proposed to process data from accelerometers including wear time algorithms and valid days analysis introduce bias, and limit the generalizability of the findings and comparability between studies.[14] In a recent narrative review with commentary on the methodology of prospective observational studies determining the relationship between physical activity levels determined by accelerometer and risk profiles, measurement problems stemming from missing data were highlighted.[15] The reviewers highlighted the inability to compare results between studies because of each study using different definitions of wear time (eg, the number of days and hours per day of monitoring required).[15] A lack of harmonization resulted in different amounts of missing data between the studies thereby changing the interpretation of the study results.[15]

Analyses that Include Only Complete Data May Lead to Inaccurate and Biased Results

For example, in a retrospective analysis of accelerometer data available from the 2002 to 2003 National Health and Nutrition Examination Survey differences in demographic and biologic characteristics of participants who provided valid accelerometer data and invalid accelerometer data were explored.[16] Data were considered valid if 4 or more days of 10 or more hours were available. Those with invalid data between the ages of 20 and 59 years were more likely to have higher body mass index, less likely to be a non-Hispanic white, and less likely to have a high school diploma.[16] Furthermore, those with invalid data were more likely to smoke and to do street drugs and reported a greater number of days inactive because of poor health.[16] Cardiovascular risk factors, such as low high-density lipoprotein and C-reactive protein, were also different in those with invalid compared with those with valid accelerometer data.[16] Findings from this study suggest that bias may be introduced when excluding accelerometer data from the analyses resulting in a change in the interpretation of the findings dependent on the wear time algorithm or valid day inclusion criteria used.

Children participating in the Millennium Cohort Study, a health survey study conducted in British children, found that compared with those who provided study consent, those with disability or illness were half as likely to provide consent.[17] Furthermore, those who reported exercise less than once per week were also less likely to consent to participate in the survey.[17] Characteristics of 12,625 children ages 7 to 8 years who consented and provided sufficient accelerometry data consisting of greater than 2 days of 10 or more hours were compared with those who did not meet the data processing requirements.[17] A little more than half of the population provided sufficient data (50.5%). Differences between those who provided and did not provide reliable data included gender, overweight or obesity status, race, maternal age of the participants mother, educational level of mother, number of siblings, maternal occupation, and presence of a disease or disability.[17,18]

Missing Data May Affect the Reliability of Outcome Measurement Tools

For example, the effects of missing data on the reliability of estimates based on accelerometer data were determined by calculating reliability coefficients using generalizability theory.[18] Furthermore, the mechanism behind the missing data was determined using Little's chi-square test.[18] Seven-day physical activity data from 1042 children collected as a part of a longitudinal study were used to conduct the analyses.[18] Different wear time algorithms were also studied with minimum wear time criteria of 6, 8, 10, or 12 hours compared across five distinct age groups: 9, 11, 12, and 15 years.[18] Findings suggested that with increasing wear-time there was a decrease in the percentage of the total sample meeting the criteria for inclusion in the analysis.[18] The chi-square test for determining the missingness mechanism indicated, with some exceptions, that missing data were not MCAR suggesting that those with "valid" data were different from those with invalid data, that is, that the mechanism was either MAR or NMAR.[18] Differences in the amount of moderate to vigorous physical activity (MVPA) calculated when using different wear time criteria were noted with absolute percentage errors ranging from 11% to 20% across the age groups when 6 hours was compared with 12-hour criteria.[18] Reliability coefficients for those with 7 complete days ranged from 0.74 to 0.84 and 0.52 to 0.67 in those with incomplete days (from 1 to 7 days).[18] Few participants provide complete physical activity data. The variability of physical activity from day to day has, until this point, only been calculated in those with complete data, limiting the external validity and generalizability. Findings from this study suggest that when all data are taken into account, the reliability of the estimates are reduced. How imputing missing data in those with incomplete data impacts the reliability of physical activity estimates needs further study.

The findings from these studies suggest that analyses that include only a certain proportion of the total sample of a study introduce bias through issues with reliability, interpretation, and generalizability of the findings. Importantly, problems with bias are present regardless of the outcome measurement tool. Imputation of missing data may provide a method to ameliorate some of these issues, but to date the application of different imputation techniques that have been applied to accelerometer data has not been collated and reviewed.

DISCUSSION

A scoping review of medical and health databases for articles regarding imputation approaches for dealing with missing accelerometer data was conducted. Findings suggest that there is wide variation in how missing data are treated once they are identified. We identified a wide range of treatments of missing data including listwise deletion, single imputation, maximum likelihood techniques, and multiple imputation. There are advantages and disadvantages to the use of each of these techniques that should be considered before being applied to missing physical activity data.

Listwise deletion was cited in several studies as the technique used to deal with missing accelerometer data. The advantage of this technique is its simplicity in terms of data management and may be appropriate under certain conditions. Listwise deletion is appropriate when data are considered to be MCAR and when a small percentage of the data are missing.

Several assumptions are made including that cases similar to the excluded cases are equally represented in the sample population, although this condition rarely exists in practice and thus limits the use of this technique.[19] Disadvantages to listwise deletion include decreasing sample size thereby affecting the power to detect true differences in outcomes, exaggerating standard errors, and limiting the generalizability of the study.

Single Imputation Methods

Single imputation techniques identified in this study included last observation carried forward, mean replacement, regression, and an individual-centered approach. Those that used mean replacement took the average of the desired accelerometer information (eg, counts) from the entire sample and used it to replace any missing data. Regression substitution involved taking the existing accelerometer data and related characteristics from a sample population (eg, height, weight) and deriving a regression equation to provide a substitute value for the missing data.[20,21] An individual-centered approach involved replacing missing data from either the mean of all valid remaining days or from the mean of valid remaining days based on the type of day missing (eg, weekday or weekend day) for a particular participant.[22,23] Finally, last observation carried forward involves using the last recorded outcome measure to replace missing data.[24]

Advantages and Disadvantages of Single Imputation

Mean replacement and regression improve on listwise deletion in that they seek to use all available data by replacing missing values. Both techniques are simple to perform; however, the disadvantages of these techniques relate to the fact that they do not provide any new information regarding the distribution of the sample under analysis. This results in an underestimate of the variances from the missing data.[19] Furthermore, both of these techniques lead to underestimates of standard errors and overly small *P* values and can lead to inaccurate conclusions.[19]

Kang and colleagues[23] suggested that an individual-centered replacement of missing data might perform better than a group-centered approach (mean replacement) and would be advantageous in terms of its simplicity to carry out as well as being applicable to small sample sizes in comparison with maximum likelihood methods, such as expectation maximization. Results of a simulation study that compared group-centered versus individual-centered replacement of missing data found smaller root mean squared errors when using the individual approach indicating less bias in the estimate. Standard errors of the estimated outcomes were also unchanged when this technique was used in addition to mean substitution in another study.[25,26] However, the group-centered and individual-centered approach resulted in negative mean signed differences (an indicator of accuracy) suggesting an overestimation of the predicted values.[23] Despite improvements over a mean replacement approach, the limitation of an individual-centered approach is that it also does not provide any new information and gives a false impression that the analyses are conducted on a complete data set, which would lead to similar problems in interpreting the results as that of mean replacement or regression. Despite this, it would be worthwhile to investigate the merits of the individual-centered technique using a simulation study to compare it with expectation maximization or multiple imputation techniques given its applicability to small sample sizes.

Maximum Likelihood Methods

The most commonly cited maximum likelihood technique used to account for missing accelerometer data was the expectation maximization algorithm, followed by the full information maximum likelihood (FIML) estimator used in conjunction with factor analyses, multilevel or mixed modeling, and finally Kriging, a geostatistical technique.

The expectation maximization algorithm was first introduced as a statistical strategy for dealing with missing accelerometry data in a simulation study using data from the trial of activity in adolescent girls.[13] The expectation maximization algorithm involves a two-step approach: the E-step and the M-step.[13] The E-step involves finding an estimate of a likelihood function based on combining information from the distribution of the observed data and a theoretic distribution of the unobserved or missing values. The M-step involves maximizing the estimated likelihood function dependent on the observed data.[13] This process continues until the system stabilizes, usually based on a small difference between the log likelihoods of the different models.

In a simulation study determining the effectiveness of the expectation maximization algorithm, it was reported that imputing missing physical activity data resulted in unbiased estimates of missing physical activity data with an average mean squared difference of −5.9 MET-minutes when data where imputed for an entire weekday versus −2.1 MET-minute difference when data were imputed in time blocks.[13] The findings of unbiased estimates were true when data where tested under the assumption of MCAR; however, the estimates were positively biased when data where imputed assuming the data were NMAR.[13] There were no significant differences in the estimates provided by the expectation maximization algorithm when it was compared with multiple imputation techniques. Furthermore, it was pointed out that the expectation maximization algorithm had increased precision and better correlations with the true values than multiple imputation.

Several studies cited use of the FIML estimator to account for missing accelerometer data in their studies.[27,28] The FIML estimator does not actually impute missing data values but rather uses all information, complete or partial, and includes it in the modeling to provide unbiased parameter estimates.[29] The use of partial data rather than excluding it allows for better estimates because it allows for a better understanding of the distribution patterns across all variables.[29]

Multilevel or mixed modeling has also been used to account for missing data. The concept of mixed modeling for handling missing data is similar in function to the FIML estimator because it also involves using partial data to provide unbiased parameter estimates. These procedures are considered preferable to listwise deletion and provide unbiased and more accurate estimates when the missing data meet the condition of MCAR or MAR.[29]

In their study, Paul and colleagues[26] studied adherence rates for wearing accelerometers and the effect of missing accelerometer data on estimating the physical activity levels in a group of healthy older adults using simulation techniques. Their group introduced a robust geostatistical technique for imputing missing data called Kriging. Kriging is often used with spatial data and involves predicting a missing location from the average of the distances between the nonmissing neighboring locations and is also derived from information from the covariance structure of the existing data. Findings from this study suggest that omitting even 1 hour of missing data from an analysis would result in significant differences in predicted physical activity levels (P>.0001) and a coefficient of variation of up to 21%.[26] Imputing using the Kriging technique resulted in an unbiased estimate of physical activity levels and was found accurate (based on identifying the appropriate covariance structure) 68.5% of the time when up to 1 hour of missing data was imputed, but decreased to 39% when 10 hours was imputed.[26]

Advantages and Disadvantages of Maximum Likelihood Methods

Maximum likelihood approaches are advantageous in comparison with single imputation because all available data (partial or complete) are used to build a variance-covariance matrix to estimate a regression model to impute the best estimate for missing data based on maximizing its likelihood. Maximum likelihood methods also have certain advantages over multiple imputation, including efficiency, consistency in giving the same results each time it is performed, and less uncertainty in terms of the number of decisions required to perform the analysis and to determine the appropriate model.[30]

Specific disadvantages related to the expectation maximization algorithm include the requirement for a large sample size, and also the need for statistical expertise.[23] However, others argue that upgrades to statistical software make the later disadvantage obsolete.[19,30] It has been suggested that maximum likelihood methods also have the potential to give biased parameter estimates and underestimate standard errors, because of a decrease in the amount of true variance, and because new information is not added to the study.[23,31] In other words, you are conducting the analysis as if you are working with a complete data set when in fact you are not, and this could potentially result in misleadingly small P values and standard errors.[30] It has also been suggested that this approach does not maximize existing available data from days where the accelerometer was worn but did not meet the minimum requirement to be included in the analysis, thus lowering the accuracy of expectation maximization.[32] No other study to date has provided further data regarding the effectiveness of the expectation maximization algorithm in the replacement of missing accelerometer data. However, in statistical papers it has been suggested that bootstrapping could be used to better estimate the standard errors and *P* values to get more accurate parameter estimates from the expectation maximization algorithm.[30]

Advantages to the Kriging approach have been previously summarized. Specific limitations to the Kriging approach include the inability to impute smaller portions of time (minute by minute) and the lack of precision in estimating physical activity levels because the amount of missing data increases beyond 1 hour.[26] Another disadvantage to this technique is the complexity of the approach. No other studies have reported on the effectiveness of this approach for replacement of missing accelerometer data.

Multiple Imputation Methods

Several multiple imputation approaches have been used to deal with missing accelerometer data. Van Dyck and colleagues[33] conducted a cross-sectional study looking at the relationships between physical activity, neighborhood walkability, and adiposity in a sample of 1200 adults living in Ghent, Belgium. Multiple imputation was used to account for an 8.7% rate of missing accelerometer data in their study.[33] Sensitivity analyses comparing the original analysis with the analysis using the imputed data set resulted in similar results; however, the authors noted that the imputed analysis resulted in smaller standard errors. In a randomized trial of geriatric patients to determine the effect of a behavioral intervention on improving physical activity levels, multiple imputation was also used to account for missing data.[34] A sensitivity analysis was not presented; however, the authors mention that a significant effect of the intervention was determined after adjustment for baseline values and once missing data were accounted for using imputation.[34]

A new imputation approach termed the "combined" approach was developed to address using all available accelerometer data from valid and invalid days to better impute missing accelerometer data.[32] To impute a missing value using this approach a two-step interchangeable process is invoked. The expected number of wear hours and the counts per minute by subject and day are imputed using multiple imputation by using additive regression and bootstrapping.[32] The imputed values are combined with any existing observed accelerometer data in the final step of the process. A simulation study was conducted to determine the effectiveness of the "combined" approach using accelerometer data from the National Health and Nutrition Examination Survey study conducted in the United States between 2003 and 2006.[32] The combined approach was compared with other imputation approaches (single imputation) under several different conditions to understand the effect on the accuracy of the imputed data when there were varying levels of missing data and number of required valid hours. Accuracy was tested by determining the root mean square error; bias was calculated by *z* scores with a score greater than 1.96 indicating the presence of bias. Differences in root mean square error between the combined approach and single imputation were tested using Student *t* tests. Results of the simulation study suggested that the combined approach could produce unbiased estimates of counts per minute and that it had significantly lower root mean square errors when compared with data imputed using single imputation methods.[32] A significant decrease in imputation error and estimated effect size error ranging from 12% to 17% and 20% to 33%, respectively, was reported.[32] The combined approach imputation was found to be more accurate when there were less missing data and when there were greater amounts of wear time available.

Advantages and Disadvantages of Multiple Imputation Methods

The main advantages to multiple imputation techniques are that estimates are imputed multiple times and an error term is added to each estimate, which allows one to estimate the uncertainty in the imputed parameter values. This helps to account for the fact that missing data distribution is estimated rather than directly represented by measured data.[19] To obtain more accurate estimates of parameters, several (usually up to 10) imputed data sets are formed from a random draw of possible data. Regression coefficients and their standard errors are derived by taking the average of the estimates from the different imputed data sets.[19]

Disadvantages to this approach include the requirement for a large sample size, different estimates are obtained with each use (because of random draws of imputed values), and statistical complexity. Also, note that these data treatments are only useful in the case that the missing data are MCAR or MAR. Despite these disadvantages, currently available simulation studies using multiple imputation approaches and data from studies using a sensitivity analysis suggest that this technique results in accurate estimates and standard errors.[32–34] To date no simulation studies have compared multiple imputation techniques, such as the combined approach with anything other than single imputation. Future work is needed to compare multiple imputation with other maximum likelihood techniques, such as expectation maximization with bootstrapping, to test the combined approach and perhaps Kriging.

SUMMARY/RECOMMENDATIONS

Missing data should be dealt with and not ignored. Consideration to the type and amount of missing data can help in the selection of the appropriate imputation method to use. However, based on available simulation study data, multiple imputation techniques should be used to impute missing accelerometer data because this method considers the level of uncertainty in imputed estimates. Simulation studies should compare different imputation techniques under assumptions of MCAR, MAR, and even NMAR and test the accuracy of the estimates with different sample sizes. Imputation techniques should be used to maximize data utilization, minimize bias, expand generalizability, and allow for comparison of studies using accelerometers in the future. Missing data poses a threat to the validity and interpretation of trials using physical activity data from accelerometry. Appropriately applying imputation techniques to missing data will enhance the validity of trials and allow for direct comparison of studies allowing for a better understanding of the contribution of physical activity on health outcomes in youth and adults with rheumatologic conditions.

REFERENCES

1. Lelieveld OT, Armbrust W, van Leeuwen MA, et al. Physical activity in adolescents with juvenile idiopathic arthritis. Arthritis Rheum 2008;59(10):1379–84.
2. Takken T, Van Brussel M, Engelbert R, et al. Exercise therapy in juvenile idiopathic arthritis: a Cochrane review. Eur J Phys Rehabil Med 2008;44(3):287–97.
3. Iversen MD, Frits M, von Heideken J, et al. Physical activity and correlates of physical activity participation over three years in adults with rheumatoid arthritis. Arthritis Care Res (Hoboken) 2017;69(10):1535–45.

4. Limentis E, Grosbein HA, Feldman BM. The relationship between physical activity levels and pain in children with juvenile idiopathic arthritis. J Rheumatol 2014; 41(2):345–51.
5. Takken T, Van der Net J, Kuis W, et al. Physical activity and health related physical fitness in children with juvenile idiopathic arthritis. Ann Rheum Dis 2003;62(9): 885–9.
6. Stephens S, Takken T, Esliger DW, et al. Validation of accelerometer prediction equations in children with chronic disease. Pediatr Exerc Sci 2016;28(1):117–32.
7. Pfeiffer KA, McIver KL, Dowda M, et al. Validation and calibration of the actical accelerometer in preschool children. Med Sci Sports Exerc 2006;38(1):152–7.
8. Little R, Rubin DB. Statistical analysis with missing data. 2nd ed. Hoboken (NJ): John Wiley and Sons Inc; 2002.
9. Payau MR, Adolph AL, Vohra FA, et al. Prediction of activity energy expenditure using accelerometers in children. Med Sci Sports Exerc 2004;36(9):1625–31.
10. Treuth MS, Sherwood NE, Butte NF, et al. Validity and reliability of activity measures in African-American girls for GEMS. Med Sci Sports Exerc 2003;35(3): 532–9.
11. Trost SG, Way R, Okely AD. Predictive validity of three ActiGraph energy expenditure equations for children. Med Sci Sports Exerc 2006;38(2):380–7.
12. Esliger DW, Copeland JL, Barnes JD, et al. Standardizing and optimizing the use of accelerometer data for free-living physical activity monitoring. J Phys Act Health 2005;3:366–83.
13. Catellier DJ, Hannan PJ, Murray DM, et al. Imputation of missing data when measuring physical activity by accelerometry. Med Sci Sports Exerc 2005; 37(11 Suppl):S555–62.
14. Masse LC, Fuemmeler BF, Anderson C, et al. Accelerometer data reduction: a comparison of four algorithms on select outcome variables. Med Sci Sports Exerc 2005;37(11 SUPPL):S544–54.
15. Tarp J, Bronda J, Andersen LB, et al. Physical activity, sedentary behavior and long-term cardiovascular risk in young people: a review and discussion of methodology in prospective studies. J Sport Health Sci 2016;5(2):145–50.
16. Loprinzi PD, Cardnal BJ, Crespo CJ, et al. Differences in demographic, behavioral, and biological variables between those with valid and invalid accelerometry data: implications for generalizability. J Phys Activity Health 2013;10(1):79–84.
17. Rich C, Cortina-Borja M, Dezateux C, et al. Predictors of non-response in a UK-wide cohort study of children's accelerometer- determined physical activity using postal methods. BMJ Open 2013;3 [pii: e002290].
18. Wickel EE. Reporting the reliability of accelerometer data with and without missing values. PLoS One 2014;9(12):e114402.
19. Donders AR, Ven Der Heijden GJ, Stijnen T, et al. Review: a gentle introduction to imputation to missing values. J Clin Epidemiol 2006;59:1087–91.
20. Warren JM, Ekelund U, Besson H, et al. Assessment of physical activity - a review of methodologies with reference to epidemiological research: a report of the exercise physiology section of the European Association of Cardiovascular Prevention and Rehabilitation. Eur J Cardiovasc Prev Rehabil 2010;17(2):127–39.
21. Poudevigne MS, O'Connor PJ. Physical activity and mood during pregnancy. Med Sci Sports Exerc 2005;37(8):1374–80.
22. Ishikawa S, Stevens SL, Kang M, et al. Reliability of daily step activity monitoring in adults with incomplete spinal cord injury. Top Spinal Cord Inj Rehabil 2011;16:77.

23. Kang M, Rowe DA, Barreira TV, et al. Individual information-centered approach for handling physical activity missing data. Res Q Exerc Sport 2009;80(2):131–7.
24. Samuels TY, Raedeke TD, Mahar MT, et al. A randomized controlled trial of continuous activity, short bouts, and a 10,000 step guideline in inactive adults. Prev Med 2011;52(2):120–5.
25. van Hees VT, Renstrom F, Wright A, et al. Estimation of daily energy expenditure in pregnant and non-pregnant women using a wrist-worn tri-axial accelerometer. PLoS One 2011;6(7):e22922.
26. Paul DR, Kramer M, Stote KS, et al. Estimates of adherence and error analysis of physical activity data collected via accelerometry in a large study of free-living adults. BMC Med Res Methodol 2008;8:38.
27. Motl RW, Weikert M, Suh Y, et al. Symptom cluster and physical activity in relapsing-remitting multiple sclerosis. Res Nurs Health 2010;33:398–412.
28. Motl RW, McAuley E. Longitudinal analysis of physical activity and symptoms as predictors of change in functional limitations and disability in multiple sclerosis. Rehabil Psychol 2009;54(2):204–10.
29. Enders CK, Bandalos DL. The relative performance of full information maximum likelihood estimation for missing data in structural equation models. Structural Equation Modeling 2001;8:430–57.
30. Allison P. Handling missing data by maximum likelihood. Paper presented at: SAS Global Forum 2012 Conference; Cary, NC, April 22-25, 2012.
31. Staudenmayer J, Zhu WM, Catellier DJ. Statistical considerations in the analysis of accelerometry-based activity monitor data. Med Sci Sports Exerc 2012;44: S61–7.
32. Lee PH. Data imputation for accelerometer-measured physical activity: the combined approach. Am J Clin Nutr 2013;97(5):965–71.
33. Van Dyck D, Cerin E, Cardon G, et al. Physical activity as a mediator of the associations between neighborhood walkability and adiposity in Belgian adults. Health Place 2010;16(5):952–60.
34. McMurdo ME, Sugden J, Argo I, et al. Do pedometers increase physical activity in sedentary older women? A randomized controlled trial. J Am Geriatr Soc 2010; 58(11):2099–106.

Use of Administrative Databases to Assess Reproductive Health Issues in Rheumatic Diseases

Evelyne Vinet, MD, PhD[a,b,*], Eliza F. Chakravarty, MD, MSc[c], Julia F. Simard, ScD[d,e], Megan Clowse, MD, MPH[f]

KEYWORDS

- Administrative databases • Reproductive health • Rheumatic diseases
- Adverse pregnancy outcomes • Epidemiology

KEY POINTS

- Administrative databases used in epidemiologic research are large datasets collected as part of the billing and administrative components of clinical care that can be used to study health care delivery and outcomes.
- Administrative databases offer several advantages for the study of reproductive issues in women with rheumatic diseases: they provide large sample size to assess rare outcomes and/or exposures, provide population-based samples allowing generalizability of findings, and facilitate selection of control groups.
- However, several methodologic issues should be addressed when using administrative databases for the study of reproductive health outcomes, such as timing of pregnancy onset, mother-child linkage failure, incomplete capture of early fetal loss, and correlated observations.

Disclosure: Dr E. Vinet: Fonds de Recherche Santé Québec (FRQS) Career award; Dr E.F. Chakravarty: None; Dr J.F. Simard: NIH NIAMS K01-AR066878; Dr M. Clowse None.

[a] Division of Rheumatology, Montreal General Hospital, A6.123, 1650 Cedar Avenue, Montreal, Quebec H3G 1A4, Canada; [b] Division of Clinical Epidemiology, McGill University Health Centre, 5252 Maisonneuve Boulevard West, Room 3D-57, Montreal, Quebec H4A 3J1, Canada; [c] Clinical Immunology Research Program, Oklahoma Medical Research Foundation, 825 Northeast 13th Street, Oklahoma City, OK 73104, USA; [d] Epidemiology, Health Research and Policy, Stanford School of Medicine, HRP Redwood Building, Room T152, 259 Campus Drive, Stanford, CA 94305-5405, USA; [e] Immunology and Rheumatology, Medicine, Stanford School of Medicine, HRP Redwood Building, Room T152, 259 Campus Drive, Stanford, CA 94305-5405, USA; [f] Medicine, Duke University School of Medicine, Box 3535 Trent Drive, Durham, NC 27710, USA

* Corresponding author. Division of Rheumatology, Montreal General Hospital, A6.123, 1650 Cedar Avenue, Montreal, Quebec H3G 1A4, Canada.

E-mail address: evelyne.vinet@mcgill.ca

Rheum Dis Clin N Am 44 (2018) 327–336
https://doi.org/10.1016/j.rdc.2018.01.008
0889-857X/18/

INTRODUCTION

Because of the relative infrequency of pregnancy in women with rheumatic diseases, collecting datasets of sufficient size with reliable data can be challenging. Administrative databases, registers, and other sources of big data can be interesting data sources to address important research questions on reproduction in women with rheumatic diseases. There are many different types of administrative datasets worldwide, and it is important to understand the type of data present and unavailable in each dataset, validity and potential misclassification of data, and the ability to link maternal data with infant data. This article discusses the advantages and methodologic issues associated with administrative database use for the conduct of observational studies on reproductive issues in women with rheumatic diseases.

ADMINISTRATIVE DATABASES

Administrative databases used in epidemiologic research are large datasets collected as part of the billing and administrative components of clinical care that can be used to study health care delivery and outcomes. The collection of these data is not primarily for research purposes. However, the increased availability of such data has fueled research by allowing for more rapid collection of data on subjects with rare diseases in sufficiently large numbers. Some administrative data sources (ie, population-based registers) are representative of a large population of individuals, unlike subjects who may voluntarily participate in a clinical cohort or subjects who are seen exclusively at tertiary care medical centers and must often provide informed consent to be included. Similarly, large numbers of control subjects can be identified within the dataset who may represent nondiseased individuals as comparators, whose data are collected in the same fashion as cases of interest. Additionally, as the data are generated at the time of the encounter, it is systematic and prospectively collected, without the inherent biases of recall of past exposures, or self-selection by volunteer status. Of course, differences in health care utilization may affect the appropriate selection of control populations. Similarly, confounding by indication may influence the extent of resources used based on the individual's underlying disease status. For example, a systemic lupus erythematosus (SLE) patient may be more likely to be hospitalized than a similarly aged healthy individual for a given set of symptoms.

CLAIM-BASED DATABASES

Because the United States does not have a nationwide health system or systematic capture of medical data, the ability to collect comprehensive medical data on a truly population-based cohort is necessarily limited. However, several datasets are available that may be relevant to research into pregnancy outcomes in rheumatic disease populations. Perhaps the most commonly used are administrative data based on medical claims, either by publicly funded insurers (eg, Medicaid) or private insurers (eg, MarketScan commercial databases). These data are quite valuable in that they often contain inpatient and outpatient visits listing diagnoses and procedures and prescription medication data linked to individuals. Unfortunately, because of the fragmentation of health care in the United States, individuals may not retain extended enrollment with any specific insurer, making long-term evaluation across multiple pregnancies more difficult. Numerous algorithms are currently used to maximize sensitivity and specificity of diagnoses made on claims data.[1,2] Additionally, important variables may not be captured in claims data, including lifestyle variables (eg, smoking, alcohol, exercise), reproductive history, results of laboratory studies, and variables on disease activity or severity.

More granularity of data in the United States and elsewhere may be obtained by using electronic medical record (EMR) data, which can complement administrative data with laboratory and imaging data. Access to EMR for research purposes can vary considerably across institutions. The government-sponsored Patient Centered Outcomes Research Institute has funded multiple large collaborative projects working to synchronize EMR data from a range of health systems, which may provide access to useful data in the future. The collaborative work from a Common Data Model is a limited dataset including billing, prescribing, and laboratory data. Additionally, data fields and key word searches may include information regarding vital signs, body mass index, lifestyle variables, reproductive history, and even data regarding gestational age and other antepartum pregnancy variables. In general, patient-reported outcomes and standardized assessments of disease activity and severity remain unavailable, as they are specific composite measures of disease that are not routinely captured for administrative or billing purposes. Using such datasets is complex and requires sophisticated analyses and cautious interpretation, thus increasing the cost, time, and required expertise of performing such studies.

POPULATION-BASED REGISTERS

Population-based registers are a type of administrative databases that offer a systematic data collection on specific outcomes, usually based on mandatory reporting within a country or region. These may contain data on all outpatient visits, hospitalizations, deaths, and filled drug prescriptions for a given population over some period of time. Such registers may also be supplemented with self-reported information, which may capture important potential confounders, exposures of interest, and comorbidities. Regions with such registers also often collect data on vital statistics, census, employment, immigration and emigration.

One example of population-based surveillance registers is the Nordic Birth Registers, which cover Denmark, Finland, Iceland, Norway, and Sweden, encompassing approximately 25 million births.[3,4] Each of the Nordic countries has kept medical birth registers for decades, all with compulsory notification with identifiers for mother and neonate and, in some cases, for fathers. Linkage to other registers and national health care databases is possible, often using a personal identification number, such as outpatient, hospitalization, and prescription databases. Collectively, this means that researchers can potentially identify some exposures of interest and outcomes from patients with rheumatic disease and a representative comparator sample of births.

The Canadian administrative health care databases can also be considered a population-based surveillance register, with each Canadian province having its own register. For example, Quebec's administrative databases cover all residents in the province (>8 million) and collect information on all hospitalizations, physician visits, and procedures. In addition, they include data on drug prescriptions filled for residents on the public drug plan, which covers recipients of social assistance and workers and their family without access to a private drug plan, representing about a third of the population. Quebec's Institute of Statistics monitors important vital statistics, including live birth and stillbirth rates, with a mandatory reporting of gestational age at birth (based on date of last menstrual period) and cause of stillbirth. All these databases can be linked to provide a rich source of information to assemble a population-based cohort of pregnancies or deliveries, with available mother and child linkage, creating a cohort of offspring with antenatal exposure of interest. One such cohort, the Offspring of Systemic Lupus Erythematosus (SLE) Mother Registry (OSLER), has been assembled to assess the risk of long-term health outcomes and stillbirths in children born to women with SLE.[5,6]

ADVANTAGES OF ADMINISTRATIVE DATABASES FOR REPRODUCTIVE STUDIES

Administrative databases offer several advantages for the study of reproductive issues in women with rheumatic diseases. The large sample size makes it possible to study outcomes associated with rare exposures, such as SLE, which only affects 0.1% women of childbearing age.[7,8] This is particularly true for the assessment of rare outcomes (such as neurodevelopment disorders), which is not feasible in clinic-based prospective cohort studies. Such data have been collected in a systematic manner, facilitating the conduct of observational studies rapidly and at relatively low cost. Population-based register data cover the entire population of a geographic region, thereby improving the generalizability of findings. Because informed consent is generally not required for selection of a subject in the study, study designs using these data sources are less prone to selection bias from nonresponse. Moreover, the use of administrative databases also eases the selection of a control group from the same source population. In the case of population-based registers, data are available to estimate baseline risks of outcomes of interest to understand the true general population risks.

CHALLENGING ISSUES SPECIFIC TO PREGNANCY IN ADMINISTRATIVE DATABASES

Differences Between Pregnancy and Birth

Several published studies examining pregnancy complications and outcomes in women with rheumatic diseases have used data from birth registers, birth certificates, and labor and delivery admissions. All of these data sources required that a birth be registered therefore missing information on first- and second-trimester losses. In some instances, losses after 20 gestational weeks are registered as stillbirths and therefore can be found, but this is not universally true. When reviewing the literature or conducting a study, it is therefore critical to define how the data were identified. Is the study looking at adverse outcomes among those pregnancies that lasted at least 20 weeks? Or is the study identifying pregnancies early on and capturing all outcomes? Most administrative databases have access to delivery admissions and birth characteristics.

Some initiatives, such as the Swedish Pregnancy Register, are collecting data from a woman's first visit to the midwife to capture clinically recognized pregnancies.[9] Using EMR, it may also be possible to search clinic notes, human chorionic gonadotropin testing, genetic testing, ultrasound records, and other clinical interactions indicating a pregnancy to assemble a group of pregnant patients.

The distinction is critical because if a researcher asks about adverse pregnancy outcomes and then only restricts to births, a significant portion of the most unwanted outcomes (ie, pregnancy loss) will necessarily be excluded, underestimating the true prevalence of the outcome. This could lead to inadvertent conclusions that there were no losses when in fact they selected a population that did not have losses. Interpretation of these data and the underlying selection of patients must take this into account.

Early Pregnancy Complications and Loss

Just as pregnancy onset is challenging to define precisely using administrative data, complications of early pregnancy can be difficult to ascertain. Approximately 99%

of fetal deaths occurring at greater than 20 weeks gestational age identified in administrative databases using International Classification of Diseases - Ninth revision (ICD-9 codes) were confirmed by medical record review; however, it is unknown how many cases were not ascertained within the datasets.[10] Furthermore, pregnancy losses that occur before 15 weeks are likely not captured in administrative datasets, as many of these losses do not require hospitalization, surgical intervention, or even medical attention if uncomplicated and early in gestation. Indeed, some early pregnancy losses may not even be clinically recognized, particularly in women who are not actively attempting to conceive. There are no validation studies available to understand the degree of incomplete ascertainment of early pregnancy losses.

Timing of Pregnancy

Understanding the timing of pregnancy using administrative data presents its own set of challenges, particularly as they relate to the time of conception and exposures related to specific gestational ages. This can be extremely important when considering issues of potential teratogenicity, in which there is often a specific window of days to weeks during organogenesis when embryos are most vulnerable in early pregnancy. Given that maternal rheumatic diseases often rely on chronic use of medications to manage symptoms, the timing of pregnancy onset with the discontinuation of chronic medications can be critical. Additionally, short-term exposures to medications during early pregnancy (steroid courses, infusion therapeutics, antibiotics, and vaccines) may potentially affect pregnancy outcomes and need to be captured accurately.

To estimate onset of pregnancy, several algorithms have been developed to maximize precision, and the algorithm is selected based on the availability of variables within the dataset and the statistical expertise available for complicated algorithms using linked datasets.[11] The simplest algorithm assigns a uniform length of delivery—270 days for full-term delivery and 245 days for a preterm delivery. Onset of pregnancy is dated by subtracting the appropriate number of days from the delivery date. This works with even the most limited dataset but is subject to misclassification of extremely premature or postterm pregnancies. This calculation requires that a birth is registered and will not capture pregnancies that do not end in a birth.

Furthermore, caution must be advised when looking at medication exposure in early pregnancy, as estimates are necessarily imprecise. More complicated algorithms include all available data from EMR, often assigning first trimester of pregnancy to the first prenatal visit, using birth weight from birth certificates to assign gestational age based on race and sex-specific standards, using standardized prenatal testing to further date pregnancies (ie, α-fetoprotein screening at 11–14 weeks), and dating by ultrasound scan during pregnancy.

Parity and Repeated Events

Because pregnancy outcomes, and even the decision to proceed with additional pregnancies, depend heavily on the outcome of previous pregnancies, classifying pregnancies into first birth versus subsequent births is of the utmost importance.[12,13] Pregnancy outcome studies have dramatically different results when only first births are included in the analysis compared with subsequent births, even in cases in which only one birth per woman is included. In the United States, outside of EMR, administrative datasets do not always include variables about parity, and it cannot be assumed (in most circumstances) that the first pregnancy during the period of data captured in a dataset is necessarily the first pregnancy for that woman, as enrollment periods in health insurance do not cover the entire reproductive history. In these cases, stratifying data on first versus subsequent births may lead to misclassification. Datasets from countries with more complete birth data capture are less likely to misclassify first versus subsequent births.

Further complications in analysis and interpretation arise when multiple births per woman are included in the dataset, as each birth is not independent of the others. The generalized estimating equation approach can be used to account for this lack of independence, as long as the pregnancies can be appropriately clustered according to mother.[14] If the autocorrelation in the data is not appropriately handled, it will make the findings appear more precise than they actually are (eg, narrower confidence intervals).

Measuring Drug Exposures

Most electronic databases capture drug exposure based on either an ordered prescription or a filled prescription. As with all pharmacoepidemiologic studies, neither receiving a prescription nor filling it guarantees compliance. In other words, this does not guarantee that the patient actually takes the drug and might lead to drug exposure misclassification in analyses. However, as patients often need to pay a minimal portion of their medications in most public drug plans, it is likely that patients who fill their prescription intend to take at least some of the prescribed drug. Unfortunately, data are rarely collected on over-the-counter medications. This is a particular concern for the study of vitamins (such as folic acid), aspirin, and/or nonsteroidal anti-inflammatory drugs (NSAIDs) in pregnancy, as these are frequently obtained without a prescription. Furthermore, most such databases provide data only on outpatient-prescribed drugs or pharmacy dispensings and do not provide information on drugs dispensed during hospitalizations or as infusions. Thus, if pregnant women are hospitalized during pregnancy (and most are at least for delivery), drug exposures during the hospitalization cannot be measured, producing what is called an *immeasurable period of exposure*.[15] This can lead to differential misclassification of exposure in mothers with rheumatic diseases as opposed to unaffected mothers, as women with rheumatic diseases are more likely to be hospitalized during pregnancy and have longer hospitalization stay for delivery. As an example, the mean length of stay for delivery within the OSLER cohort was 5.4 ± 6.7 days for SLE mothers as opposed to 3.3 ± 2.6 days for mothers from the general population.[5,6] Studies of pregnancy outcomes in the United States similarly find more frequent antenatal hospitalizations and increased length of stay for delivery hospitalizations for mothers with rheumatoid arthritis and SLE.[16] Statistical methods have been described by Suissa,[15] which use a time-varying exposable period to circumvent this potential limitation.

Ascertaining Congenital Malformations

With increasing use of polypharmacy (inadvertently or intentionally to treat maternal illness) during the periconceptional period and into pregnancy comes increasing concerns for identifying any associations with congenital malformations and medication exposure. The large numbers of subjects available through administrative datasets can be ideal for studying rare outcomes of uncommon antenatal exposures. However, several issues regarding the use of administrative datasets for teratogenicity studies must be addressed. The first issue is the ability to link mother's records to those of their infants. In the United States, state birth certificate data are often the only infant data available to determine infant outcomes, and the ability and ease of linking these data to maternal data depend on the specific datasets and user access to such data.[17] Neonatal outcomes are limited to those that could be diagnosed at birth. In other cases, infant medical records can be linked to maternal records. Comprehensive medical records for infants will contain more detailed data on neonatal outcomes and complications identified beyond the delivery period than will data obtained solely from birth certificates. As described above, there are inherent difficulties in accurately determining the onset of pregnancy to a precision of days to weeks for early antenatal exposure to medications.

Once maternal medical records are linked to infant data, the diagnostic accuracy and completeness of ascertainment of congenital anomalies from these records becomes critical. A major concern of using administrative databases is related to the validity of the diagnostic information, because diseases are primarily coded for billing and not for research purposes. One can try to use previously validated case definitions. However, they are not always available and, when available, none are 100% sensitive and specific. One recent study comparing birth certificate data with administrative health plan data found a high positive predictive value (PPV) for demographic and some pregnancy outcome data on birth certificates, including gestational age, birth weight, race/ethnicity, and prior maternal obstetric history.[18] Unfortunately, PPVs for selected congenital anomalies were much lower for both birth certificate data and administrative claims data. For example, using medical record review as the gold standard, the PPV for cardiac defects in the Tennessee Medicaid population was only 35.7% for birth certificate data, increasing to 74.5% for claims data.[19] Arguably, this is unacceptably low to make meaningful interpretations regarding teratogenicity.

To address the issue of imperfect case ascertainment, one can use Bayesian latent class models, which use various case definitions with each contributing some information about the latent case status of each individual instead of trying to identify a disease case (or outcome) with certainty.[20] Subjects are thus assigned a probability of being a disease case. This method can be used to correct for all sources of uncertainty related to case ascertainment.

The last, and perhaps most challenging, aspect to studying teratogenicity is the issue of the appropriate sample size to determine associations with reasonable power. Power calculations are influenced both by the prevalence of the specific congenital anomaly (estimates of the overall birth defect rate in the general population are 3%–5% of pregnancies) and the magnitude of the effect, or the increase risk of the anomaly in the exposed compared with the unexposed group that is considered clinically significant. Given the low prevalence of specific congenital anomalies in the general obstetric population, tens to hundreds of thousands of pregnancies must be analyzed to detect even a large increase in risk.[21] And this is before adjusting for relevant covariates, confounders, and multiple comparisons. The need for such large sample sizes to do this type of research is among the greatest strengths of administrative data. However, the tremendous increase in sample size often comes with a loss of granularity regarding the reliability and precision of data capture in settings in which large-scale validation and potential for more careful data scrutiny are largely unavailable.

Because the ramifications of publishing associations between specific manifestations and congenital anomalies can be profound and affect the management of serious maternal conditions before and during conception, researchers must be careful to address all of the relevant issues regarding exposure and outcome data. These include (1) accurate timing of antenatal exposure, (2) the potential for concomitant medication exposures and other potential causes of congenital malformations, (3) rigorous definitions and accurate ascertainment of congenital anomalies, and (4) adequate sample sizes of both exposed and unexposed pregnancies.

UNMEASURED CONFOUNDERS

As with all observational research, unmeasured confounders may be present. For instance, administrative databases may not record information on smoking, alcohol use, and obesity, which all have been associated with adverse reproductive outcomes. To account for this, one can use sensitivity analyses of unmeasured confounders using previously developed formulas.[22]

As an example, if we wanted to study the effect of maternal SLE on the risk of birth defects in the offspring, maternal alcohol intake could be an important unmeasured confounder. Using previously described formulas, one can determine how large the maternal SLE-alcohol association in the cohort would have to be so that adjusting for the presence of the maternal confounder (ie, alcohol intake) during pregnancy would remove an apparent maternal SLE-birth defect association.[22]

Immortal Time Bias

Observational studies using administrative databases might also be plagued by immortal time bias (**Fig. 1**). *Immortal time* refers to a period over cohort follow-up during which, by design, subjects could not have died (or have the outcome/event). As an example, Daniel and colleagues[23] described the potential for immortal bias in assessing the effect of maternal NSAID exposure in pregnancy on fetal death before 20 weeks of gestation. If NSAID exposure is based on at least one prescription filled before 20 weeks of gestation, exposed fetuses are necessarily immortal during the time

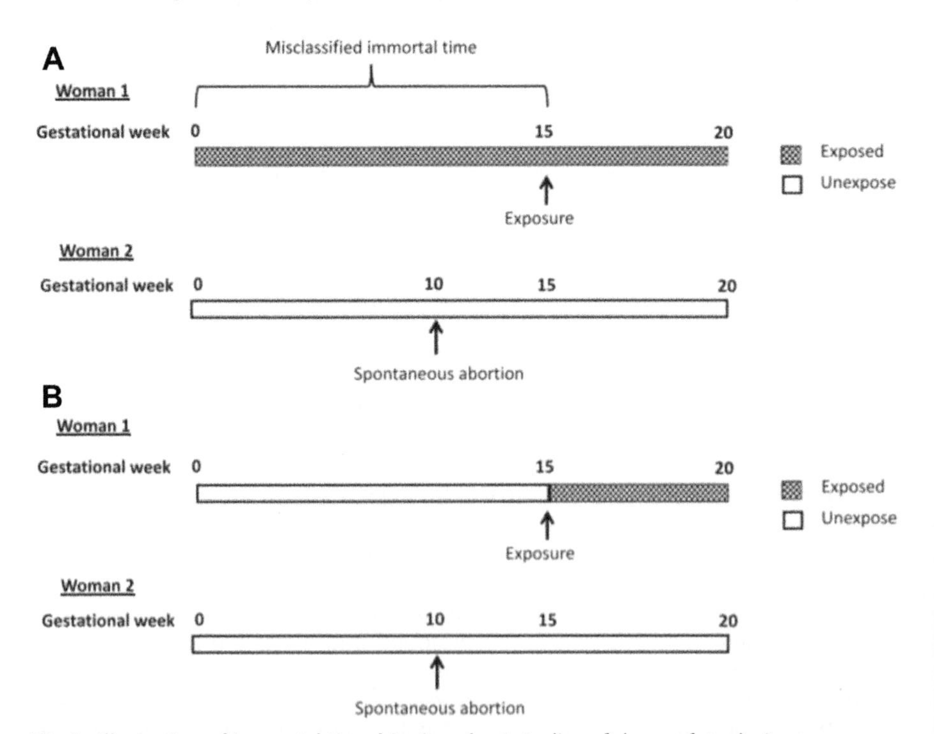

Fig. 1. Illustration of immortal time bias in cohort studies of drug safety during pregnancy. Definition of exposure *A*, not controlling vs *B*, controlling for immortal time bias. (*From* Daniel S, Koren G, Lunenfeld E, et al. Immortal time bias in drug safety cohort studies: spontaneous abortion following nonsteroidal antiinflammatory drug exposure. Am J Obstet Gynecol 2015;212(3):307.e1-6; with permission.)

span between conception and exposure. By contrast, fetuses in the unexposed group have no such advantage because they could have had the outcome fetal death at any time during follow-up.[23] To avoid introducing immortal time in our analysis, the solution is simply to categorize follow-up time for each subject according to exposure category.

SUMMARY

Administrative databases are a useful and powerful data source for the conduct of rheumatic diseases research, such as investigating reproductive issues in which infrequent outcomes in rare diseases limit the ability to accrue adequate sample sizes for meaningful interpretation and analysis. Furthermore, temporal changes in management of rheumatic diseases and changes in prenatal monitoring and management make it imperative to compare pregnancies that occur in relatively short timeframes. However, the increase in sample size and availability of data on relevant control populations come with a degree of loss in granularity of detail and restricted ability to validate outcomes. Therefore, we must be aware of the potential limitations and use different strategies to minimize potential biases.

REFERENCES

1. Moores KG, Sathe NA. A systematic review of validated methods for identifying systemic lupus erythematosus (SLE) using administrative or claims data. Vaccine 2013;31(Suppl10):K62–73.
2. Hanly JG, Thompson K, Skedgel C. Identification of patients with systemic lupus erythematosus in administrative healthcare databases. Lupus 2014;23:1377–82.
3. Langhoff-Roos J, Krebs L, Klungsøyr K, et al. The Nordic medical birth registers–a potential goldmine for clinical research. Acta Obstet Gynecol Scand 2014;93: 132–7.
4. Furu K, Wettermark B, Andersen M, et al. The Nordic countries as a cohort for pharmacoepidemiological research. Basic Clin Pharmacol Toxicol 2010;106:86–94.
5. Vinet É, Pineau CA, Scott S, et al. Increased congenital heart defects in children born to women with systemic lupus erythematosus: results from the offspring of Systemic Lupus Erythematosus Mothers Registry Study. Circulation 2015;131: 149–56.
6. Vinet É, Pineau CA, Clarke AE, et al. Increased risk of autism spectrum disorders in children born to women with systemic lupus erythematosus: results from a large population-based cohort. Arthritis Rheumatol 2015;67:3201–8.
7. Dall'Era M, Cisternas MG, Snipes K, et al. The incidence and prevalence of systemic lupus erythematosus in San Francisco County, California: the California Lupus surveillance project. Arthritis Rheumatol 2017;69:1996–2005.
8. Izmirly PM, Wan I, Sahl S, et al. The incidence and prevalence of systemic lupus erythematosus in New York County (Manhattan), New York: the Manhattan Lupus surveillance program. Arthritis Rheumatol 2017;69:2006–7.
9. Palmsten K, Simard JF, Chambers CD, et al. Medication use among pregnant women with systemic lupus erythematosus and general population comparators. Rheumatol 2017;56:561–9.
10. Likis FE, Sathe NA, Carnahan R, et al. A systematic review of validated methods to capture stillbirth and spontaneous abortion using administrative or claims data. Vaccine 2013;31:K74–82.
11. Margulis AV, Palmsten K, Andrade SE, et al. Beginning and duration of pregnancy in automated health care databases: review of estimation methods and validation results. Pharmacoepidemiol Drug Saf 2015;24:335–42.

12. Wallenius M, Salvesen KÅ, Daltveit AK, et al. Systemic lupus erythematosus and outcomes in first and subsequent births based on data from a national birth registry. Arthritis Care Res 2014;66:1718–24.
13. Hernandez-Diaz S, Toh S, Cnattingius S. Risk of pre-eclampsia in first and subsequent pregnancies: prospective cohort study. BMJ 2009;338:b2255.
14. Ziegler A, Vens M. Generalized estimating equations. Notes on the choice of the working correlation matrix. Methods Inf Med 2010;49:421–5 [discussion: 426–32].
15. Suissa S. Immeasurable time bias in observational studies of drug effects on mortality. Am J Epidemiol 2008;168:329–35.
16. Chakravarty EF, Nelson L, Krishnan E. Obstetric hospitalizations in the United States for women with systemic lupus erythematosus and rheumatoid arthritis. Arthritis Rheum 2006;54:899–907.
17. Johnson KE, Beaton SJ, Andrade SE, et al. Methods of linking mothers and infants using health plan data for studies of pregnancy outcomes. Pharmacoepidemiol Drug Saf 2013;22:776–82.
18. Andrade SE, Scott PE, Davis RL, et al. Validity of health plan and birth certificate data for pregnancy research. Pharmacoepidemiol Drug Saf 2013;22:7–15.
19. Cooper WO, Hernandez-Diaz S, Gideon P, et al. Positive predictive value of computerized records for major congenital malformations. Pharmacoepidemiol Drug Saf 2008;17:455–60.
20. Joseph L, Gyorkos TW, Coupal L. Bayesian estimation of disease prevalence and the parameters of diagnostic tests in the absence of a gold standard. Am J Epidemiol 1995;141:263–72.
21. Tinker SC, Carmichael SL, Anderka M, et al. Birth defects study to evaluate pregnancy exposures. Next steps for birth defects research and prevention: the birth defects study to evaluate pregnancy exposures (BD-STEPS). Birth Defects Res A Clin Mol Teratol 2015;103:733–40.
22. Greenland S. Basic methods for sensitivity analysis of biases. Int J Epidemiol 1996;25:1107–16.
23. Daniel S, Koren G, Lunenfeld E, et al. Immortal time bias in drug safety cohort studies: spontaneous abortion following nonsteroidal antiinflammatory drug exposure. Am J Obstet Gynecol 2015;212:307.e1-6.

Measuring Patient Preferences

An Overview of Methods with a Focus on Discrete Choice Experiments

Glen S. Hazlewood, MD, PhD[a,b,*]

KEYWORDS

• Patient preference • Discrete choice experiment • Rheumatoid arthritis
• Rheumatic disease • Review • Method • Bias

KEY POINTS

- Patient preference measures differ from patient-reported outcomes. The latter measures a patient's health status, while the former measures the value patients place on a health outcome.
- Patient preferences can be quantified either in absolute (eg, 0–1, where 0 is death and 1 is full health) or relative terms.
- A discrete choice experiment quantifies the relative importance of treatment attributes by asking patients to choose between treatments that differ in their attributes.
- A discrete choice experiment is a powerful tool for understanding patient preferences that is growing in popularity. Like any measurement tool, it requires careful consideration and understanding of potential biases, which we review in this article.

INTRODUCTION

To understand how patient preferences can be measured, we must first define what patient preferences are. Broadly speaking, a preference is an expression of desirability of one alternative over another. In a health care context, this can be clarified as the relative importance of alternative management options or outcomes related to health.[1] These alternative options will often be different treatments or treatment strategies, but

Disclosure: G.S. Hazlewood has no potential conflict of interest to declare. G.S. Hazlewood is supported by a CIHR New Investigator Salary Award and The Arthritis Society Young Investigator Salary Award.

[a] Department of Medicine, University of Calgary, 3280 Hospital Drive NW, Calgary, Alberta T2N4Z6, Canada; [b] Department of Community Health Sciences, University of Calgary, 3280 Hospital Drive NW, Calgary, Alberta T2N4Z6, Canada
* Department of Medicine, University of Calgary, 3280 Hospital Drive NW, Calgary, Alberta T2N4Z6, Canada.
E-mail address: gshazlew@ucalgary.ca

Rheum Dis Clin N Am 44 (2018) 337–347
https://doi.org/10.1016/j.rdc.2018.01.009
rheumatic.theclinics.com
0889-857X/18/

can also be diagnostic alternatives or other choices that patients face. Anytime a choice exists, a preference can be stated.

Patient preferences should be distinguished from patient-reported outcome measures (PROMs) and patient-reported experience measures that are widespread in rheumatic disease research and clinical care.[1] The use of PROMS and patient-reported experience measures in rheumatic diseases have been recently reviewed in an issue of *Rheumatic Disease Clinics of North America*.[2] PROMs measure a patient's health state in 1 or more domains at a given point in time. In contrast, patient preferences seek to understand the importance of this health (or any other) outcome relative to something else. For example, the Health Assessment Questionnaire Disability Index is a PROM that measures a patient's functional status. A measure of patient preferences would ask whether a patient would prefer a given functional state (or improvement in function) over, for example, an improvement in pain. Alternatively, the value of both function and pain could be elicited on an absolute scale (eg, 0–1, where 0 is death and 1 is full health) and then compared.

WHY SHOULD WE MEASURE PATIENT PREFERENCES?

Shared decision making is a model whereby patients and clinicians work together to reach a decision aligned with patients' values, and is widely regarded as the preferred medical decision-making approach.[3] The shared decision-making model recognizes that, although physicians are experts in disease diagnosis and management, patients have unique preferences that should be elicited and considered in treatment decisions. Measuring the preferences for a population of patients is not necessary for the individual encounter, because each patient will have their own preferences that should be considered. Measuring patient preferences, however, can identify which decisions are most preference sensitive and, therefore, most critical for shared decision making. Studies routinely demonstrate that physicians are poor judges of patients' preferences.[4] Understand patient preferences through objective measurement can help to clarify these misconceptions.

Patient preferences also often vary, and understanding the factors that are associated with risk aversion or risk seeking can inform decision making. Preferences for rheumatoid arthritis treatment have been associated with both disease characteristics (including disease severity,[5] disease duration,[5] and prior treatment experience[6,7]) and sociodemographics (including age,[8] employment status,[9] education level,[10] income,[8] and ethnicity[9,10]). This knowledge may help to inform the development or implementation of strategies to promote shared decision making. The association between preferences and sociodemographics also highlights the importance of tailoring decisions to the patient as a whole, rather than just their disease severity.

Understanding patient preferences can also help to inform policy decisions and treatment recommendations. Patient preferences are a critical step in the Grading of Recommendations, Assessment, Development and Evaluation (GRADE) process,[11] which has been adopted by the American College of Rheumatology (ACR). Under the GRADE approach, strong recommendations are reserved for situations in which most patients, on the balance of benefits and harms, would choose a particular treatment approach. Fraenkel and colleagues[12] provided an example of how incorporating patient preferences may impact treatment recommendations for rheumatoid arthritis. In a pilot study, they presented the same evidence on treatment risks and benefits used by the physician dominated ACR guideline panel to a patient panel trained in the GRADE approach. For 3 of 16 treatment recommendations, the patient panel recommended a different treatment, and the strength of the recommendation (confidence that most patients would prefer the treatment) varied in an additional 3 recommendations.[12] The reason for these differences were in how the patient and physician-dominated panels valued the tradeoffs.

Finally, there is also a growing interest in using methods of preference elicitation with individual decision making. Decision aids can include exercises that elicit patient preferences, and help patients to clarify their preferences and communicate these to their health care team.[13] These tools are promising, although as with all decision aids, barriers to implementation (eg, time pressure/constraints) exist and use in practice is rare.

MEASURING PATIENT PREFERENCES

Patient preferences can be elicited using various methods. Health state utilities measure patient values for a certain health condition in absolute terms, typically on a scale from 0 (death) to 1 (full health). This can be done using several different methods. In the standard gamble method, patients are asked to make a choice between staying in a given health state or taking a gamble of either returning to full health or immediate death. The probability of death is varied to find the patient's threshold of indifference, which defines his or her utility for the health state. In time tradeoff, patients conduct a similar exercise, but the tradeoff is between full health and a shortened life expectancy. A visual analogue scale is often used as well, although is not considered a utility-based measure, as it does not require any trade-off.

With utility-based valuation, the perspective of the health state elicited is critical in the interpretation of the findings. If patients are asked to consider their current health state, then the utility provides a measure of health-related quality of life, that is, the value patients place on their current health state. Alternatively, patients' preferences may be elicited for a defined health state or outcome. For example, in a study of patients with rheumatoid arthritis, investigators presented scenarios wherein they described varying levels of an ACR response (ACR20/50/70) and adverse effects (none, mild, moderate, or severe).[14] They then had patients value these outcomes with a visual analog scale. One of their findings was that the utilities for ACR50 and ACR70 were considerably higher than ACR20, suggesting the latter is a less important outcome for patients. By valuing defined treatment outcomes, the results can be used by guideline panels who need to balance tradeoffs that may exist in the evidence. In comparison, health-related quality of life is an outcome that can be used to compare treatment approaches within an individual study or through modeling studies.

DISCRETE CHOICE EXPERIMENTS

Instead of asking patients to directly value each attribute relevant to a decision, preferences can be estimated by asking people to choose between 2 or more treatment options. These exercises are collectively known as conjoint analysis (*con*sidered *joint*ly).[15] In conjoint analysis exercises, patients are asked to express their preferences for scenarios that involve the consideration of at least 2 differences in the treatments (thus providing a tradeoff between the attributes). The methods differ in how many attributes of the full set considered are presented at once (either a complete or partial set) and in how the preferences are elicited (choice, ratings, or rankings). Discrete choice experiments are a form of conjoint analysis in which patients choose their preferred treatment in a series of hypothetical choice tasks, where 2 or more treatment choices are presented. The treatments are described in terms of attributes, each of which has a set of possible levels (eg, a dose administration attribute, with levels of weekly tablets or weekly injections). An example of a discrete choice experiment, adapted and simplified from a published example,[7] is presented in **Fig. 1**.

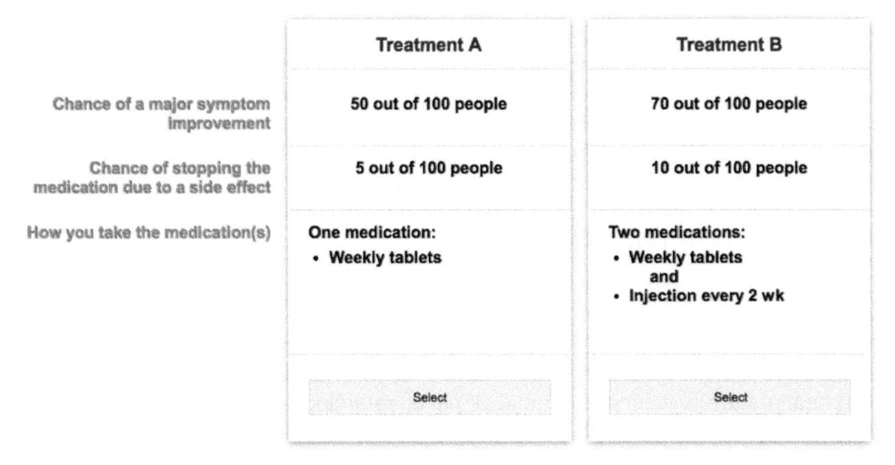
If these 2 treatment options were presented to you by your rheumatologist, which would you choose?
Treatment A
Treatment B
Chance of a major symptom improvement
50 out of 100 people
70 out of 100 people
Chance of stopping the medication due to a side effect
5 out of 100 people
10 out of 100 people
How you take the medication(s)
One medication:
• Weekly tablets
Two medications:
• Weekly tablets
and
• Injection every 2 wk
Select
Select

Fig. 1. Example of a discrete choice experiment.

In this example (see **Fig. 1**), patients are asked to make a choice between treatment A and treatment B. Treatment A provides a lower chance of benefit, but requires fewer medications and has a lower chance of side effects. By analyzing participants' responses across a series (often 10–12) of these tasks, where the levels for each treatment are varied, the relative importance of the attribute levels can be estimated.

A major advantage of conjoint analysis is that it allows an estimation of the relative importance of multiple attributes at once, without having to value each separately. The tasks are also more realistic to treatment decision making than traditional standard gamble or time tradeoff exercises. As such, they may have greater face validity. They are also typically easier to administer and are often administered online. These advantages have contributed to the rapid growth of discrete choice experiments in health care evaluation.[16]

CONDUCTING A DISCRETE CHOICE EXPERIMENT

Conducting a discrete choice experiment is an iterative process and requires a number of steps.[15] The process typically begins by framing the research question and deciding which attributes and levels to include.[15] A full list of attributes and levels is first identified, then reduced to a final list. The selection of attributes should be guided by the research question and may be informed by experts, prior studies, or qualitative research.[15]

After the selection of the attributes and levels, the tasks are constructed and the experiment is designed. This involves deciding which treatment options to include in each task, and how many tasks to present to each patient. The goal is to elicit unbiased preferences with maximal efficiency. Various methods exist to determine the most efficient experimental design.[17] The most statistically efficient designs will be orthogonal (no correlation between the appearance of any attribute level), have level balance (each level shown the same number of times), and have minimal level overlap (different levels in each treatment option).[18] Designs that are the most efficient statistically, however, may be more challenging for patients to complete. For example, if the treatments options are different for every attribute (minimal level overlap), patients are required to consider more tradeoffs. Thus, determining the most efficient design for any application requires balancing the statistical efficiency with the response efficiency.[15] Pilot testing and data simulations can help to inform these decisions before field testing the survey by providing estimates for the standard errors of the part-worths with different survey designs.

Once a discrete choice experiment has been designed, it is necessary to develop the final survey, administer it to the target population, collect the data, and perform the analysis. Throughout this entire process, it is important to understand the assumptions made and potential biases that can result.

POTENTIAL BIASES AND ASSUMPTIONS

When eliciting preferences with discrete choice experiments, certain assumptions are required, and violation of these assumptions can lead to potential biases.[19] Most of these assumptions are common to all methods of stated preference research, and many apply to any survey research.

Hypothetical Bias

With any method of measuring patients' preferences, we assume that patients' choices in the choice tasks reflect their true underlying preferences if faced with an actual treatment decision. Certain strategies may be used to try to reduce the hypothetical bias. One approach is to explain this potential bias to participants and encourage them to deliberate more carefully than they would otherwise. This method is commonly referred to as "cheap talk" and is often used in research assessing willingness to pay, where it has been shown to lead to greater discrimination between the willingness to pay between attribute levels.[20,21] Patients may also have incentives to intentionally misrepresent their true preferences.[19] For example, a patient may believe that they are "supposed" to prefer a certain medication and, therefore, choose treatments that do not align with their true preferences. Conducting the survey anonymously can help to minimize this type of bias.

Scenario Misspecification

A misspecification bias may exist if patients do not interpret the task in the way that the researchers intended.[19] Minimizing this type of bias requires patients to understand the instructions for the overall choice task, as well as the meaning of each level. Piloting the study can help to identify potential misunderstandings and is recommended before fielding the study.[15]

The phrasing of attributes involving uncertainty (risk) requires careful consideration, because risk can be challenging to convey to patients, particularly for rare events. Guidelines exist for presenting risk to patients in decision aids, and similar principles regarding survey design apply with discrete choice experiments.[22] A framing effect is well-known, whereby patients may respond differently if the chance of a good outcome is presented, versus the chance of a poor outcome.[22] Thus, it is recommended to present risk in different ways, and display the probability of both the event and the nonevent (**Fig. 2**).[22] People may also "recode" continuous attributes into discrete categories, without considering the absolute magnitude of the options. For example, when considering the "chance of a symptom improvement," patients may read options of 30%, 50%, and 70% as low, medium, or high, respectively, without considering the absolute magnitude of the risk. Including cheap talk or graphics to represent the risks may help to reduce this potential bias.[23]

Other decisions made during the design can affect patients' responses. An ordering effect in discrete choice experiments is well-known, whereby participants'

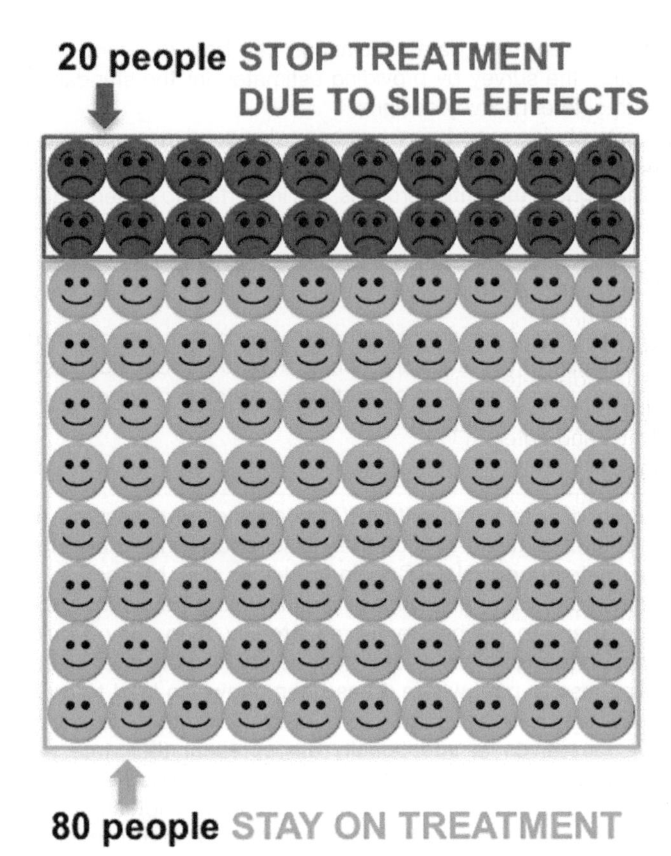
20 people STOP TREATMENT
DUE TO SIDE EFFECTS
80 people STAY ON TREATMENT

Fig. 2. Example of a graphical representation of risk displaying both the event and nonevent.

responses may be biased by the position of the attribute within the choice task. Attributes that are at the top of the screen are usually prescribed more importance.[24] Randomizing the attribute order can minimize this phenomenon. The levels included for an attribute may also affect the preferences elicited. Attributes with more levels will tend to have a greater overall importance. Similarly, including a wider range for continuous attributes (eg, risk, cost) can lead to higher importance.[19] The appropriate selection of levels in discrete choice experiments is an ongoing area of investigation. In general, it is recommended that the levels should encompass the range of plausible options.[15]

In a discrete choice experiment, we assume that patients choose their preferred treatment according to the overall value they place on each treatment, which is defined as a sum of the value (part-worth) of each attribute level that defines the treatment. Some patients may focus on a subset of the attributes, using simplifying heuristics to simplify choices.[25] This method is appropriate if patients have considered all attributes and decided that some are unimportant, regardless of the level. However, if patients do not tradeoff between some attributes for other reasons, the responses will be potentially biased. This bias may occur if patients do not understand a particular attribute or if the range of levels does not include appropriate options that are important to them.[26]

Sampling Biases

As with any survey, the sampling method may bias the results.[19] A nonresponse bias may exist if the patients who do not respond are systematically different from those who do respond. The sample may also be biased if the sample population is not representative of the intended population. Including measures to maximize response rates are, therefore, important to ensure the validity of the results.

ASSESSING THE VALIDITY OF A DISCRETE CHOICE EXPERIMENT

The validity of a survey or instrument is the extent to which it measures what it is intended to measure. The principles of assessing the validity of any survey instrument can be applied to discrete choice experiments. In general, validity as it applies to discrete choice experiments can be grouped into 3 broad types: face validity, construct validity, and criterion validity.[19]

Face validity refers to the degree to which the discrete choice experiment seems to appropriately measure patients' preferences in the way it is intended. It is a subjective decision that requires an assessment of the survey, including the attributes and levels chosen, the wording of the discrete choice experiment, and the entire survey. Ensuring face validity requires the input of the relevant experts (including patients) during the design and testing of the instrument.

Construct validity is the extent to which the survey measures the construct it intends to measure (in this case, patients' preferences).[19] The potential biases discussed can all affect the construct validity. Several methods can be used to investigate the construct validity. The overall pattern of part-worths observed can be examined, where a natural ordering exists to determine whether they are in the expected direction of effect. For example, as the risk of a side effect increases, the part-worths should decrease. Consistency tests can also be included, in which 1 treatment option is worse than the other options across all attributes. If patients choose this task, it suggests they did not understand the choices involved. The results of a discrete choice experiment can also be compared with patients' preferences elicited using other methods within the same study or to different studies (convergent validity). Some differences will naturally exist, so it is important to establish an a priori hypothesis about the expected correlation. Finally, the association between patient characteristics and preferences can also be explored. If expected associations are found between certain patient variables and patterns of risk preferences, it adds confidence to the construct validity.

Criterion validity is the extent to which the construct measured agrees with another measure that could be considered the gold standard. In patient preference research, this is often taken as the true choice that someone makes (revealed preferences). However, actual choice behavior is often driven by physicians' preferences.[27] Therefore, comparing patients' stated preferences with their choice of treatment would not reveal their preferences. Instead, a comparison of stated and revealed preferences would require a prospective study in which patients' stated preferences were elicited and compared with their choice of treatment when presented with a choice using a decision aid or similar tool.

ANALYSIS

Theoretic Basis

The theoretic basis of conjoint analysis is derived from random utility theory, which assumes that people choose something based on the overall good or value of the item or service, which is a function of the underlying properties, or attributes of the treatment.[28]

Variations on the analytical method exist and have been reviewed recently.[29] The probability that a patient will chose a given treatment within a set of alternatives can be related to the utilities of each treatment, which are exponentiated to ensure they are on a positive scale (0 to infinity):

$$P(\text{choosing } A,\ \text{given } A \text{ and } B) = \frac{e^{\text{utility treatment } A}}{e^{\text{utility treatment } A} + e^{\text{utility treatment } B}} \quad (1)$$

The utility is a latent (unobserved) variable, which is assumed to be a function of the part-utilities of the attribute levels that define the treatment choice. In a main effects model (no interactions), these are assumed to be a linear sum. The utility of any treatment (*i*) for any patient (*j*) can be expressed mathematically:

$$Utility_{i,j} = \beta_j X_i + \varepsilon_{i,j} \quad (2)$$

Where β_j is a vector of the part-worths for the *j*th patient, X_i is a vector of the attribute levels that define the *i*th treatment, and $\varepsilon_{i,j}$ is a random error term. The part-utilities are the estimates of interest; they measure the strength of preferences for each attribute level.

Sample Size Considerations

Sample sizes for discrete choice experiments are based on reducing the standard error of the part-worths of each attribute level and therefore depend on the complexity of the survey. A rule of thumb, based on the number of respondents and task complexity, has been proposed: ($nta/c \geq 500$, where n = patients, t = number tasks, a = number alternatives, and c = largest number of levels for any attribute), but this is somewhat arbitrary.[24] To help inform the sample size calculations, data simulations can be conducted to estimate the standard error around the attribute part-worths. Using these data simulations, researchers found that, for typical survey designs, the precision of the estimates tends to level off at around 150 patients.[17]

Interpretation of the Findings

The part-utilities from a discrete choice experiment are only meaningful relative to each other. As such, it is common to compare their values and express the results in more meaningful terms (**Table 1**). In this respect, it is helpful to have an attribute that can be expressed on a linear scale. In the example in **Fig. 1** (adapted from a published discrete choice experiment),[7] the part-utilities could be scaled relative to the "chance of a major symptom improvement." If major symptom improvement is modeled as a linear attribute (after determining this is valid), the marginal rate of substitution can be expressed. Cost is also popular in this regard, and if preferences are scaled to a monetary unit, it is known as the willingness to pay.

Treatment Predictions

Once the part-utilities in a discrete choice experiment have been estimated, they can also be used to make treatment predictions. The theoretic basis is the same as described for the discrete choice experiment analysis, but applied in reverse. First, the utility of each treatment for each patient is calculated as a sum of the part-worths of each attribute level that defines the treatment (Equation 2). By calculating utilities of 2 or more treatments and entering the results into Equation 1, the probability that each treatment will be chosen can be calculated. These predictions can be useful for relating the part-utilities to actual treatment decisions that patients may face.

Table 1
Common ways to express the results from discrete choice experiments

Term	Meaning	Illustration From Published Discrete Choice Experiment[7]
Part utility	A quantification of the preference for a particular attribute.	The part utility for an increase in the chance of a major symptom improvement from 30% to 70% was 10 (95% CI, 9.1–10.9) The part utility for a decrease in the chance of side effects from 20% to 2% was 2.4 (95% CI, 1.6–3.2)
Relative importance	The ratio of part utilities for any 2 attributes.	Major symptom improvement was 10/2.4 = 4.17 times more important than side effects, across the range of levels considered.
MRS	The relative importance of an attribute per unit of another attribute. If cost is used, then the MRS is the willingness to pay.	A 1% point absolute increase in the chance of a major symptom improvement was 1.9 times more important than a 1%-point increase in the chance of side effects. $=\frac{\frac{10}{70-30}}{\frac{2.4}{20-2}}=\frac{0.25}{0.13}=1.9$

Abbreviations: CI, confidence interval; MRS, Marginal rate of substitution.

Assessing Heterogeneity in Patient Preferences

Patient preferences can, and often do, vary considerably. Multiple approaches exist for modeling this variability. Latent class models group patients into 2 or more subgroups with similar patterns of responses. Using latent class analysis in a discrete choice experiment of patients with early rheumatoid arthritis, we identified a group of patients that was more risk averse, particularly for a "small risk of serious infections and possible increased risk of certain cancers."[7] This more risk averse group had lower levels of education, lower rates of current smoking, lower incomes, and were more likely to be taking disease-modifying antirheumatic drug monotherapy, although only the latter held in multivariate analyses. Hierarchical Bayesian models and mixed logit models model individual variability and may more fully account for differences between patients.[29,30]

SUMMARY

Discrete choice experiments, as a form of conjoint analysis (and the broader field of stated preference methods), provide a method for quantifying patients' preferences for tradeoffs that need to be balanced. It is a powerful tool that is growing in popularity, but as with any measurement tool, it requires careful attention to the assumptions made and potential biases that can affect the validity of findings.

REFERENCES

1. Bridges JFP, Onukwugha E, Johnson FR, et al. Patient preference methods—a patient centered evaluation paradigm. ISPOR Connections 2007;13:4–7.
2. Barton JL, Katz P. The patient experience: patient-reported outcomes in rheumatology. Rheum Dis Clin North Am 2016;42:xv–xvi.
3. Elwyn G, Frosch D, Thomson R, et al. Shared decision making: a model for clinical practice. J Gen Intern Med 2012;27:1361–7.

4. Muhlbacher AC, Juhnke C. Patient preferences versus physicians' judgement: does it make a difference in healthcare decision making? Appl Health Econ Health Policy 2013;11:163–80.
5. O'Brien BJ, Elswood J, Calin A. Willingness to accept risk in the treatment of rheumatic disease. J Epidemiol Community Health 1990;44:249–52.
6. Fraenkel L, Bogardus S, Concato J, et al. Unwillingness of rheumatoid arthritis patients to risk adverse effects. Rheumatology (Oxford) 2002;41:253–61.
7. Hazlewood GS, Bombardier C, Tomlinson G, et al. Treatment preferences of patients with early rheumatoid arthritis: a discrete-choice experiment. Rheumatology (Oxford) 2016;55:1959–68.
8. Augustovski F, Beratarrechea A, Irazola V, et al. Patient preferences for biologic agents in rheumatoid arthritis: a discrete-choice experiment. Value Health 2013;16:385–93.
9. Fraenkel L, Cunningham M, Peters E. Subjective numeracy and preference to stay with the status quo. Med Decis Making 2015;35:6–11.
10. Constantinescu F, Goucher S, Weinstein A, et al. Racial disparities in treatment preferences for rheumatoid arthritis. Med Care 2009;47:350–5.
11. Andrews JC, Schunemann HJ, Oxman AD, et al. GRADE guidelines: 15. Going from evidence to recommendation-determinants of a recommendation's direction and strength. J Clin Epidemiol 2013;66:726–35.
12. Fraenkel L, Miller AS, Clayton K, et al. When patients write the guidelines: patient panel recommendations for the treatment of rheumatoid arthritis. Arthritis Care Res (Hoboken) 2016;68:26–35.
13. Fraenkel L. Incorporating patients' preferences into medical decision making. Med Care Res Rev 2013;70:80S–93S.
14. Chiou CF, Weisman M, Sherbourne CD, et al. Measuring preference weights for American College of Rheumatology response criteria for patients with rheumatoid arthritis. J Rheumatol 2005;32:2326–9.
15. Bridges JF, Hauber AB, Marshall D, et al. Conjoint analysis applications in health-a checklist: a report of the ISPOR good research practices for conjoint analysis task force. Value Health 2011;14:403–13.
16. Marshall D, Bridges JF, Hauber B, et al. Conjoint analysis applications in health - how are studies being designed and reported? An update on current practice in the published literature between 2005 and 2008. Patient 2010;3:249–56.
17. Reed Johnson F, Lancsar E, Marshall D, et al. Constructing experimental designs for discrete-choice experiments: report of the ISPOR Conjoint Analysis Experimental Design Good Research Practices Task Force. Value Health 2013;16:3–13.
18. Street D, Burgess L. The construction of optimal stated choice experiments: theory and methods. Hoboken (NJ): A John Wiley & Sons, Inc; 2007.
19. Kjaer T. A review of the discrete choice experiment - with emphasis on its application in health care. Health Economics Papers 2005;1:1–139.
20. Cummings RG, Harrison GW, Rutström EE. Homegrown values and hypothetical surveys: is the dichotomous choice approach incentive-compatible? Am Econ Rev 1995;85:260–6.
21. Ozdemir S, Johnson FR, Hauber AB. Hypothetical bias, cheap talk, and stated willingness to pay for health care. J Health Econ 2009;28:894–901.
22. Elwyn G, O'Connor A, Stacey D, et al. Developing a quality criteria framework for patient decision aids: online international Delphi consensus process. BMJ 2006; 333:417.
23. Johnson FR, Mohamed AF, Ozdemir S, et al. How does cost matter in health-care discrete-choice experiments? Health Econ 2011;20:323–30.

24. Orme B. Getting started with conjoint analysis: strategies for product design and pricing research. Madison (WI): Research Publishers LLC; 2005.
25. Lloyd AJ. Threats to the estimation of benefit: are preference elicitation methods accurate? Health Econ 2003;12:393–402.
26. Cairns J, van der Pol M, Lloyd A. Decision making heuristics and the elicitation of preferences: being fast and frugal about the future. Health Econ 2002;11:655–8.
27. Harris JA, Bykerk VP, Hitchon CA, et al. Determining best practices in early rheumatoid arthritis by comparing differences in treatment at sites in the Canadian Early Arthritis Cohort. J Rheumatol 2013;40:1823–30.
28. Ben-Akiva M, Bierlaire M. Discrete choice methods and their applications in short term travel decisions. In: Hall R, editor. Handbook of transportation science. New York: Springer Science + Business Media; 1999. p. 5–33.
29. Hauber AB, Gonzalez JM, Groothuis-Oudshoorn CG, et al. Statistical methods for the analysis of discrete choice experiments: a report of the ISPOR Conjoint Analysis Good Research Practices Task Force. Value Health 2016;19:300–15.
30. Hazlewood GS, Bombardier C, Tomlinson G, et al. A Bayesian model that jointly considers comparative effectiveness research and patients' preferences may help inform GRADE recommendations: an application to rheumatoid arthritis treatment recommendations. J Clin Epidemiol 2018;93:56–65.

Cluster and Multiple Correspondence Analyses in Rheumatology

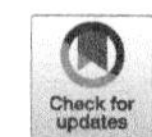

Paths to Uncovering Relationships in a Sea of Data

Lu Han, PhD[a], Susanne M. Benseler, MD, PhD[b], Pascal N. Tyrrell, PhD[a,c,*]

KEYWORDS

- Cluster analysis • Multiple correspondence analysis • Rheumatic disease
- Systematic review

KEY POINTS

- There is an increase over time in studies adopting cluster and multiple corresponding analyses in rheumatic disease since the year 2000. This increase parallels the increase in available clinical data from electronic research databases, repositories, and registries.
- Researcher experience and expertise was determined to be one of the main barriers to considering the use of cluster or multiple correspondence analyses.
- As both cluster and multiple correspondence analyses are data driven, methodologies are often underpowered in this field of research, and they are best suited to exploratory/hypothesis-generating studies.

INTRODUCTION

Rheumatic diseases encompass a wide range of conditions caused by inflammation and dysregulation of the immune system, often leading to damage of bones, joints, cartilage, and internal organs. As the most prevalent rheumatic disease, arthritis (and related conditions) is the second most common cause of days off work in both men and women. Because of the complexity and heterogeneity of rheumatic diseases

[a] Department of Medical Imaging, University of Toronto, 263 McCaul Street, Toronto, Ontario M5T 1W7, Canada; [b] Department of Paediatrics, Alberta Children's Hospital, Cumming School of Medicine, University of Calgary, 2888 Shaganappi Trail NW, Calgary, Alberta T3B 6A8, Canada; [c] Department of Statistical Sciences, University of Toronto, 100 St George Street, Toronto, Ontario M5S 3G3, Canada

* Corresponding author. Department of Medical Imaging, University of Toronto, Toronto, Ontario M5T 1W7, Canada.

E-mail address: pascal.tyrrell@utoronto.ca

Rheum Dis Clin N Am 44 (2018) 349–360
https://doi.org/10.1016/j.rdc.2018.01.013
rheumatic.theclinics.com

with many associated categorical variables, making sense of so many relationships between variables that are often correlated is at the same time a challenge but also an incredible opportunity for discovery. This type of research often benefits from dimension reduction: the creation of a smaller and more interpretable dataset and acquisition of equivalent analytical results of the original representation.[1] Cluster analysis (CA) and multiple correspondence analysis (MCA) are 2 multivariate methods that can assist in identifying rheumatic disease causes, patterns, severity, or the association between different diseases or with drug/treatment response.[2]

CA reveals hidden structures by grouping entities or objects with similar characteristics (similarity measurement) into homogenous groups while maximizing heterogeneity across groups. It is a process used to determine similar groups of interests based on the combined values of their measured characteristics, without knowledge of outcomes. In performing this approach, it is important to identify groups when it is not clear which entity belongs to which group, and how many groups may best be used to cluster the entities.[3–5] However, because of the hierarchical complexity of rheumatic diseases, there are no obvious means for forming clusters. In addition, the complexity of the data coupled with investigators needing to deal with outliers, overlapping clusters, and potential overfitting often deters investigators from embarking on CA adventure.[6]

On the other hand, MCA (an extension of correspondence analysis where there are 3 or more variables) is an exploratory nonparametric statistical method that represents a complex nominal categorical dataset in a low-dimensional graphical form (called a biplot). It can simplify complex data from a large table into a simpler display of categorical variables while preserving all of the valuable information in the dataset.[7–10] However, there is no theoretic distribution to which the observed distances can be compared, which implies that MCA does not support significance testing and is instead a more appropriate exploratory method.

Researchers will often refer to previously published articles when planning a new study because of the above stated challenges to perform successful CA and MCA in rheumatic diseases studies. For this reason, it is important to correctly and clearly report methodology so that others may replicate and/or follow the existing study. The trick, of course, is deciding on which article to use as a correct template![11] Because available information for the clinical researcher is often difficult to understand and apply, the purpose of this review is to develop recommendations for the application of these 2 methods in rheumatic disease research. The objectives of this review are to (1) describe and evaluate the application of CA and MCA in rheumatic disease research (systematic review), (2) evaluate the cluster/correspondence analysis based on reporting standards relevant to the field of rheumatic disease research, (3) make recommendations for when and how cluster/correspondence analysis can be applied in the field of rheumatic disease.

SYSTEMATIC REVIEW

In order to assist them in writing this review, the authors chose to perform a systematic review of the rheumatology literature with the following inclusion criteria for articles that (1) focused on a rheumatic disease, (2) used CA or correspondence analysis as the statistical analysis method.

Methods

The authors conducted a search for CA and MCA in rheumatology. The search was done at University of Toronto using MEDLINE (OVID), and the methods used to perform the systematic review were based on the Prisma guidelines[12] with information from included articles extracted by 2 authors; a third author resolved any disagreement. A detailed search was conducted with the title, abstract, and keyword terms found in **Table 1** and was limited to journal articles in the English language from 2000 to late October 2017 on diseases more commonly found in research. In total, 181 articles were retrieved and 101 studies were suitable for review (**Fig. 1**). For details of data extraction, please refer to Table S1 in the supplementary material.

Results

All articles reviewed were published after the year 2000, with most articles (72.3%) published between the years 2009 and 2017 (**Fig. 2**). An increasing trend in studies for both cluster and corresponding analyses was observed over the study period. Of the 101 articles, the top 3 publication journals were *Arthritis Research and Therapy* (12 of 101, 11.9%), *Arthritis and Rheumatism* (9 of 101, 8.9%), *Annals of Rheumatic Disease* (8 of 101, 7.9%), and *Arthritis Care and Research* (8 of 101, 7.9%). The remaining articles were retrieved from 39 other journals. The top 3 out of 22 countries of the corresponding authors were the United States (21 of 101, 22.8%), Netherlands (14 of 101, 13.8%), and Canada (7 of 101, 6.9%). When considering journal impact factors and study sample size of the articles, the median impact factor of reviewed articles was 3.3 (interquartile range [IQR] 2.8), the median H-index of reviewed articles was 21 (IQR 30), and the median study sample size was 105 (IQR 415).

Rheumatic diseases

The most common rheumatic diseases studied were arthritis (43 of 101, 42.5%) followed by lupus (21 of 101, 20.8%) and pediatric rheumatic disease (15 of 101, 14.8%).

Multivariate methods and standards used

Of all the reviewed articles, 12 of 101 (11.9%) used MCA, whereas 91 of 101 (88.1%) used CA. Among the studies that used CA, the vast majority (88.3%) had less than 6 clusters in the final formation of cluster partitions, 22 (28.6%) had 2 clusters, 29 (37.7%) had 3 clusters, 8 (10.4%) had 4 clusters, and 9 (11.7%) had 5 clusters.

Cluster analysis

When considering the 5 standards from Aldenderfer and Blashfield[11,13] (**Table 2**), 33 of 91 (36.2%) of the CA articles reviewed correctly reported all 5 criteria:

- *Criteria 1 (software used):* Considering all the articles in both cluster and correspondence analysis, 26 of 101 (25.7%) of the articles used SPSS, 16 of 101 (15.8%) used R, 13 of 101 (12.9%) used SAS, 7 of 101 (6.9%) used Cluster

Table 1
Search terms from MEDLINE (OVID) queries

Query	Results
(Arthritis.ti,ab,kw or lupus.ti,ab,kw or dermatomyositis.ti,ab,kw or polymyositis.ti,ab,kw or scleroderma.ti,ab,kw or systemic sclerosis.ti,ab,kw or Sjogren's syndrome.ti,ab,kw or Raynaud's.ti,ab,kw or vasculitis.ti,ab,kw) AND (cluster analysis.ti,ab,kw or k means.ti,ab,kw or hierarchical analysis.ti,ab,kw)	167 items
(Arthritis.ti,ab,kw or lupus.ti,ab,kw or dermatomyositis.ti,ab,kw or polymyositis.ti,ab,kw or scleroderma.ti,ab,kw or systemic sclerosis.ti,ab,kw or Sjogren's syndrome.ti,ab,kw or Raynaud's.ti,ab,kw or vasculitis.ti,ab,kw or inflammatory marker*.ti,ab,kw or autoinflammatory.ti,ab,kw) AND (correspondence analysis.ti,ab,kw)	16 items

* The inflammatory marker* will search for words with marker as prefix, and was used to avoid missing terms that are phrased differently. Therefore, it is a wildcard symbol used by search engine syntax.

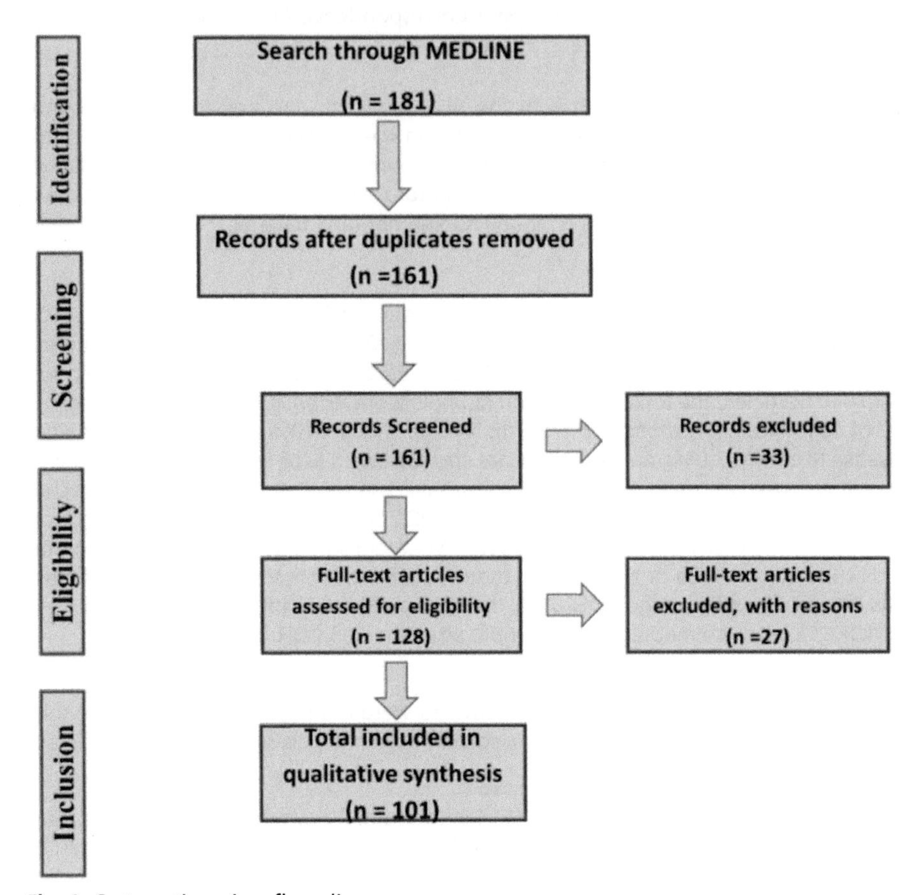

Fig. 1. Systematic review flow diagram.

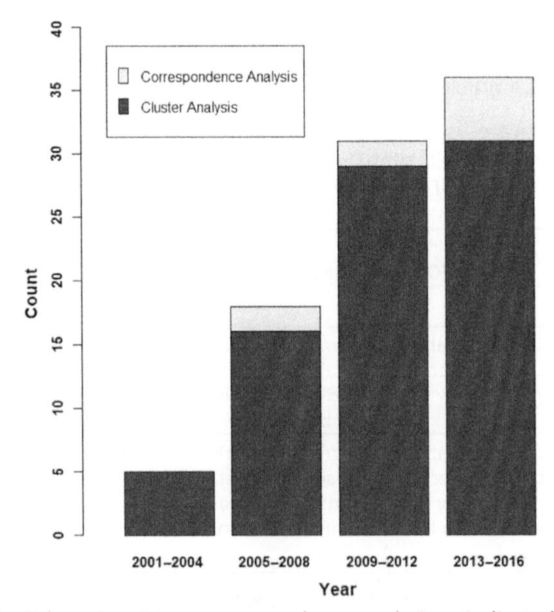

Fig. 2. Count of articles using CA or correspondence analysis as indicated in the legend by 4 years from 2001 to 2016.

Table 2
Reporting standards for cluster analysis and multiple correspondence analysis

Methods	CA[a]	MCA[b]
Description	A multivariate technique that reveals hidden structures by grouping objects with similar characteristics into homogenous groups while maximizing heterogeneity across groups. It is important to identify groups when it is not clear which entity belongs to which group, and how many groups may best be used to cluster the entities	A multivariate technique that represents a complex nominal categorical dataset in a low-dimensional graphical form. It can simplify complex data from a large multiway table into a simpler display of categorical variables while preserving all of the valuable information in the dataset
Assessment criteria	1. *Software reported* (R, SAS, SPSS) 2. *Similarity measurements* (Euclidean distance, Pearson's correlation) 3. *CA methods* (hierarchical or nonhierarchical) 4. *How to determine the number of clusters* (criterion such as pseudo-F statistic) 5. *Statistical methods for validation clusters* (such as sensitivity analysis)	1. *Significance of dependencies* (χ^2 statistic can be used to examine whether there is a significant dependency between rows and columns of the contingency table) 2. *Dimensionality of solution* (determine the appropriate number of dimensions that can explain the most variability [called inertia] in the model.) 3. *Interpreting the axes* (interpret by way of the contribution that each element makes toward the total inertia accounted for by the axis) 4. *The quality of representation* (determining the quality of representation of a row or column provides additional richness to the interpretation of the relationships)

[a] Aldenderfer and Blashfield,[13] 1984.
[b] *Adapted from* Bendixen,[9] 2003.

3.0, and 6 of 101 (5.9%) used JMP. Other software included Java Treeview; TibcoSportfire; Matlab, and Python, and so forth. Nineteen of 101 (17.9%) articles did not report the software used.

- *Criteria 2 (similarity measurements):* Among all the articles that performed CA, 40 of 91 reported similarity measurements with 25 using Squared Euclidean distance and 9 using other metrics like Pearson correlation (4 of 101, 3.9%), Log likelihood distance (4 of 101, 3.9%), and Jaccard index (1 of 101, 0.9%).
- *Criteria 3 (CA methods):* Among these articles that use CA, 72 of 91 (79.1%) reported hierarchical clustering methods; 35 of 91 (38.5%) reported nonhierarchical clustering methods. Finally, among these 35 articles, 34 of 35 (97.1%) clearly stated they used k-means as nonhierarchical clustering methods.
- *Criteria 4 (how to determine the number of clusters):* About half (51 of 101) the articles wrote the criteria of how to identify the number of clusters, with more than 30% using dendrogram and about 20% using clinical features to estimate the appropriate number. Most conducted a hypothesis test to describe the association or mean difference between the clusters, like χ^2 tests or *t* tests. Less than 10% of the articles conducted a sensitivity analysis, such as bootstrap or leave-one-out cross-validation.

- *Criteria 5 (statistical methods for the validation clusters)*: Criteria 5 is primarily explained by clinical meanings while also recommended to use sensitivity analysis such as randomly dividing the study sample into 2 halves to repeat the CA on each, or to repeat the CA in a different sample drawn from the same population. More than half of the articles performed postanalysis (80 of 101, 79.9%) to validate the number of clusters and partitions of the clusters. The common postanalysis methods are similar as those criteria, such as χ^2 test, Fisher's exact test, *t* test, and analysis of variance. Therefore, except for the way the validation was reported, there was no distinct difference between postanalysis and criteria for the validation of the clusters. For example, 10 of 33 articles (30.3%) that used χ^2 clearly stated it as criterion. Two of 18 (11.1%) articles that used Fisher's exact test clearly stated it as one criterion.

Multiple correspondence analysis

According to the criteria the authors have adopted from previous research[7,9] to evaluate the quality of reporting MCA (see **Table 2**), only 1 of 12 articles met all 4 criteria:

- *Criterion 1 (*Significance of Dependencies: *χ^2 statistics can be used to examine whether there is a significant dependency between rows and columns of the contingency table)*. Only 1 of 12 (8.4%) articles reported the cutoff threshold in the dependency test.
- *Criterion 2* (Dimensionality of the Solution: *determine the appropriate number of dimensions that can explain the most variability [called inertia] in the model*). *Consider including in the solution any dimensions contributing (as a percent) more than the maximum of 100% per number of columns or number of rows. The sum of the percentages of the solution is called retention (where the higher the better)*. There were 10 of 12 (83.33%) articles reporting the dimensionality of the solution, most in terms of the total percentages of retention with some also reported as the contributed inertia of one variable to each dimension.
- *Criterion 3* (Interpreting the Axes: *decide whether to interpret the axes in terms of rows or columns and then interpret by way of the contribution that each element makes toward the total inertia accounted for by the axis)*. There were 10 of 12 (83.33%) articles able to interpret the factors by graphical visualization in the biplot, indicating the more distant a point is from the origin, the higher its contribution is.
- *Criterion 4* (the Quality of Representation: *Determining the quality of representation of a row or column provides additional richness to the interpretation of the relationships. It can be measured by the contributions to the total χ^2 statistic or further a standardized Pearson's residual*[14]). There were 2 of 12 (16.6%) articles able to report Pearson's residual to check the strength of the associations.

DISCUSSION

This review has revealed an increase over time in studies adopting cluster and multiple corresponding analyses in rheumatic disease after the year 2000. This increase parallels the increase in available clinical data from electronic research databases, repositories, and registries. Data are fundamentally changing the way research is done and creating new opportunities to learn things that were either unlearnable or would not have been feasible.[15] With sophisticated new approaches to analyzing data comes the need for statistical oversight. Not surprisingly, this systematic review found that there is a need for better standardized reporting of CA and MCA in the rheumatic disease research literature.

The major use of the CA and correspondence analysis was for both grouping patients and variable selection. It was common to use these 2 methods to identify phenotypic groups of patients by various factors related to rheumatic diseases.[16–18] Patients can be characterized on either feature variables that were relating to clinically assessed symptoms or laboratory-recorded measurements[19–21] or features based on the findings of groups of genes that had similar biological functions.[22,23] Many studies worked on identifying medical patient groups in need of targeted interventions or drug response or medical prognosis.[24,25] MCA was also used for the verification of developed diagnostic criteria for rheumatic diseases.[26,27] Although there is an increasing number of investigators who are choosing to use these methods, many studies were not reporting these analyses with sufficient rigor.

Based on the authors' systematic review, the median sample size in the reviewed articles was just more than 100, reflecting the limitation and dimension of rheumatic disease studies. Formann[28] suggests the minimal sample size to include is no less than 2^m (m being the number of clustering variables). For example, if there are 7 variables involved in the clustering, a minimum of 128 patients would be required. In MCA, there are fewer clear guidelines relating to sample size requirements. Given the strong sensitivity of MCA to small changes, it has been recommended to include 20 cases per active category (levels across all variables).[29] For example, an analysis of 10 active categories would require at least 200 cases. However, it is easier to remember that more is better, always. If underpowered, the risk of spurious results increases, and one needs to consider this when interpreting and generalizing findings. Most of these studies were performed in North America and Europe which may be due to the higher intensity of research in rheumatology among these countries. The relatively high median corresponding investigators' H-index and impact factors of the publishing journals suggest a need for more experienced and senior-level researchers. The barrier researchers face is the requirement for statistical expertise to undertake these types of multivariate analyses and very often it is easier to overlook such methods than it is to find a collaborator to engage in them.

EVALUATION OF CLUSTER ANALYSIS/MULTIPLE CORRESPONDENCE ANALYSIS BASED ON REPORTING STANDARDS

Most studies used CA as opposed to MCA. CA is more like a general task than a specific algorithm that can be achieved by various approaches. The way to constitute the cluster can differ significantly. Clustering using distance functions requires formation in such a way that any 2 objects within a cluster have a minimum and any 2 objects across different clusters have a maximum distance value. The distance functions can differ significantly depending on the choice of similarity measurement.

The reporting on similarity measurements was found to be the most commonly missing standard. A similarity measurement needed to be identified before the cluster method was conducted to form the group. Most reported distance functions included Euclidean distance, Pearson correlation, and log likelihood distances in the authors' review. Among the articles that reported the choice of similarity measurement, it was not clear whether the researchers intended to choose the similarity measurement by the nature of the study or by the default of the software they were using, because very rare articles reported the reason to decide which one to use. It is suggested to consider Euclidean distance with uncorrelated and equal variance measurements, and other metrics such as Pearson's correlation or log likelihood distance when adjusting for correlation and unequal variance.[30] Once the distance function has been chosen, one then needs to decide on the approach.

RECOMMENDATIONS FOR THE APPLICATION OF CLUSTER ANALYSIS/MULTIPLE CORRESPONDENCE ANALYSIS

Cluster Analysis

Clustering algorithms can be categorized broadly into the following categories: hierarchical clustering, nonhierarchical clustering, and density-based clustering (such as 2-step clusters). Hierarchical clustering can be either agglomerative or divisive. Agglomerative is more commonly used, which includes the different linkages (single, complete, and average, for example) and is used to merge a dataset into a sequence of nested partitions from each case. Nonhierarchical clustering method such as k-means iteratively estimates the cluster means and assigns each case to the cluster for optimized partition. It is always required to know the number of clusters before performing k-means. Many studies reported using nonhierarchical k-means without hierarchical cluster methods to form the clusters. It might be partially because of the researchers having prior clinical knowledge to determine the number of clusters, more possibly to reflect the lack of knowledge to perform CA in a rigorous manner to deal with the complexity and unforeseen classifications. Based on the authors' review, it is suggested to perform a hierarchical cluster method to determine the optimized number of clusters before a nonhierarchical cluster method to obtain the optimized partitions under the obtained the optimized number of clusters. Two-step cluster method is also encouraged to use with mixed continuous and categorical analysis. Besides the necessity to choose which method to use, how to determine the number of clusters is very important in CA.

When performing CA, number of clusters less than 2 may not be meaningful to reflect the reasonable characteristics in distinct groups, whereas a large number of clusters is harder to interpret and is sometimes confusing. This reason was probably why 3 clusters were found to be reported most commonly in the articles of the authors' systematic review. Most of the studies explained clinical foundations for the obtained clusters in the postanalysis to validate the cluster partitions, as supported by further statistical tests such as χ^2/Fisher's exact test/Mann-Whitney U test, dendrograms/heat map, AIC/BIC, t test, F test. In addition, although the goal of CA is to have distinct clusters with the distance as separate as possible, it is common to see overlap between the clusters. It is interesting to look for patients who are very close and associated with another cluster as a means to better understand the abnormality and mechanism. Therefore, the procedures used to determine the number of clusters and to validate the clusters should include insight from clinical evidence. Therefore, the procedures used to determine the number of clusters and to validate the clusters should include insight from clinical evidence as this helps to explain the clinical significance of cluster partitions. Clearly, clinical knowledge can reduce the complexity of a CA and provide guidance for the form of clusters, but it may, if one is not careful, also bring some bias to the cluster partitions. Specifically, it is not recommended to directly use prior clinical knowledge to decide the number of groups without performing clustering techniques objectively ahead of time. Clinical insight is best used to lay the groundwork for an objective statistical analysis and then again when validating results. In addition, one should see that clinical expertise plays a fundamental role throughout the whole study from beginning to end for MCA.

Multiple Correspondence Analysis

MCA is an exploratory nonparametric statistical method that represents a complex nominal categorical dataset in a low-dimensional graphical form. Rows (often assigned to a disease type, for example) and/or columns (often assigned to predictors) with comparable patterns of counts will have points that are close together on the biplot. The goal of MCA is to explain the most variance (called inertia) in the model in the least number of dimensions (also referred to as decomposition). The inertia determines the spatial representations, and dimension that has higher inertia coordinates will be heavily weighted in the graphs. The distance between the points in the graphs, defined according to a χ^2 metric, indicates the dissimilarities between categories.

Based on the authors' review, the quality of reporting the correspondence analysis lacked consistency in various ways. Dependency test and the strength of the association between the categories were frequently missing; this may be because researchers were not aware of its importance. When reporting the dimensionality of solution, it is suggested to provide the significance of the dependency test, or the explanation of the cutoff threshold to form the solutions, which is a percentage of the maximum between the 100% divided by the row or column number. Meanwhile, although determining the quality of representation of a particular row or column can be graphically visualized by the distance of the variable between the centroid, it would be better to test the strength of these associations using a χ^2 test and then report a Pearson residual of the table, which was equal to the deviation between the observed conditional frequency and expected frequency. These residuals allow for one to use a simple test to determine those cells that deviate from what is expected under independence: the larger the absolute value of residuals, the stronger than expected association between the categories.

Value Added

Although the above discussions were more focused on the statistical aspects to perform and validate both analyses, it should be noted that when conducting either method, clinical expertise and direct involvement are beneficial throughout the analysis. Clinicians need to decide from the beginning in CA the selection of factors of interest, help in determining the number of clusters that is at the same time clinically relevant and easily interpretable, and finally, validate the resulting clusters and provide insight to their meaning and generalizability. Similarly, clinicians play a fundamental role in MCA in deciding the number of dimensions to be considered in the solution, interpreting the meaning of the axes (dimensions) and quality of representation. As both of these methodologies are data driven and often underpowered in this field of research, they are best suited to exploratory/hypothesis-generating studies.

ILLUSTRATED EXAMPLE OF CLUSTER ANALYSIS AND MULTIPLE CORRESPONDENCE ANALYSIS

To illustrate the proper reporting of the studies from CA and correspondence analysis, the following 2 articles are selected as examples that separately followed the standards well.

Cluster Analysis Example

Background

The article by Mahr and colleagues[31] is a CA to investigate the classification of clinical phenotypes of antineutrophil cytoplasmic antibody-associated vasculitis (AAV). The study was based on 673 patients diagnosed as having granulomatosis with polyangiitis (GPA) and microscopic polyangiitis (MPA) between 1995 and 2003. GPA and MPA were subgroups of antibody-associated vasculitis (AAV), which were heterogeneous entities with overlapping phenotypes. There were not exclusive associations, and there was substantial overlap in the expression of GPA and MPA. Because of the nature of heterogeneous entities with overlapping phenotypes of GPA and MPA, it is challenging to subcategorize GPA and MPA as well as to reconcile the classification with the broader concept of AAV.

Cluster analysis methods (with similarity measurement and software)
To build homogeneous clusters of patients, a 2-step CA with agglomerative hierarchical clustering based on the Ward method followed by K-means was conducted in SAS and R. A total of 11 characteristics at trial entry were used as input variables: renal, lung, ear/nose/throat, eye, skin, neurologic, cardiovascular (CV) and gastrointestinal (GI) disease, sex, and ANCA status and type (PR3-ANCA or MPO-ANCA). Input variables were coded as present or absent. The metric used to assess the proximity between 2 classes was the Euclidian distance.

How to determine the number of clusters
The clustering process was plotted as a dendrogram, and 2 distinct approaches were used for estimating the optimal number of clusters: a visual distance criterion by cutting the dendrogram horizontally at the level of highest dissimilarity (ie, where the vertical branches were the longest) and the gain in within-cluster inertia achieved at each clustering step.

Validation for the classification
Survival and relapse analyses were performed to test whether the classes had prognostic value and to describe the patient population and GPA and MPA characteristics and CV and GI manifestations. Classification trees were manually constructed based on the most discriminant characteristics of the obtained classes to test how accurately class membership could be predicted. Predictive accuracy (the observed number [%] of individuals allocated to the predicted classes) and model parsimony were both considered in selecting the best classification trees.

Reproducibility of the classification
Two sensitivity analyses were performed to evaluate the stability of the cluster partitions. First, the cluster algorithm was repeated 5 times by excluding data from one trial at a time. Second, 1000 iterations of the clustering process performed randomly to select subsets to 50% of the entire dataset.

It should be noted that the recommendation of sensitivity analysis is not necessary.

Correspondence Analysis Example

The above article conducted MCA to use the coordinates of the observations on the retained factorial axes as new variables for the CA. It was not enough detail reported for the selection and interpretation of the obtained solutions. The article by Kuemmerle-Deschner and colleagues[27] had a better description of the interpretation of the correspondence analysis.

In this study, MCA was performed in SAS to assess the multidimensional relationship between putative diagnosis variable for a rare and heterogenous autoinflammatory disease, cryopyrin-associated periodic syndrome and patient diagnoses.

When reporting the findings of the MCA, the study reported the dimensionality of the solution as a retention of 78.8% total inertia (dimensionality of the solution) for a 2-dimensional solution (see supplementary Table S3 in Ref.[27]) as determined by trace analysis for dependencies ($\chi^2 = 2696.6$, $df = 78$, $P<.0001$) and test for dimensionality (axis inertia >16.7%). The study also provided the graphic interpreting of the axes. The quality of representation of a specific row or column has been provided as contributions to the total χ^2 statistic and Pearson's residuals.

SUMMARY

This review has revealed an increase in studies making use of both cluster and MCA in rheumatic disease research since the millennium. There is a need for standardization in the way CA and MCA are reported in rheumatology journals. Clear guidelines for conducting and reporting CA in this area were suggested in this review.

ACKNOWLEDGMENTS

The authors thank Hua Lu, BSc for his valuable assistance in preparing and performing the database searches as well as for his help in data collection, validation, and management.

REFERENCES

1. Ghodsi A. Dimensionality reduction a short tutorial. 2006. Available at: https://www.math.uwaterloo.ca/aghodsib/courses/f06stat890/readings/tutorial_stat890.pdf. Accessed March 21, 2018.
2. Johnson SR, Goek ON, Singh-Grewal D, et al. Classification criteria in rheumatic diseases: a review of methodologic properties. Arthritis Care Res 2007;57(7):1119–33.
3. Mclachlan GJ. Cluster analysis and related techniques in medical research. Stat Methods Med Res 1992;1(1):27–48.
4. Liao M, Li Y, Kianifard F, et al. Cluster analysis and its application to healthcare claims data: a study of end-stage renal disease patients who initiated hemodialysis. BMC Nephrol 2016;17. https://doi.org/10.1186/s12882-016-0238-2.
5. Hennig C, Meila M, Murtagh F, et al. Handbook of cluster analysis. Boca Raton (FL): CRC press; 2015. p. 753.
6. Steinbach M, Ertöz L, Kumar V. The challenges of clustering high dimensional data. In: Steinbach M, Ertöz L, Kumar V, editors. New directions in statistical physics. Berlin: Springer Berlin Heidelberg; 2004. p. 273–309. https://doi.org/10.1007/978-3-662-08968-2_16.
7. Greenacre M. Correspondence analysis in medical research. Stat Methods Med Res 1992;1(1):97–117.
8. Yelland PM. An introduction to correspondence analysis. Math J 2010;12:1–23.
9. Bendixen M. A practical guide to the use of correspondence analysis in marketing research. Mark Bull 2003;14(1):16–38. Available at: http://davide.eynard.it/noustat/papers%20ontology%20learning/A%20practical%20guide%20to%20the%20use%20of%20correspondence%20analysis%20in%20marketing%20research.pdf. Accessed March 20, 2018.
10. Sourial N, Wolfson C, Zhu B, et al. Correspondence analysis is a useful tool to uncover the relationships among categorical variables. J Clin Epidemiol 2010. https://doi.org/10.1016/j.jclinepi.2009.08.008.
11. Clatworthy J, Buick D, Hankins M, et al. The use and reporting of cluster analysis in health psychology: a review. Br J Health Psychol 2005;10(3):329–58.
12. Liberati A, Altman DG, Tetzlaff J, et al. The PRISMA statement for reporting systematic reviews and meta-analyses of studies that evaluate health care interventions: explanation and elaboration. PLoS Med 2009;6(7):e1000100.

13. Aldenderfer MS, Blashfield RK. Cluster analysis. Thousand Oaks (CA): Sage Publications; 1984.
14. Beh EJ, Lombardo R. Correspondence analysis: theory, practice and new strategies.
15. IDC/EMC. The digital universe of opportunities. IDC/EMC Rep. 2014. p. 17. Available at: https://www.emc.com/collateral/analyst-reports/idc-digital-universe-2014.pdf. Accessed December 22, 2017.
16. Mehta J, Lin J. Phenotypic cluster analysis of juvenile idiopathic arthritis: relationship to international leagues of associations for rheumatology classification criteria. Arthritis Rheum 2013;65:S126.
17. Cellucci T, Tyrrell PN, Twilt M, et al. Distinct phenotypical clusters in childhood inflammatory brain diseases: implications for diagnostic evaluation. Arthritis Rheum 2011;63(10 SUPPL. 1):750–6.
18. Soler ZM, Hyer JM, Ramakrishnan V, et al. Identification of chronic rhinosinusitis phenotypes using cluster analysis. Int Forum Allergy Rhinol 2015;5(5):399–407.
19. Lipkovich IA, Choy EH, Van Wambeke P, et al. Typology of patients with fibromyalgia: cluster analysis of duloxetine study patients. BMC Musculoskelet Disord 2014;15(1):450.
20. Verra ML, Angst F, Staal JB, et al. Differences in pain, function and depression between subgroups of patients with chronic musculoskeletal pain classified by the multidimensional pain inventory. Physiother (United Kingdom) 2011;12:145.
21. Núñez M, Núñez E, Sanchez A, et al. Patients' perceptions of health-related quality of life in rheumatoid arthritis. Clin Rheumatol 2009;28(10):1157–65. Alegre C, Arasa X, Campillo MA, Carandell M, Centelles M, Clavaguera T, Figueiras L, Llopart E, Ordonez S, Oriach MR, Trabado C, Alzaga X BD, ed.
22. Batliwalla FM, Baechler EC, Xiao X, et al. Peripheral blood gene expression profiling in rheumatoid arthritis. Genes Immun 2005;6(5):388–97.
23. Jarvis JN, Jiang K, Frank MB, et al. Gene expression profiling in neutrophils from children with polyarticular juvenile idiopathic arthritis. Arthritis Rheum 2009;60(5): 1488–95.
24. Heard BJ, Martin L, Rattner JB, et al. Matrix metalloproteinase protein expression profiles cannot distinguish between normal and early osteoarthritic synovial fluid. BMC Musculoskelet Disord 2012;13:126.
25. van Leeuwen N, Bossema ER, Knoop H, et al. Psychological profiles in patients with Sjogren's syndrome related to fatigue: a cluster analysis. Rheumatology (Oxford) 2015;54(5):776–83.
26. Ingegnoli F, Galbiati V, Boracchi P, et al. Reliability and validity of the Italian version of the hand functional disability scale in patients with systemic sclerosis. Clin Rheumatol 2008. https://doi.org/10.1007/s10067-007-0785-9.
27. Kuemmerle-Deschner JB, Ozen S, Tyrrell PN, et al. Diagnostic criteria for cryopyrin-associated periodic syndrome (CAPS). Ann Rheum Dis 2016. https://doi.org/10.1136/annrheumdis-2016-209686.
28. Formann AK. Constrained latent class models: theory and applications. Br J Math Stat Psychol 1985;38(1):87–111.
29. Di Franco G. Multiple correspondence analysis: one only or several techniques? Qual Quant 2016;50:1299–315.
30. Irani J, Pise N, Phatak M. Clustering techniques and the similarity measures used in clustering: a survey. Int J Comput Appl 2016;134(7):975–8887.
31. Mahr A, Katsahian S, Varet H, et al. Revisiting the classification of clinical phenotypes of anti-neutrophil cytoplasmic antibody-associated vasculitis: a cluster analysis. Ann Rheum Dis 2013;72(6):1003–10.

Applied Bayesian Methods in the Rheumatic Diseases

Sindhu R. Johnson, MD, PhD[a,b,c,*], George A. Tomlinson, PhD[b,d,e], John T. Granton, MD[f,g], Gillian A. Hawker, MD, MSc[b,h], Brian M. Feldman, MD, MSc[i,j]

KEYWORDS

- Bayesian • Statistics • Scleroderma • Systemic sclerosis
- Juvenile inflammatory arthritis • Rheumatoid arthritis

KEY POINTS

- Bayesian methods permit simple, intuitive, and meaningful statements of statistical inference.
- They provide a transparent framework for combining new information with preexisting information and knowledge.
- Importantly, to the study of uncommon rheumatic diseases, the Bayesian paradigm allows for inferences to be made from a limited number of subjects.

Disclosure Statement: None of the authors have any commercial or financial conflicts of interest to disclose.
Dr S.R. Johnson has been awarded a Canadian Institutes of Health Research New Investigator Award. Dr G.A. Hawker is supported as the Sir John and Lady Eaton Chair of Medicine. Dr B.M. Feldman holds the Ho Family Chair in Autoimmune Diseases.
[a] Division of Rheumatology, Department of Medicine, Toronto Western Hospital, Mount Sinai Hospital, 155 College Street, Toronto, Ontario M5T 3M6, Canada; [b] Institute of Health Policy, Management and Evaluation, University of Toronto, Toronto, Ontario, Canada; [c] Toronto Western Hospital, 399 Bathurst Street, Toronto, Ontario M5T 2S8, Canada; [d] Dalla Lana School of Public Health, University of Toronto, 155 College Street, Toronto, Ontario M5T 3M7, Canada; [e] Department of Medicine, Division of Support Systems and Outcomes, Toronto General Hospital Research Institute, University Health Network, Mount Sinai Hospital, Eaton North, 13th Floor, Room 238, 200 Elizabeth Street, Toronto, Ontario M5G 2C4, Canada; [f] Division of Respirology, Department of Medicine, Toronto General Hospital, University Health Network, MUNK Building, 11-1170, 200 Elizabeth Avenue, Toronto, Ontario M5G 2C4, Canada; [g] Division of Critical Care Medicine, Department of Medicine, Toronto General Hospital, University Health Network, MUNK Building, 11-1170, 200 Elizabeth Avenue, Toronto, Ontario M5G 2C4, Canada; [h] Division of Rheumatology, Department of Medicine, Women's College Hospital, 76 Grenville Street, 8th Floor East, Room 815, Toronto, Ontario M5S 1B2, Canada; [i] Institute of Health Policy, Management and Evaluation, Dalla Lana School of Public Health, University of Toronto, Toronto, Ontario, Canada; [j] Division of Rheumatology, Department of Paediatrics, Hospital for Sick Children, 555 University Avenue, Toronto, Ontario M5G 1X8, Canada
* Corresponding author. Division of Rheumatology, Toronto Western Hospital, Ground Floor, East Wing, 399 Bathurst Street, Toronto, Ontario M5T 2S8, Canada.
E-mail address: Sindhu.Johnson@uhn.ca

Rheum Dis Clin N Am 44 (2018) 361–370
https://doi.org/10.1016/j.rdc.2018.01.003
0889-857X/18/

INTRODUCTION

The ability to make precise estimates using observational data in uncommon diseases has historically faced several challenges. The first challenge relates to patient numbers. In the setting of uncommon diseases, small numbers of patients are available for study recruitment. The number of accrued patients (sample size) influences the amount of sampling error in a statistical test result. A low sample size will decrease the probability of concluding a treatment is effective when there is actually a treatment effect (referred to as the power of a statistical test).[1] As they often recruit relatively small numbers of patients, studies of uncommon diseases often have inadequate power to detect important effects.[2,3] One potential methodologic solution to the challenges of small sample sizes involves the use of the Bayesian statistical inference.

Science and Statistical Inference

According to some philosophers, science is based on forming models of the world from sensory input (or instrumentation). We use the models that are most successful at explaining events and assume that the models match reality.[4] The discipline of statistics, in part, describes the way people learn as they make observations.[5] Investigators try to understand the world by making mathematical models, say for example, the relationship between smoking and lung cancer. Each model represents our understanding of the process or phenomenon we are studying.[1] Statistical inferences are based on mathematical models.[1] In the long run, we retain models based on their validity, reliability, predictability, and perceived match to reality.[4] Statistics facilitate the description of the average person, ascertain how well the idealized model fits the sample on which it is based, and allow us to generalize from this sample to another group of people or the population.[6] Furthermore, statistics is a science of making inferences about unknown quantities. Unknown quantities can include important outcomes, such as measures of effectiveness, adverse events, and diagnostic test results.[7]

Models posit a relationship between observable data and some underlying set of mathematical functions and a set of constants in those functions that determine the values of the functions. A clinical example is the evaluation of the impact of male sex on survival in systemic sclerosis, whereby there is an exponential distribution for time to the event.[8] The true values of the constants in the model are referred to as parameters, inherent properties of nature. Because the complete population is usually not fully observable, the parameter is not known with certainty. Observations are most often restricted to a sample from the population.[1] Statistical inferences are based on observations and involve a description of uncertainty. There are philosophic differences in how uncertainty is conceptualized and handled that characterize the various schools of statistical inference.

Schools of statistical inference differ in their approach to truth and uncertainty. The frequentist statistical method (also referred to as classic statistics) is one method of making inferences from observations. Frequentist inference uses methods developed by Ronald A. Fisher, Egon Pearson, and Jerzy Neyman. Observations are treated as one of an infinite set of possible instances of data that could have come from a given probability distribution.[9] Hypothesis testing is based on the frequency of obtaining a result (data), as extreme or more extreme, if the experiment was repeated many times, under certain fixed conditions.[10] In fact, all inferential probability statements (*P* values, coverage percentages of confidence intervals) refer to these hypothetical replications of the data collection and analysis. Under the frequentist approach, it is not possible to represent uncertainty about parameter values in the sense that we could say *there is a 90% chance that the mean is between 40 and 70*.

By contrast, in the Bayesian paradigm, uncertainty about the values of parameters is represented directly by probability distributions, whereas data, once observed, are treated as fixed.[9] Probability is used to measure uncertainty. That which is unknown has a probability distribution. Everything that is known is taken as given, and probabilities are calculated conditionally on known values.[1]

These fundamental differences in the conceptualization of truth and uncertainty not only affect how investigators think about research and evidence but also how we learn from our observations over time.

Bayesian Versus Frequentist Inference

Bayesian statistical inference began with the work of Reverend Thomas Bayes.[11,12] The Bayesian statistical paradigm uses probability as the measure of one's uncertainty about an unknown quantity. In its simplest terms, one may begin with a probability of the truth of a hypothesis, for example, that a parameter is equal to a specific value. Using Bayes theorem, observations can be used to update the probability that this hypothesis is true. Preexisting data or knowledge about the hypothesis are quantifiably expressed as a prior probability or prior.[13] New observations are made, and their information content is expressed through the likelihood (ie, the likelihood of the data under a given hypothesis).

For example, an investigator may test 2 point hypotheses. Under hypothesis 1, the probability of response is 0.5. Under hypothesis 2, the probability of response is 0.6. The data will be a collection of measured scores and the likelihoods.

Through incorporation of the new observations, the probability of the truth of the original hypotheses is recalculated. Bayes theorem (also known as Bayes rule or the rule of inverse probabilities)[1] indicates how probabilities change in view of new data.

Formula 1: Bayes theorem. The probability of the hypothesis, given the data, is equal to the probability of the data, given that particular hypothesis, multiplied by the probability of the hypothesis before obtaining the data divided by the averaged probability of the data.[10]

$$P(H|D) = P(D|H) \times P(H)/P(D)$$

where P is probability, H is hypothesis, and D is data; $P(H|D)$ = probability of the hypothesis given the data also called the posterior probability distribution or posterior; $P(D|H)$ = probability of the data given the hypothesis, also called the likelihood function for the data; $P(H)$ = probability of the hypothesis, also called the prior probability distribution or prior; $P(D)$ = probability of the data over all k possible competing hypotheses, where

$$P(D) = P(D|H_1)P(H_1) + P(D|H_2)P(H_2) + \ldots + P(D|H_k)P(H_k)$$

The application of the Bayesian paradigm confers potential advantages. First, the use of priors confers the ability to incorporate external knowledge, beliefs, and data into models estimating treatment effects.[13] Often there is some form of preliminary knowledge preceding the conduct of a study. The knowledge may take the form of published clinical observations, such as case reports, case series, observational studies, or randomized trials. The knowledge may also take the form of expert opinion. In the absence of published data, clinicians frequently look to experts to inform therapeutic decision-making. The expert's knowledge is usually the result of years of training and observations treating patients. In clinical reality, when new data are published, it is considered in the context of preexisting knowledge. Instead of limiting preexisting knowledge only to the background and discussion sections of an article, Bayesian methods allow the investigator to incorporate all sources of information in the estimation of the probability of a hypothesis.[14] Thus, the Bayesian process of making inferences mirrors clinical practice.

In contrast, frequentist inference requires investigators to blind themselves to existing information because of concerns that it might bias their conclusions.[10] Indeed, it has been argued that when interpreting new data, frequentist statistical inference ignores the past.[10] Preexisting information is only considered after the conclusions of a given study are presented.

Bayesian inference also allows direct probability statements to be made (eg, there is a 95% probability that ibuprofen use will reduce headache pain). The probability statement can be revised as more data are gathered. This inference contrasts with frequentist inference, which takes the following approach.

Before the initiation of a study, an alternative hypothesis that a treatment effect of some magnitude exists and a null hypothesis of no effect is specified. The alternative hypothesis typically has no further role in the analysis of data using the frequentist paradigm and is used mainly to help decide on the sample size. A permissible false-positive rate (level of significance) is typically set somewhat arbitrarily at 5%, wherein a therapy is said to be beneficial if the *P* value is less than .05 or the 95% confidence interval for the therapy effect does not include the null value. If the *P* value is greater than .05, the investigators must conclude that there is insufficient evidence to reject the null hypothesis of no treatment effect (even if the data suggest there is evidence of a beneficial treatment effect).[2,3] The use of the frequentist paradigm in the setting of uncommon diseases can result in studies with low power against important effects and that have conclusions that are meaningless for practicing clinicians.

A serious and pragmatic limitation of the frequentist method is that clinicians and investigators, even those with some statistical experience, misinterpret the *P* value and 95% confidence interval.[10] A *P* value of less than .05 is frequently interpreted as *there is a treatment effect*, whereas a *P* value greater than .05 is frequently interpreted as evidence of *no treatment effect*. In reality, the *P* value is the probability of observing data as extreme or more extreme than the observed data assuming the null hypothesis is true (ie, the treatment is ineffective), if the study were to be repeated a countless number of times.[3] The 95% confidence interval is also frequently misunderstood.[3] The 95% confidence interval indicates that if the same study were repeated an infinite number of times, 95% of the confidence intervals formed would include the true treatment effect.[15] The confidence interval does not report what clinicians are interested in, a fixed range of values that has a 95% probability of including the true treatment effect.[16] In fact, the probabilities in frequentist inference do not refer to uncertainty in the treatment effect but to the uncertainty in behavior of the intervals based on hypothetical samples of data from the same population.

Clinicians regularly use the Bayesian framework when considering the utility of a diagnostic test. Using information from a patient history and physical examination, clinicians construct a pretest probability of disease (equivalent to a prior). Information is gained from a diagnostic test (equivalent to a likelihood) and used to construct the posttest probability of disease (equivalent to the posterior).

The use of Bayesian inference in the interpretation of new data in the context of preexisting knowledge parallels this way of thinking. The widespread use of Bayesian inference in daily experiences can be seen in weather forecasting (eg, 40% probability of precipitation) or information technology (80% probability that an e-mail is spam and should be removed).[17]

Bayesian Inference in Rheumatology

The following examples show that Bayesian methods have increasingly been applied in rheumatology research.[17]

Amitriptyline use in juvenile inflammatory arthritis

A synthesis of the evidence evaluating amitriptyline in juvenile inflammatory arthritis for pain reduction used Bayesian methods to combine N-of-1 trials from multiple patients.[18] The investigators demonstrated a mean reduction in pain with amitriptyline use of 0.67 (standard deviation 0.89, 95% credible interval [CrI] −0.99, 2.55). The probability that the treatment effect was beneficial, in that there were reductions in pain, was 16%. This use of applied Bayesian methods allowed data from a small number of patients (n = 6) to estimate the probability of treatment benefit and the population average effect. This early stage trial did not incorporate prior information in the analysis, so the analysis was agnostic about the amount of benefit conferred by amitriptyline. The Bayesian approach confers important value before embarking on a potentially costly, multicenter trial. In this case, the investigators reported a small probability of a beneficial treatment effect thereby preventing the initiation of a clinical trial that would likely have been futile.[18]

Warfarin use in systemic sclerosis associated pulmonary arterial hypertension

In contrast to the amitriptyline example, the Bayesian paradigm has been used to quantify and illustrate international experts' beliefs about the effect of warfarin for improving survival in systemic sclerosis (SSc)–associated pulmonary arterial hypertension (PAH).[19] This paradigm had 2 important applications. First, investigators were able to scientifically demonstrate the presence of community equipoise, a necessary prerequisite before the conduct of a clinical trial. Second, in a setting where good-quality data are scarce (or absent), clinicians readily rely on experts in the field to guide clinical practice. The quantification of expert knowledge was used in combination with observational data from longitudinal cohorts to evaluate evidence of clinical benefit and evaluate if investigators should proceed with a clinical trial to answer this question (**Fig. 1**). In the evaluation of warfarin in SSc-PAH, the authors demonstrated a low probability of a beneficial effect of warfarin on survival[20] (**Fig. 2**).

Certolizumab in rheumatoid arthritis

Bayesian methods for meta-analysis were applied to evaluate the noninferiority of certolizumab compared with other biological agents (infliximab, etanercept, adalimumab, golimumab, anakinra, tocilizumab) in the treatment of rheumatoid arthritis.[21] The investigators used Bayesian methods to make indirect comparisons to evaluate treatments that have been compared against placebo in other studies and made inferences about specific treatment contrasts.[22] Indirect comparisons allow measures of treatment effects that have never been directly observed.[22] This point is true of non-Bayesian indirect comparisons too, although Bayesian methods for indirect comparisons (and especially for mixtures of direct and indirect comparisons) are more fully established and more widely used than their frequentist counterparts.

In this example, the primary outcome was the American College of Rheumatology (ACR) 20, defined as a 20% improvement in tender and swollen joint counts and 20% improvement in at least 3 of the following 5 ACR core set measures: pain, patient and physician global assessments, self-assessed physical disability, and acute-phase reactant.[23] The analysis demonstrated that the ACR20 response of certolizumab (odds ratio [OR] 11.82; 95% CrI 5.98, 21.71) was superior to that of infliximab (OR 3.31; 95% CrI 2.05, 5.03), adalimumab (OR 3.72; 95% CrI 2.35, 5.93), and anakinra (OR 2.40; 95%

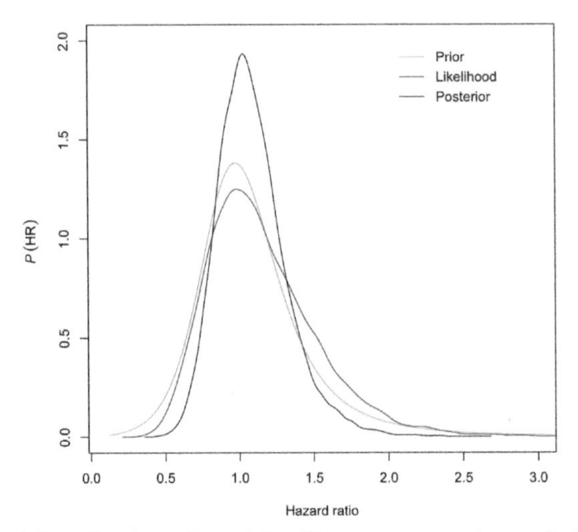

Fig. 1. Bayesian triplot. The Bayesian triplot illustrates the prior probability distribution (preexisting information, in *green*), the likelihood (new data, in *red*), and the posterior probability distribution (revised estimate based on preexisting information and new data, in *blue*). Hazard ratio (HR) greater than 1 indicates increased mortality; HR less than 1 indicates decreased mortality. Note: In this example, the agreement of the prior and likelihood leads to a posterior that is more sharply located around values supported by the data. In this study, the information in the prior and data are similar in magnitude. (*Reprinted from* Johnson SR, et al. J Rheumatol 2012;39(2); with permission.)

CrI 0.96, 5.03) and equivalent or superior to that of etanercept (OR 8.07; 95% CrI 3.34, 16.75), golimumab (OR 3.62; 95% CrI 1.62, 6.97), and tocilizumab (OR 4.13; 95% CrI 2.64, 6.19). This analysis provided evidence regarding the efficacy of different treatments' effect in a setting where no head-to-head trial evidence exists.

Abatacept in rheumatoid arthritis

Bayesian methods for a meta-analysis were also applied to evaluate the noninferiority of abatacept compared with other biological agents (infliximab, etanercept, adalimumab, golimumab, certolizumab) in the treatment of patients with methotrexate nonresponsive rheumatoid arthritis. The primary outcome was the change in the health assessment questionnaire disability index at 6 months after initiation of therapy. The expected absolute health assessment questionnaire disability index change from baseline for abatacept (−0.57, 95% CrI −0.69; −0.43) was superior to placebo (−0.27, 95% CrI −0.30; −0.24) and comparable with the other biologics (expected mean between −0.46 and −0.65). This analytical approach demonstrated that abatacept is an effective, alternative option in the treatment of methotrexate nonresponsive patients in the absence of a placebo-controlled trial.[24]

Prevalence of systemic autoimmune rheumatic diseases

Bayesian methods have also been applied in the estimation of the prevalence of inflammatory myositis (polymyositis and dermatomyositis) using administrative data.[25] Ascertainment of cases depended on accurate *International Classification of Diseases, Ninth Revision* coding and different diagnostic algorithms. The administrative data sources were potentially susceptible to measurement error resulting in misclassification. The investigators used a Bayesian latent class regression model to account for uncertainty in prevalence estimates due to patient demographics and

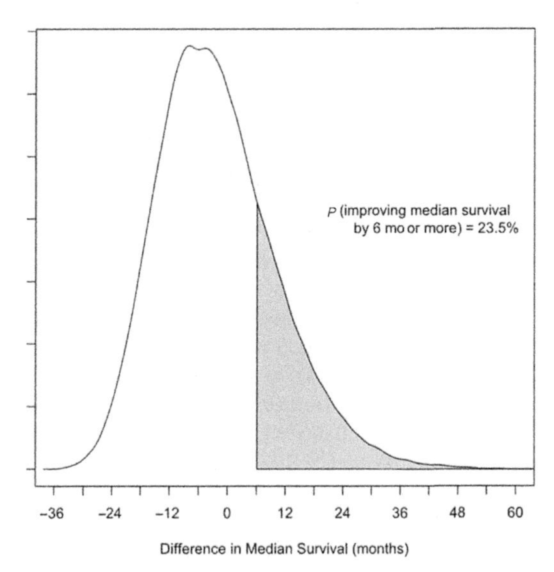

Fig. 2. Density plot for difference in median survival times in patients with SSc-associated PAH untreated and treated with warfarin, using an informative group prior. Differences in median survival greater than 0 indicate improved survival associated with warfarin exposure. Differences in median survival less than 0 indicate worsened survival associated with warfarin exposure. The y-axis indicates relative probability. Note: The Bayesian approach allows direct probability statements to be made from the data. In this example, the probability that warfarin improves survival in SSc-PAH by 6 months or more is 23.5%. (*From* Johnson SR, Granton JT, Tomlinson GA, et al. Warfarin in systemic sclerosis-associated and idiopathic pulmonary arterial hypertension. a bayesian approach to evaluating treatment for uncommon disease. J Rheumatol 2012;39(2); with permission.)

sensitivity and specificity of the diagnostic algorithms. The investigators demonstrated the prevalence of inflammatory myositis to be 21.5 per 100,000 (95% CrI 19.4, 23.9). The prevalence was highest in older, urban women (70 per 100,000, 95% CrI 61.3–79.3) and lowest in young, rural men (2.7 per 100,000, 95% CrI 1.6, 4.1). The sensitivity of case ascertainment was lower for older versus younger individuals. Hospitalization data were more sensitive in ascertaining cases in rural regions. In contrast, rheumatology billing data were more useful in urban areas. These applied Bayesian methods allowed the researchers to make population-level estimates of inflammatory myositis prevalence despite imperfect data and variable case ascertainment algorithms. Furthermore, this example and the examples on indirect comparisons illustrate an additional benefit of Bayesian analysis. The software that is most widely used (OpenBUGS, JAGS, and Stan) allows the user to specify and fit models for nonstandard data analyses.

Based on this work, Bayesian latent class regression models have been used to comparatively evaluate the prevalence of systemic autoimmune rheumatic diseases (SARDs) (systemic lupus erythematosus, SSc, Sjögren syndrome, polymyositis, dermatomyositis) across 3 Canadian provinces accounting for regional and demographic variations.[26] The investigators demonstrated the prevalence of SARDs to be 2 to 3 cases per 1000. The prevalence in older women was approximately 1 in 100 (possibly related to the presence of Sjögren syndrome in this subset of patients), and there was a greater prevalence in urban regions. Again, applied Bayesian methods allowed the researchers to make population-level estimates of SARDs' prevalence despite imperfect data and variable case ascertainment algorithms. This research provided important information about regional and demographic variations and suggests that surveillance of SARDs using administrative data is feasible.

Development of classification criteria in systemic sclerosis

Classification criteria are used to identify more homogeneous groups of subjects for inclusion into clinical trials.[27] These criteria are particularly useful in diseases that do not have a single diagnostic test. The development of the ACR–European League Against Rheumatism Classification Criteria for SSc required the evaluation of the discriminant validity of the candidate criteria to distinguish SSc cases from conditions that could mimic SSc.[28] Bayesian statistics were used to calculate the pooled mean OR and 95% CrI. This approach was taken, as it provides the reader the interval for which there is a 95% probability that the true OR falls within. For example, the presence of puffy fingers had an OR of 34.9 (95% CrI 24.0, 49.2), whereas a reduced forced vital capacity had an OR of 0.9 (95% CrI 0.6, 1.3).[28]

Methotrexate use in systemic sclerosis

Using the example of the efficacy of methotrexate in SSc, Bayesian inference was used to make inferences about treatment effects in an uncommon disease whereby the sample size was small and the study had insufficient power to detect a treatment effect using the frequentist inference.[16] Data from the SSc trial indicated that treatment with methotrexate improved the skin score.[2] However, because of the small sample size and limited power, the researchers concluded that there was insufficient evidence to reject the null hypothesis of no treatment effect. This finding supported the (potentially false) belief that methotrexate is ineffective in SSc. A survey of general rheumatologists and scleroderma experts, conducted after the publication of the methotrexate trial, found only 22% frequently use methotrexate for SSc skin involvement.[29] Reanalysis of the same study data with Bayesian methods demonstrated that methotrexate has a high probability of a beneficial treatment effect on the skin score.[16] The probability that methotrexate resulted in improvement is 94% for the modified Rodnan skin score, 96% for University of California, Los Angeles skin score, and 88% for physician global assessment. There is 96% probability that at least 2 of 3 primary outcomes improved with methotrexate. These findings have contributed to an improved perception of the utility of methotrexate, as it is presently considered a treatment option in patients with SSc.[30] Bayesian methods facilitated clinically useful inferences to be made with the data from a small clinical trial.[31]

SUMMARY

Given the issues that challenge research in uncommon diseases (small samples sizes resulting in limited power), Bayesian inference has several potential advantages. Bayesian methods permit simple, intuitive, and meaningful statements of statistical inference.[32] They provide a transparent framework for combining new information with preexisting knowledge.[32] Although there are many standardized Bayesian model fitting approaches, the current software for Bayesian modeling allows the specification of customized models that reflect the relationships between data that are available in a particular study. Most importantly to the study of uncommon diseases, Bayesian inference allows for inferences to be made from a limited number of patients, providing an escape from the confines of strict hypothesis testing or arbitrary levels of significance.

REFERENCES

1. Berry DA. Bayesian clinical trials. Nat Rev Drug Discov 2006;5(1):27–36.
2. Pope JE, Bellamy N, Seibold JR, et al. A randomized, controlled trial of methotrexate versus placebo in early diffuse scleroderma. Arthritis Rheum 2001; 44(6):1351–8.
3. Burton PR, Gurrin LC, Campbell MJ. Clinical significance not statistical significance: a simple Bayesian alternative to p values. J Epidemiol Community Health 1998;52(5):318–23.
4. Hawking S, Mlodinow L. The grand design. Belmont (CA): Bantam Books; 2010.
5. Berry DA. Statistics: a Bayesian perspective. New York: Wadsworth Publishing Company; 1996.
6. Streiner DL, Norman GR. Health measurement scales. A practical guide to their development and Use 4th edition. Oxford (United Kingdom): Oxford Universit Press; 2008.
7. Campbell G. Guidance for the use of Bayesian statistics in medical device clinical trials. Rockville (MD): Division of Dockets Management, US Food and Drug Administration; 2010.
8. Hussein H, Lee P, Chau C, et al. The effect of male sex on survival in systemic sclerosis. J Rheumatol 2014;41(11):2193–200.
9. Kadane JB. Prime time for Bayes. Control Clin Trials 1995;16(5):313–8.
10. Malakoff D. Bayes offers a 'new' way to make sense of numbers. Science 1999; 286(5444):1460–4.
11. Bayes T. An essay towards solving a problem in the doctrine of chances. Philos T Roy Soc 1763;53:370–418.
12. Barnard G, Bayes T. Studies in the history of probability and statistics: IX. Thomas Bayes's essay towards solving a problem in the doctrine of chances. Biometrika 1958;45(3/4):293–315.
13. Johnson SR, Tomlinson GA, Hawker GA, et al. Methods to elicit beliefs for Bayesian priors: a systematic review. J Clin Epidemiol 2010;63(4):355–69.
14. Wijeysundera DN, Austin PC, Hux JE, et al. Bayesian statistical inference enhances the interpretation of contemporary randomized controlled trials. J Clin Epidemiol 2009;62(1):13–21.e15.
15. Burton PR. Helping doctors to draw appropriate inferences from the analysis of medical studies. Stat Med 1994;13(17):1699–713.
16. Johnson SR, Feldman BM, Pope JE, et al. Shifting our thinking about uncommon disease trials: the case of methotrexate in scleroderma. J Rheumatol 2009;36(2): 323–9.
17. Johnson SR. Bayesian inference: statistical gimmick or added value? J Rheumatol 2011;38(5):794–6.
18. Huber AM, Tomlinson GA, Koren G, et al. Amitriptyline to relieve pain in juvenile idiopathic arthritis: a pilot study using Bayesian meta-analysis of multiple N-of-1 clinical trials. J Rheumatol 2007;34(5):1125–32.
19. Johnson SR, Granton JT, Tomlinson GA, et al. Effect of warfarin on survival in scleroderma-associated pulmonary arterial hypertension (SSc-PAH) and Idiopathic PAH. Belief elicitation for Bayesian priors. J Rheumatol 2011;38(3):462–9.
20. Johnson SR, Granton JT, Tomlinson GA, et al. Warfarin in systemic sclerosis-associated and idiopathic pulmonary arterial hypertension. A Bayesian approach to evaluating treatment for uncommon disease. J Rheumatol 2012;39(2):276–85.

21. Launois R, Avouac B, Berenbaum F, et al. Comparison of certolizumab pegol with other anticytokine agents for treatment of rheumatoid arthritis: a multiple-treatment Bayesian meta-analysis. J Rheumatol 2011;38(5):835–45.
22. Spiegelhalter DJ, Abrams KR, Myles JP. Bayesian approaches to clinical trials and health care evaluation. Chichester (United Kingdom): John Wiley and Sons Ltd; 2004.
23. Felson DT, Anderson JJ, Boers M, et al. American College of Rheumatology. Preliminary definition of improvement in rheumatoid arthritis. Arthritis Rheum 1995; 38(6):727–35.
24. Guyot P, Taylor PC, Christensen R, et al. Indirect treatment comparison of abatacept with methotrexate versus other biologic agents for active rheumatoid arthritis despite methotrexate therapy in the United Kingdom. J Rheumatol 2012;39(6): 1198–206.
25. Bernatsky S, Joseph L, Pineau CA, et al. Estimating the prevalence of polymyositis and dermatomyositis from administrative data: age, sex and regional differences. Ann Rheum Dis 2009;68(7):1192–6.
26. Bernatsky S, Lix L, Hanly JG, et al. Surveillance of systemic autoimmune rheumatic diseases using administrative data. Rheumatol Int 2011;31(4):549–54.
27. Johnson SR, Goek ON, Singh-Grewal D, et al. Classification criteria in rheumatic diseases: a review of methodologic properties. Arthritis Rheum 2007;57(7): 1119–33.
28. Johnson SR, Fransen J, Khanna D, et al. Validation of potential classification criteria for systemic sclerosis. Arthritis Care Res (Hoboken) 2012;64(3):358–67.
29. Pope JE, Ouimet JM, Krizova A. Scleroderma treatment differs between experts and general rheumatologists. Arthritis Rheum 2006;55(1):138–45.
30. Kowal-Bielecka O, Distler O. Use of methotrexate in patients with scleroderma and mixed connective tissue disease. Clin Exp Rheumatol 2010;28(5 Suppl 61):S160–3.
31. Abrahamyan L, Feldman BM, Tomlinson G, et al. Alternative designs for clinical trials in rare diseases. Am J Med Genet C Semin Med Genet 2016;172(4):313–31.
32. Willan A. Why a Bayesian be? In: SSo, editor. Wolfville (Canada): 2011.

Moving?

Make sure your subscription moves with you!

To notify us of your new address, find your **Clinics Account Number** (located on your mailing label above your name), and contact customer service at:

Email: journalscustomerservice-usa@elsevier.com

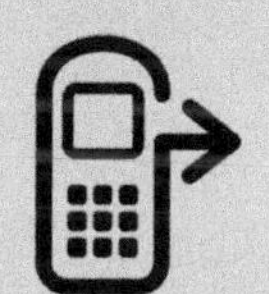

800-654-2452 **(subscribers in the U.S. & Canada)**
314-447-8871 **(subscribers outside of the U.S. & Canada)**

Fax number: 314-447-8029

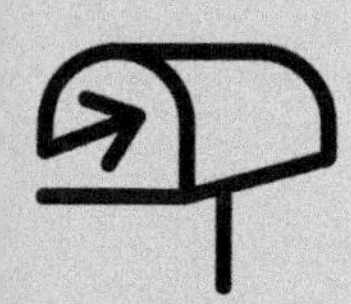

Elsevier Health Sciences Division
Subscription Customer Service
3251 Riverport Lane
Maryland Heights, MO 63043

*To ensure uninterrupted delivery of your subscription, please notify us at least 4 weeks in advance of move.

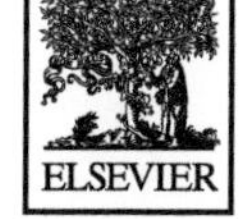

Printed and bound by CPI Group (UK) Ltd, Croydon, CR0 4YY

11/05/2025

01866590-0001